DYNAMICAL
DISEASE

Mathematical Analysis
of Human Illness

DYNAMICAL DISEASE

Mathematical Analysis of Human Illness

Editors

JACQUES BÉLAIR
University of Montréal, Montréal, Canada

LEON GLASS
McGill University, Montréal, Canada

UWE AN DER HEIDEN
University of Witten-Herdecke, Witten, Germany

JOHN MILTON
The University of Chicago Hospitals, Chicago, Illinois

81122

AIP PRESS

American Institute of Physics

Woodbury, New York

©1995 by American Institute of Physics.
All rights reserved.
Printed in the United States of America.

Reproduction or translation of any part of this work beyond that permitted by Section 107 or 108 of the 1976 United States Copyright act without the permission of the copyright owner is unlawful. Requests for permission or further information should be addressed to the Rights and Permissions Department, American Institute of Physics.

AIP Press
American Institute of Physics
500 Sunnyside Boulevard
Woodbury, NY 11797-2999

Library of Congress Cataloging-in-Publication Data
Dynamical disease : mathematical analysis of human illness / edited by Jacques Bélair... [et al.].
  p. cm.
 "Papers based on a NATO advanced research workshop held in Mont Tremblant, Québec, Canada in February, 1994"--Pref.
 ISBN 1-56396-370-1
 1. Medicine--Research--Mathematical models--Congresses.
2. Dynamics--Congresses. 3. Nonlinear theories--Congresses.
I. Bélair, Jacques.
R853. M3D96 1995   95-18267
610'. 1'185 --dc20   CIP

10 9 8 7 6 5 4 3 2 1

To the memories of
G. R. Mines, W. Mobitz, and H. A. Reimann,
pioneers in the study of dynamical diseases

CONTENTS

PREFACE

This collection of papers surveys the interface between the mathematical field of nonlinear dynamics and the clinical treatment of human disease. The papers are based on a NATO Advanced Research Workshop held in Mont Tremblant, Québec, Canada in February 1994. The workshop brought together approximately 100 scientists and physicians with a common interest in dynamics associated with disease.

One distinguishing feature of the workshop was the diverse backgrounds of the participants. Workers with primary training in medicine came from a variety of backgrounds including neurology, cardiology, respirology, and endocrinology. On the mathematical side, primary interests ranged from time series analysis to mathematical modeling of disease and theoretical analysis of nonlinear equations. Although most workers were not familiar with research outside their narrow disciplines, it was striking how similar problems emerged naturally in different settings. For example, the time series that can be obtained from human tremor, heart rate variability, respiration, and circulating levels of hormones, might be mistaken for one another if plotted on similar scales with axes labels removed. Compelling problems that arise are: How can the time series be characterized? What dynamical processes lead to the time series? Are there differences between normal and diseased individuals? Can therapies be initiated to normalize control of physiological function?

As documented in the following papers, progress is taking place along broad fronts. However, few individuals have both the clinical and the mathematical skills that appear to be essential for progress. Consequently, there is widespread formation of interdisciplinary research teams. Although once it was unusual to find collaborations between physicists or mathematicians and physicians, such research is now common.

We have two main goals in collecting these papers. The first is to provide a survey of the state of the field circa 1994. Perhaps more important, we hope that talented physicists and applied mathematicians will recognize the enormous intellectual challenges in the study of human disease and devote their skills to these problems. We hope that the current volume helps stimulate research into human rhythms and disease.

We would like to thank the many organizations and individuals who provided assistance in organizing the workshop and editing the proceedings. Financial support was obtained from NATO, the National Institutes of Health, the Field Institute for Research in Mathematical Sciences (Waterloo, Ontario), the Centre de recherches mathématiques (Montréal), and Medtronic Corporation (Québec). Louis Pelletier and Josée Laferrière of the Centre de recherches mathématiques carried out essential administrative work prior to the workshop with skill and good cheer. The Foundation for International Nonlinear Dynamics (Bethesda) cosponsored the meeting and suggestions of its president, Kathleen Madden, were particularly useful. Club Tremblant provided a gracious environment for the workshop, complete with delicious food and a beautiful setting. Candace Taylor, Centre for Nonlinear Dynamics in Physiology and Medicine, McGill University, and Janis Bennett, American Institute of Physics, provided indispensable assistance in sending manuscripts to referees and tracking them during the review process. Maria Taylor, American Institute of Physics, was responsible for the production of the current volume.

Jacques Bélair
Leon Glass
Uwe an der Heiden
John Milton

Dynamical disease: Identification, temporal aspects and treatment strategies of human illness

Jacques Bélair
Centre for Nonlinear Dynamics in Physiology and Medicine, McGill University, 3655 Drummond Street, Montreal, Québec H3G 1Y6, Canada; and Département de Mathématiques et de Statistique, Centre de Recherches Mathématique, Université de Montréal, Montréal, Québec H3C 3J7, Canada

Leon Glass
Centre for Nonlinear Dynamics in Physiology and Medicine, McGill University, 3655 Drummond Street, Montreal, Québec H3G 1Y6, Canada; and Department of Physiology, McGill University, 3655 Drummond Street, Montréal, Québec H3G 1Y6, Canada

Uwe an der Heiden
Department of Mathematics, University of Witten/Herdecke, Stockumer Strasse 10, D 5810 Witten, Germany

John Milton
Centre for Nonlinear Dynamics in Physiology and Medicine, McGill University, 3655 Drummond Street, Montréal, Québec H3G 1Y6, Canada; and Department of Neurology and Committee on Neurobiology, The University of Chicago Hospitals, 5841 South Maryland Avenue, Room B 206, Chicago, Illinois 60637

(Received 14 December 1994; accepted for publication 14 December 1994)

Dynamical diseases are characterized by sudden changes in the qualitative dynamics of physiological processes, leading to abnormal dynamics and disease. Thus, there is a natural matching between the mathematical field of nonlinear dynamics and medicine. This paper summarizes advances in the study of dynamical disease with emphasis on a NATO Advanced Research Worshop held in Mont Tremblant, Québec, Canada in February 1994. We describe the international effort currently underway to identify dynamical diseases and to study these diseases from a perspective of nonlinear dynamics. Linear and nonlinear time series analysis combined with analysis of bifurcations in dynamics are being used to help understand mechanisms of pathological rhythms and offer the promise for better diagnostic and therapeutic techniques. © *1995 American Institute of Physics.*

I. INTRODUCTION

Physicians have long recognized the importance of considering the temporal dimension of illness for arriving at a diagnosis and deriving treatment strategies. Diseases can be distinguished by their onset (acute versus sub-acute) and by their subsequent clinical course (self-limiting, relapsing-remitting, cyclic, chronic progressive). Recognition of the temporal rhythms, combined with the knowledge that certain temporal rhythms respond best to certain treatment strategies, often provides a basis for therapy.

The recent and dramatic advances in molecular medicine have shifted the attention of the medical community away from considerations of temporal phenomena. At the current time, a strong impetus for studying disease dynamics is coming from the mathematics and physics communities. Advances in our understanding about the nature of oscillatory phenomena in the discipline of nonlinear dynamics offer the possibility of applying this new knowledge to gain insights into the etiology and treatment of diseases. The mathematical methods for understanding the origin, stability, and bifurcations of dynamical behavior in nonlinear equations appear to be ideally suited for the analysis of complex rhythms confronted by the physician on a daily basis.

Although the origins for the application of nonlinear dynamics to the study of human disease can be traced back to the analyses of certain cardiac arrhythmias in the 1920s,[1,2] the concept of a *dynamical disease* was first proposed by Mackey and Glass.[3,4] Dynamical diseases arise because of abnormalities in the underlying physiological control mechanisms. The hallmark of a dynamical disease is a sudden, qualitative change in the temporal pattern of physiological variables. Such changes are often associated with changes in physiological parameters or anatomical structures. The significance of identifying a dynamical disease is that it should be possible to develop therapeutic strategies based on our understanding of dynamics combined with manipulation of the physiological parameters back into normal ranges. Progress in this direction requires the careful documentation of the temporal aspects of disease combined with suitable theoretical analyses. Several books, conferences and reviews have focused on nonlinear dynamics and human disease.[5-10]

A workshop held in Mont Tremblant, Québec, Canada, February 1994 provided an opportunity to review recent advances in the study of dynamical disease. The meeting attracted a multidisciplinary audience of physicians, physiologists, mathematicians, and physicists. Topics included the identification of dynamical diseases, methods for analyzing the temporal aspects of diseases, onset and offset of rhythms, mechanisms of oscillatory phenomena, and the design of treatment strategies. In this article we provide an overview of our current understanding of dynamical disease. Although we emphasize material covered at the workshop, we also mention other work in order to provide a more balanced overview of the field.

II. DYNAMICAL DISEASES

In a typical medical clinic, a significant proportion of patients present abnormalities in the dynamics of a physiological process. Easily identified arrhythmias are well known in cardiology, respirology, and neurology. Arrhythmias may be significant causes of patient mortality, as in cardiac arrest. Symptoms which recur frequently, such as obstructive sleep apnea or epileptic seizures, are important causes of patient morbidity.

One obstacle confronted by non-physicians studying dynamical disease is that they have little idea of the extraordinary range of dynamics that can be found in the human body. The papers in this volume provide a glimpse into what is going on. In an attempt to document dynamical disease in the nervous system, Milton and Black[11] carried out a literature survey that identified at least 32 diseases with interesting time courses in which symptoms and/or signs recur. Although many of these disorders are relatively common, for example, see the discussions in this volume of hiccups,[12] Parkinsonism,[13] tardive dyskinesia,[14] respiratory arrest,[15] there are also many obscure disorders. For example, Milton and Black[11] identify 8 different disorders associated with control of eye position and pupillary size. Even though the abnormal dynamics in these disorders are easy to observe and can be recorded noninvasively, there has been little analysis to date of the rhythms from the perspective of basic science and mathematics.

One area in which dynamical aspects are significant, but still are not well understood is endocrinology. The mammalian ovulation cycle is perhaps the most carefully studied, but there is still scant theoretical analysis.[16] Moreover, it is becoming clear that, in general, hormone secretion displays complex pulsatile secretion patterns. Since hormones are active in such small quantities, and assays are expensive, systematic studies are extremely difficult to carry out. Notable exceptions are provided by analyses of blood concentrations of parathyroid hormone,[17] insulin,[18] and growth hormone.[19] The gaps in our understanding of the control of hormone secretion are still huge. For example, although it is known that menopausal hot flashes are associated with changes in hormone secretion occurring at menopause,[20] the exact control mechanisms regulating the hot flashes are unknown. Similarly, there are many blood disorders characterized by striking dynamics, but the control circuits regulating these disorders are difficult to isolate and study.[3,6,7,21]

III. COLLECTION OF DATA

The first step towards obtaining a dynamical perspective of disease is the careful measurement of the phenomena as a function of time. Such measurements take the form of a time series, i.e. the tabulation of the phenomena as a function of time. The analysis of such time series may provide important insights into the etiology of the phenomena.

In medicine, collection and interpretation of time series always involves difficulties. Since physicians interact with patients, collection of data almost always requires the active collaboration of a physician. The physician's main interest is in identifying disorders that are associated with significant mortality and/or morbidity for which there is an adequate therapy. Collection of long time series often involves inconvenience and extra cost, and may be of little immediate benefit to the patient based on current knowledge. Studies of dynamical disease are notable for the variety of time series assembled, for the ingenuity of methodology used to collect them, and the wide range of different methods that are being developed to analyze them.

The techniques used to collect data include a variety of noninvasive and invasive techniques. Information about dynamical disease is derived from the following sources:

(1) Noninvasive methods
- patient diaries;[11]
- mechanical displacements of respiratory structures;[12]
- air flow velocities and concentrations of oxygen and carbon dioxide in expired gases;[15]
- motion of extremities using lasers and accelerometers;[13,14,22,23]
- electromyographic (EMG) activity associated with muscle;[12,15,23]
- sound waves generated by the voice;[24]
- changes in pressure on a pressure plate associated with changes in posture;[25]
- magnetic fields from the brain;[26]
- blood pressure and electrical activity associated with the heart beat.[27–30]

(2) Invasive measurements
- concentration of hormones in the blood;[17–19]
- core body temperature;[20]
- concentration of blood cells in the blood;[21]
- intracardiac electrical activity, blood pressure and wall motion.[31]

The time scales of measurements range from seconds to days. Noninvasive measurements are capable of collecting vast amounts of data but limitations arise because of the necessity of appropriate methods of data storage, retrieval and analysis.

IV. TIME SERIES ANALYSIS

Typically times series of physiological data display significant irregularities. Various issues arise. Are the irregularities associated with noise or a deterministic process or some combination of the two? Independent of any understanding of underlying dynamic mechanism, is there any way to analyze the data to distinguish between subgroups of subjects (e.g. healthy versus diseased)? To what extent can an analysis of the time series give hints about mechanisms?

The simplest way to analyze a time series is to graph it and examine the time series by eye. For example, Whitelaw et al.[12] illustrated this approach in their discussion of hiccups. They were able to conclude that the timing of hiccups is controlled by a central neural oscillator which is influenced by both the cardiac and respiratory cycles.

A slightly more sophisticated method of data analysis is to form a histogram from the time series, i.e. a graph of the frequency at which the variable attains a certain value. These histograms can be described mathematically in terms of a density function. A clinically familiar density function is the "bell-shaped" normal distribution. Density functions are very useful shorthand descriptions of a time series since they can be used to calculate measurable quantities such as the mean value, the probability that the next value will be greater than a certain value, and so on. Demongeot *et al.*[32] suggest that it may be easier to analyze mathematical models describing neurophysiological networks from the point of view of density functions and their associated invariant measures. Thus the measurement of a density function provides one method to directly compare the predictions of a mathematical model to clinical observations.

Most research involving data analysis requires computers. We briefly review several of the computer-based methods of data analysis.

Some of the methods involve traditional time series methods such as autocorrelation and power spectrum. For example, Deuschl *et al.*[22] used this approach to obtain a novel classification of tremor. They observed that in order to distinguish between the various types of tremors observed in clinical practice it was necessary to use methods based on waveform as well as frequency and amplitude of the tremor.

The role of noise in the generation of complex dynamics is being attacked at a variety of levels. At the most basic level, it is still not known whether the opening and closing of ion channels is associated with noise or a deterministic process. Guevara and Lewis[33] assume that there is a stochastic element in the opening and closing of ion channnels and investigate the effect this has on the timing of interbeat variability in a theoretical model of cardiac rhythm generation. They conclude that a significant degree of irregularity (about 3%) can arise solely as a consequence of the underlying variability in the ion channel dynamics. On a more phenomenological level, Boose *et al.*[23] modeled EMG behavior associated with tremor as sinusoidally modulated white noise. Collins and DeLuca[25] considered postural control during quiet standing from the point of view of a random walk. They concluded that both open and closed loop control is utilized by the nervous system in regulating postural sway. Finally, Paydarfar and Buerkel[15] include noise as a mechanism for switching between respiratory arrest and a normal respiratory rhythm. Analysis of experimental data in which there is a combination of both noise and deterministic chaos is a difficult issue that is treated by Schreiber and Kantz.[34]

"Nonlinear" methods for time series analysis developed in the last decade are being exercised against physiological time series. There are still significant methodological issues. Practical problems arise because of the shortness of the time series, lack of stationarity of time series, and the influence of noise on the measurements.

Probably the most commonly used nonlinear statistic for data analysis is the correlation dimension, originally used by Grassberger and Procaccia.[35] However, Kantz and Schreiber[36] describe the difficulties in applying the Grassberger–Procaccia correlation dimension algorithm to experimental data and present useful advice for novices. Newell *et al.*[14] use a measurement of the correlation dimension to demonstrate the finger tremor in patients with tardive dyskinesia is different from that measured in healthy controls. Bezerianos *et al.*[30] discuss the practical limitations during the application of the correlation dimension to heart rate time series. They find that heavy smoking and mild exercise do not alter the complexity of EKG rhythms.

Determination of the entropy or one of its variants provides an alternative method to characterize the "complexity" of a time series.[37] Using estimates of the dimension and entropy, Lipsitz[28] found that there is a decrease of complexity of heart dynamics associated with aging. Peng *et al.*[27] have examined long range fluctuations using the method of detrended fluctuation analysis. There appear to be significant differences between the fluctuations of heart rate in normal individuals and high risk cardiac patients.[27] Finally, Ding *et al.*[38] suggested that analysis of dwell times may be better than other measures of complexity for studying the dynamics of auditory perception.

If used only as a diagnostic tool, there is no need to have an interpretation of the dimension, approximate entropy, or other statistical measure of a time series. However, there is currently significant interest in using methods of nonlinear dynamics to control complex rhythms. In this enterprise, it may be useful (or essential) to understand more about the underlying dynamics. In particular, it may be important to know if the time series is generated by a deterministic or chaotic process. If a time series is generated by a deterministic process, then it should be possible to predict the dynamics (at least for short times into the future). Chang *et al.*[39] and Sauer[40] discuss prediction methods for time series analysis. If one can predict the future better for a given time series than for a suitable stochastic surrogate, then this provides good evidence that there is nonlinear determinism that can potentially be exploited in applications. For example, prediction of when clinically significant events will occur in the future would be of obvious benefit for the design of therapeutic strategies for the management of sudden cardiac death syndrome and epilepsy. Prank *et al.*[17] conclude from their computations of dimension of hormone levels that a nonlinear deterministic process is underlying the dynamics in this system. Based on theoretical modeling, Chang *et al.*[39] find that prediction is a better method to distinguish determinism from noise than other quantitative measures.

Overall, it is difficult at this time to conclude that one method or style of data analysis is better than another. There are heated debates between proponents of the various methods. Each method has its advantages and disadvantages. It is of pressing importance that the different groups make both their data and their algorithms available to facilitate convergence to common methodologies. At this stage, humility in the face of complexity is essential. Dynamics in physiological systems reflect random and deterministic processes at a variety of levels ranging from the molecular level, to the system level, to the environment. It is impossible to control all random influences and the problem of interpretation is formidable. Facile generalizations and easy answers should be viewed with skepticism.

V. BIFURCATIONS IN DYNAMICS AND ORIGINS OF DYNAMICAL DISEASE

A striking aspect of some dynamical diseases is the sudden change in qualitative dynamics. The most dramatic of these changes lead to imminent death as in respiratory or cardiac arrest or a seizure in a patient with epilepsy. From a mathematical perspective, the observations of qualitative changes in dynamics may provide a clue for the initiation of theoretical analyses. Indeed, mathematical analyses of bifurcations in nonlinear equations combined with experimental obsevations of dynamics in biological systems often provide an entry point for theoretical analyses.

A. Bifurcations in maps

One of the most extensively studied problems in nonlinear dynamics of biological systems is the periodic forcing of oscillatory and excitable biological systems.[7] Understanding of the dynamics in these systems has implications for a wide variety of phenomena ranging from generation of cardiac arrhythmias from the competition between competing pacemakers to the entrainment of the circadian rhythm by light. In the simplest cases, biological systems can be modeled by low dimensional maps. Kunysz *et al.*[41] described the effects of periodic stimulation on *in vitro* preparations of atrioventricular (AV) nodal tissue. This work is directly relevant to functioning of AV node in normal and pathological conditions. Periodic stimulation of the tissue generated rhythms similar to what is observed during AV heart block. Kunysz *et al.* found however that one dimensional maps are not adequate to interpret the entire range of phenomena observed.[41]

The effects of periodic forcing in hormonal and control systems is more difficult to analyze because of the experimental difficulties of measuring hormonal concentrations. However, Sturis *et al.*[18] analyzed the effects of periodic glucose infusion in humans and in mathematical models. They found evidence for phase locking between the glucose infusion rhythm and the insulin rhythm. The phenomena they observed are similar to bifurcations in low dimensional maps proposed for phase locking. Foweraker *et al.*[42] modeled the pulsatile release of luteinizing hormone releasing factor (LHRH) from the hypothalamus. LHRH regulates the release of two hormones from the pituitary gland which are essential for the maintenance of normal reproductive function. In their model, the external periodic forcing arises from adrenergic inputs to the hypothalamus and the oscillator is formed by a network composed of reciprocally connected LHRH neurons and gamma-aminobutyric acid containing neurons. To analyze this they carried out extensive simulations of periodically forced Fitzhugh–Nagumo equations. The bifurcations observed can be at least partially understood from bifurcations of low dimensional maps. Finally, Mayer *et al.*[21] show that periodic forcing of a simple model for the immune system can display chaotic dynamics.

These studies of different systems underscore the following observation: periodic forcing of nonlinear oscillations gives rise to a large number of different regular and irregular rhythms that can be understood based on fundamental mathematical principles related to bifurcations of low dimensional maps.[7] Because of the relevance of the dynamics in model systems to human health and disease, periodic forcing is an important technique to study physiological dynamics and control.

B. Hopf bifurcation

From a mathematical perspective, one of the best known and understood bifurcations is the Hopf bifurcation. In the Hopf bifurcation, as a parameter is changed, a stable steady state is destabilized and is supplanted by a stable oscillation. This occurs in two different ways. In the supercritical Hopf bifurcation, the amplitude of the oscillation grows gradually larger, and no parameter values lead to bistability between a steady state and an oscillation. In the subcritical Hopf bifurcation, there is a range of parameter values that gives either a stable steady state or stable oscillation, depending on the initial condition. A dynamical signature of a subcritical Hopf bifurcation is a sudden onset of a high amplitude oscillation as a parameter changes with hysteresis effects depending on whether the parameter is increased or decreased.

It is known that gradual tuning of parameters in negative feedback loops can give rise to a supercritical Hopf bifurcation.[7] An intriguing but speculative possibility is that dynamical diseases with an insidious onset may be associated with supercritical Hopf bifurcations. For example, perhaps the gradual development of abnormal tremor in tardive dyskinesia is associated with gradual modification of feedback loops for movement control.[14] Similarly, some of the altered dynamics in aging may occur as a consequence of changes in the time delays and sensitivity of physiological feedback loops.[28]

Sudden onset or offset of large amplitude oscillations is observed in many circumstances. An important case is respiratory arrest, studied by Paydarfar and Buerkel.[15] They propose that this important clinical arrhythmia may be associated with a bistability between a steady state and an oscillation where there is a perturbation that can take you from one basin of attraction to another. This analysis emphasizes an important point of direct relevance for an understanding of human disease. In dynamical systems with multiple basins of attraction, changes in dynamics can arise as a consequence of: changes in control parameters that destabilize the basins of attraction; changes in the boundary basins as a consequence of parameter modification; and perturbations that take you from one basin to the other. However, much more analysis is needed of such phenomena as paroxysmal cardiac arrhythmias, hiccups, hot flashes, and respiratory apnea in order to identify the origin of the abnormal rhythms.

Another important class of phenomena are those in which there is a sudden switch between two qualitative rhythms. A striking example is provided in the study of Beuter and Vasilakos[13] who demonstrated a sudden switch to large amplitude Parkinsonian tremor from a tremor that appeared superficially to be normal. This is similar to the subcritical Hopf bifurcation, but there is a bistability between different rhythms. Switches between physiological tremor and pathological tremor are also described by Boose *et al.*[23]

C. Skipped beat rhythms

In some biological rhythms, there appears to be a clock setting the rhythm, but there is a haphazard appearance to expressed rhythms with a seemingly random dropping of beats. As Longtin[43] discusses, such rhythms can arise from a number of different mechanisms—the simplest might be a gradual increase of a variable controlling a rhythm to an oscillating threshold combined with noise. Experimental observations of this type of rhythm are common in neurophysiology and in some types of cardiac arrhythmias. To date, these rhythms have not been studied in great detail and it is not known the extent to which they are important in basic physiology or pathophysiology.

D. Spatio-temporal bifurcations

Data consisting of a time series collected from a single site directs attention to the sorts of comparatively simple theoretical explanations based on the bifurcations in low dimensional maps and equations. However, it is important to recognize that the body is three dimensional, and understanding bifurcations in space and time may be crucial. Progress in these areas is necessarily difficult due to the necessity for collecting data from a spatially distributed system. Probably the most important clinical and theoretical applications to date have been in the mapping of spatio-temporal patterns of excitation associated with cardiac arrhythmias.[31] In the conference, an elegant demonstration of a qualitative change in spatio-temporal dynamics in the spread of neural activity in the brain was provided by the work of Kelso and Fuchs.[26] In their experiment, a human subject is asked to syncopate with a periodic tone. When the rate of the periodic tone exceeds a certain critical value, the subject is unable to perform this task. With the use of an array of SQUIDs (Superconducting QUantum Interference Devices) placed over the scalp, they were able to demonstrate that at this critical frequency the spatiotemporal pattern of brain activity changes.

Herzel *et al.*[24] showed that irregularities in voiced speech relate to intrinsic nonlinearities in the vibration of the vocal folds and provided a convincing demonstration of bifurcations involved in the production of sound in normal and pathological situations.

VI. TREATMENT STRATEGIES

To date, most research into dynamical disease has focused on simplified models, data collection, and time series analysis as sketched out above. There has been a serious absence of practical applications of the theory.

This is not to say that there is not active intervention by physicians that lead to a modification of dynamical aspects of disease. Many types of drug, surgical, and device therapies are specifically directed towards eliminating abnormal and dangerous rhythms. For example, on a daily basis cardiologists, neurologists, and endocrinologists choose among a range of different treatment strategies that alter internal rhythms. However, to date the methods of nonlinear dynamics have not played a significant role in the development of therapies.

In this section we wish to summarize the directions that now seem the most promising.

(1) Diagnosis. There is active work trying to utilize time series analysis for practical applications. These include: identification of those at high risk for cardiac death,[27] early diagnosis and classification of abnormalities of tremor[13,14,22] and postural control.[25]

(2) Therapy—drug delivery and hormone replacement therapy. There is a pressing need for understanding better the dynamics of control systems to help improve administration of drugs and hormones. For example, it is not yet known how the temporal delivery of many drugs influences their effectiveness. This is likely to be most important for hormone replacement therapies. An intriguing possibility is that theoretical insight and modeling will enable one to alter parameters. For example, Claude[44] analyzes a control-theoretic approach to alter the parameters regulating a limit cycle in a pathological regime back to a normal condition. Although technological advances have made available a number of sophisticated drug delivery apparatus,[45] there is still need for a better understanding of the global regulatory mechanisms involved in the controlled physiological systems. Also, optimization of temporal administration of prescription medicine may be possible by incorporating the findings from chronopharmacology.[46]

(3) Device design. At the current time, there are extremely sophisticated devices to control cardiac rhythm.[31] Such devices can deliver electrical impulses to the atria and/or ventricles, and can be programmed in a number of different ways. Devices exist to convert rapid tachycardias to a normal rhythm either by rapid pacing, or by delivering a shock. These devices have been developed largely by engineers working with cardiac electrophysiologists. An intriguing possibility is that future devices might be able to exploit in a more direct manner understanding of the dynamics of arrhythmias. For example, pacing might be able to avert a dangerous arrhythmia before it started. Alternatively, there is considerable interest in identifying deterministic dynamics in complex settings. In this case it might be possible to design stimulation protocols based on nonlinear dynamics. There have been suggestions that this might be important for cardiac arrhythmias, such as atrial or ventricular fibrillation[47,48] and neural rhythms found in epilepsy.[49]

VII. CONCLUSIONS

One focus in dynamical disease is on the control parameter. In this sense the strategies in the study of dynamical disease bear similarities to those of molecular medicine. However, whereas molecular medicine concerns itself with the chemical composition of biomolecules and their synthesis, in dynamical disease the emphasis is on the interrelationship between the molecule's concentration and the resulting physiological dynamics. Moreover there is the recognition that certain molecules are of more crucial importance than others.

Many present-day physicians and medical researchers are searching for the "magic bullet." They hope that by replacing molecules that are altered or made deficient by disease, or by delivering the right drug, disease will be cured. Although one cannot dispute the profound successes of this strategy (in the discovery of many miracle drugs—antibiotics, hormones, cortisone), theoretical analyses of complex systems such as presented here shift attention to system interactions and dynamics. Dynamics can be extraordinarily sensitive to minute changes in drug concentration. The cardiac arrhythmia suppression trial offers a striking example of increased mortality associated with increased sudden cardiac death in patients receiving a drug that reduced certain types of cardiac arrhythmias.[50] Another graphic example is in Sacks' recounting of the difficulties encountered in titrating the concentration of dopamine in encephalitis patients.[51] Even small changes of delivered drug can change a potential beneficial effect to an effect that causes significant patient morbidity or even mortality.

The road from the development of ideas at the benchtop to their application at the bedside is fraught with false turns and hidden pitfalls. Scientific wisdom dictates that the crucially important experiments cannot be performed without a theoretical knowledge of the properties of the underlying control mechanisms and their response to perturbations. Nonetheless, the use of empirical methods, such as drug trials involving animals and patients, is the mainstay of present-day clinical research. This meeting drew attention to the fundamental importance of carefully documenting the temporal aspects of disease and emphasized that "pencil and paper" research may have important implications for managing patients at the bedside. It is anticipated that forming an effective partnership between theorists studying dynamical disease, basic biological scientists, and clinical investigators holds great promise for treating human disease.

ACKNOWLEDGMENTS

The workshop was a NATO Advanced Research Workshop with additional support and funding provided by NIH, Centre de Recherches Mathématiques (Montréal), The Fields Institute for Research in Mathematical Sciences (Waterloo, Ontario), Foundation International for Nonlinear Dynamics (Bethesda), Medtronics (Québec). Some of the material in Sec. V on bifurcations is based on an analysis of Professor W. F. Langford (Guelph) presented at the workshop.

[1] W. Mobitz "Uber die unvollstandige Störung der Erregüngsuberleitung zwischen Vorhof und Kammer des mensclichen Herzens," Z. Gesamte Exp. Med. **41**, 189–237 (1924).

[2] B. van der Pol and J. van der Mark, "The heartbeat considered as a relaxation oscillator and an electrical model of the heart," Philos. Mag. **6**, 763–775 (1928).

[3] M. C. Mackey and L. Glass, "Oscillation and chaos in physiological control systems," Science **197**, 287–289 (1977).

[4] L. Glass and M. C. Mackey, "Pathological conditions resulting from instabilities in physiological control systems," Ann. N.Y. Acad. Sci. **316**, 214–235 (1979).

[5] L. Rensing, U. an der Heiden, and M. C. Mackey (Editors), *Temporal Disorders in Human Oscillatory Systems* (Springer-Verlag, Berlin, 1987).

[6] J. Milton and M. C. Mackey, "Dynamical diseases," Ann. N.Y. Acad. Sci. **504**, 16–32 (1987).

[7] L. Glass and M. C. Mackey, *From Clocks to Chaos: The Rhythms of Life* (Princeton University Press, Princeton, 1988).

[8] J. Jalife (Editor), "Mathematical approaches to cardiac arrhythmias," Ann. N. Y. Acad. Sci. **591**, 1–417 (1990).

[9] L. Glass, P. J. Hunter, and A. McCulloch (Editors), *Theory of Heart: Biomechanics, Biophysics, and Nonlinear Dynamics of Cardiac Function* (Springer-Verlag, New York, 1991).

[10] L. Glass (Editor), *Chaos Focus Issue on Nonlinear Dynamics of Physiological Function and Control,* Chaos **1**, 247–334 (1991).

[11] J. Milton and D. Black, "Dynamic diseases in neurology and psychiatry,"Chaos **5**, 8–13 (1995).

[12] W. A. Whitelaw, J-Ph. Derenne, and J. Cabane, "Hiccups as a dynamical disease," Chaos **5**, 14–17 (1995).

[13] A. Beuter and K. Vasilakos, "Tremor: Is Parkinson's disease a dynamical disease?" Chaos **5**, 35–42 (1995).

[14] K. M. Newell, F. Gao, and R. L. Sprague "The dynamical structure of tremor in tardive dyskinesia,"Chaos **5**, 43–47 (1995).

[15] D. Paydarfar and D. M. Buerkel, "Dysrhythmias of the respiratory oscillator,"Chaos **5**, 18–29 (1995).

[16] L. E. Meuli, H. M. Lacker, and R. B. Thau, "Experimental evidence supporting a mathematical theory of the physiological mechanism regulating follicle development and ovulation number," Biol. Reprod. **37**, 589–594 (1987).

[17] K. Prank, H. Harms, G. Brabant, R-D. Hesch, M. Dämmig, and F. Mitschke, "Nonlinear dynamics in a pulsatile secretion of parathyroid hormone in normal human subjects," Chaos **5**, 76–81 (1995).

[18] J. Sturis, C. Knudsen, N. O'Meara, J. S. Thomsen, E. Mosekilde, E. Van Cauter, and K. S. Polonsky, "Phase-locking regions in a forced model of slow insulin and glucose oscillations" Chaos **5**, 193–199 (1995).

[19] R. Lanzi and G. Tannenbaum, "Time course and mechanism of growth hormone's negative feedback effect on its own spontaneous release," Endocrinology **130**, 780–788 (1992).

[20] F. Kronenberg, "Menopausal hot flashes: Randomness or rhythmicity," Chaos **1**, 271–278 (1991).

[21] H. Mayer, K. S. Zaenker, and U. an der Heiden, "A basic mathematical model of the immune response," Chaos **5**, 155–161 (1995).

[22] G. Deuschl, M. Lauk, and J. Timmer, "Tremor classification and tremor time series analysis," Chaos **5**, 48–51 (1995).

[23] A. Boose, C. Jentgens, S. Spieker, and J. Dichgans, "Variations on tremor parameters," Chaos **5**, 52–56 (1995).

[24] H. Herzel, D. Berry, I. Titze, and I. Steinecke, "Nonlinear dynamics of the voice: Signal analysis and biomechanical modeling," Chaos **5**, 30–34 (1995).

[25] J. J. Collins and C. J. De Luca, "Upright, correlated random walks: A statistical-biomechanics approach to the human postural control system," Chaos **5**, 57–63 (1995).

[26] J. A. S. Kelso and A. Fuchs, "Self-organizing dynamics of the human brain: Critical instabilities and Šil'nikov chaos, " Chaos **5**, 64–69 (1995).

[27] C. K. Peng, S. Havlin, H. E. Stanley, and A. L. Goldberger, "Quantification of scaling exponents and crossover phenomena in nonstationary heartbeat time series," Chaos **5**, 82–87 (1995).

[28] L. A. Lipsitz, "Age-related changes in the 'complexity' of cardiovascular dynamics: A potential marker of vulnerability to disease," Chaos **5**, 102–109 (1995).

[29] J. Kurths, A. Voss, A. Witt, P. Saparin, H. J. Kleiner, and N. Wessel, "Quantitative analysis of heart rate variability," Chaos **5**, 88–94 (1995).

[30] A. Bezerianos, T. Bountis, G. Papaioannau, and P. Polydoropoulos "Nonlinear time series analysis of electrocardiograms," Chaos **5**, 95–101 (1995).

[31] D. P. Zipes and J. Jalife (Editors), *Cardiac Electrophysiology: From Cell to Bedside,* 2nd ed. (Saunders, Philadelphia, 1994).

[32] J. Demongeot, D. Benaouda, and C. Jézéque " 'Dynamical confinement' in neural networks and cell cycle," Chaos **5**, 167–173 (1995).

[33] M. R. Guevara and T. J. Lewis, "A minimal single-channel model for the regularity of beating in the sinoatrial node," Chaos **5**, 174–183 (1995).

[34] T. Schreiber and H. Kantz, "Noise in chaotic data: Diagnosis and treatment," Chaos **5**, 133–142 (1995).

[35] P. Grassberger and I. Procaccia, "Measuring the strangeness of strange attractors," Physica D **9**, 189–208 (1983).

[36] H. Kantz and T. Schreiber, "Dimension estimates and physiological data," Chaos **5**, 143–154 (1995).

[37] S. Pincus, "Approximate entropy (ApEn) as a complexity measure," Chaos **5**, 110–117 (1995).

[38] M. Ding, B. Tuller, and J. A. S. Kelso, "Characterizing the dynamics of auditory perception," Chaos **5**, 70–75 (1995).

[39] T. Chang, T. Sauer, and S. J. Schiff, "Tests for nonlinearity in short stationary time series," Chaos **5**, 118–126 (1995).

[40] T. Sauer, "Interspike interval embedding of chaotic signals," Chaos **5**, 127–132 (1995).

[41] A. M. Kunysz, A. A. Munk, and A. Shrier, "Phase resetting and dynamics in isolated atrioventricular cells," Chaos **5**, 184–192 (1995).

[42] J. P. A. Foweraker, D. Brown, and R. W. Marrs, "Discrete-time stimulation of the oscillatory and excitable forms of a FitzHugh–Nagumo model applied to the pulsatile release of luteinizing hormone releasing hormone," Chaos **5**, 200–208 (1995).

[43] A. Longtin, "Mechanisms of stochastic phase locking," Chaos **5**, 209–215 (1995).

[44] D. Claude, "Shift of a limit cycle in biology: From pathological to physiological homeostasia," Chaos **5**, 162–166 (1995).

[45] R. Langer, "New methods of drug delivery," Science **249**, 1527–1533 (1990).

[46] A. E. Reinberg, G. Labrecque, and M. H. Smolensky, *Chronobiologie et Chronothérapeutique: Heure Optimale d'Administration des Médicaments* (Flammarion, Paris, 1991).

[47] A. Garfinkel, M. L. Spano, W. L. Ditto, and J. N. Weiss, "Controlling cardiac chaos," Science **257**, 1230–1235 (1992).

[48] W. L. Ditto and L. M. Pecora, "Mastering chaos" Sci. Am. **269**(2), 78–84 (1993).

[49] S. J. Schiff, K. Jerger, D. H. Duong, T. Chay, M. L. Spano, and W. L. Ditto, "Controlling chaos in the brain," Nature **370**, 615–620 (1994).

[50] D. S. Echt *et al.*, "Mortality and morbidity in patients receiving encainide, flecainide, or placebo: The cardiac arrhythmia suppression trial," N. Engl. J. Med. **324**, 781–788 (1991).

[51] O. Sacks, *Awakenings* (Harper & Row, New York, 1974).

Dynamic diseases in neurology and psychiatry

John Milton
Department of Neurology and Committee on Neurobiology, MC-2030, The University of Chicago Hospitals, 5841 South Maryland Avenue, Chicago, Illinois 60637, and Center for Nonlinear Dynamics, McGill University, Montréal, Québec, Canada

Deborah Black
Départment de Neurologie, Hôpital Hôtel Dieu, Montréal, Québec, Canada

(Received 16 May 1994; accepted for publication 21 September 1994)

Thirty-two (32) periodic diseases of the nervous system are identified in which symptoms and/or signs recur. In 10/32, the recurrence of a symptom complex is one of the defining features of the illness, whereas in 22/32 oscillatory signs occur in the setting of an ongoing nervous system disorder. We discuss the possibility that these disorders may be dynamic diseases. © 1995 American Institute of Physics.

I. INTRODUCTION

The human nervous system is composed of a hierarchy of oscillatory processes. Self-sustained oscillations occur at the level of the single neuron,[1,2] small collections of neurons,[2–5] and in large neural populations.[6,7] In addition, the behavior of the nervous system can be influenced by external "zeitgebers," such as daylight and seasonal cycles.[8–10] Thus, it should not be surprising to observe that many diseases of the nervous system also have oscillatory features. Indeed, recurrence is a defining feature of many neurological and psychiatric illnesses, including epilepsy, migraine, manic-depressive illness, and multiple sclerosis. The clinical significance of altered neural rhythms in sleep,[11] epilepsy,[12] and depression[10] is well recognized.

The importance of considerations of the temporal pattern of illness derives from theoretical insights into the nature of oscillatory phenomena.[13–25] Mathematical studies have predicted that a single neurophysiological control mechanism, for example, a recurrent inhibitory loop,[26] is capable of generating a variety of qualitatively different periodic rhythms, as well as irregular, noise-like fluctuations. The temporal pattern that is seen depends on the value of certain critical control parameters. In patients with nervous system disorders, two patterns of recurrent disease can be recognized clinically:[18,20,23,27] (1) regular, possibly periodic recurrences; and (2) irregular, seemingly random recurrences. Is it possible that the temporal pattern of some of these disease, herein referred to as *dynamic diseases*, reflect an abnormal setting of a critical neurophysiological parameter, such as neural conduction time?[13,29] The significance of identifying a dynamic disease is that it may be possible to develop therapeutic strategies based on manipulation of the critical control parameter(s).[13,15,18,20,28]

The hallmark of a dynamic disease is a sudden, qualitative change in the temporal pattern of an illness, in response either to a therapeutic maneuver or to some endogenous factor, which presumably changes a critical control parameter.[13–15,20,29,30] It is not currently possible to apply this approach to detect a dynamic disease, since the nature of the relevant control parameters is not known. Here we identify "periodic" diseases in neurology and psychiatry. This represents a first step toward determining those diseases that are potential candidates for dynamic diseases. It is possible that longitudinal study of the diseases may help identify critical control parameters that may be susceptible to therapeutic modification.

II. METHODS

A computer-assisted (MEDLINE) search of the English and French literature from 1966 to 1994 identified ~4500 papers, which dealt with periodic phenomena in clinically related neuroscience. By restricting the search to human disease and specifically excluding the term "circadian rhythm," the number of papers was reduced to ~300. All of these papers were reviewed.

III. RESULTS

A. "Periodic" diseases

Thirty-two diseases were identified in which symptoms and/or signs recurred periodically. These disorders could be grouped into two broad categories: (1) Group I: diseases that were characterized by the recurrence of certain symptoms (10/32 diseases; Table I); and (2) group II: oscillations that appear in the context of an ongoing nervous system disease (22/32 diseases; Table II). In group I diseases, no anatomical/biochemical lesion has yet been identified that causes the recurrent symptoms. In between the episodes, the patient is well, unless the attack itself causes a structural lesion as, for example, in patients with multiple sclerosis. On the other hand, in group II diseases, an anatomical/biochemical has been identified or is presumed to exist. These abnormalities typically occur within the relevant neural feedback loop(s). Persistence of symptoms in the setting of a chronic disability is the hallmark.

Reports of patients with periodic diseases take four forms: (1) case reports; (2) analysis of patient diaries; (3) longitudinal studies of institutionalized patients; and (4) laboratory monitored time series.

B. Case reports

The most common manner in which a periodic disease is brought to the attention of the medical community is in the

TABLE I. Recurrent nervous system disease.

Disease	Time series	References
Behavioral		
Manic-depressive illness	Yes	10, 31–37
Cycloid psychoses	No	38
Kleine–Levin syndrome	Yes	39–41
Neurological		
Epilepsy	Yes	27, 42–45
Migraine and its variants	Yes	46–47
Multiple sclerosis	Yes	48–49
Periodic ataxia	No	50–52
Periodic hypothermia	No	53
Periodic dystonic choreoathetosis	No	54–56
Periodic paralysis	No	57–58

TABLE II. Oscillations in setting of neurological disease.

Disease	Time series	References
Behavior		

Repetitive movements of mentally retarded
  Head banging
  rocking
  violent
	Yes	59–64

Neuro-ophthalmology		
Nystagmus	Yes	65
Opsoclonus	Yes	65
Ping–pong gaze	Yes	66–67
Periodic alternating nystagmus	Yes	68–70
Periodic esotropia	Yes	71
Periodic mydriasis	No	72
Hippus	Yes	73
Pupil cycle time	Yes	74–78
Movement Disorders		
Tremors:		
Physiological	Yes	79
Essential	Yes	80
Cerebellar	Yes	81–82
Parkinson's	Yes	83–85
Movement disorders (continued)		
Myoclonus:		
Post-anoxic	Yes	86
Hiccups	Yes	87
Palatal	No	88
Galloping tongue	No	89
Stuttering	Yes	90
Periodic laryngospasm	No	91
Gait	Yes	92
Breathing		
Periodic	Yes	93–94
Ataxic	Yes	94
Cheyne–Stokes	Yes	94–95
Cluster	Yes	94
Electro-encephalography		
Seizures	Yes	96
Periodic complexes		
PLEDS	Yes	96–97
SSPE	Yes	96, 98–100
JC	Yes	96, 101
Electromyography		
Fibrillations	Yes	102–103
Fasiculations	Yes	102
Myotonic discharges	Yes	102
Myokimia	Yes	102

form of a case report. As might be anticipated, the publication of a case report overemphasizes patients with unusual and rare clinical presentations. The observation of the appearance or disappearance of a rhythmic process following a discrete lesion in the nervous system is evidence that this part of the nervous system is somehow involved in the genesis of the dynamic process. This tight correlation between clinical observation and anatomical abnormality is most clear in the setting of disorders of ocular motility[65–72]

In many cases the clinical phenomena are so fascinating that they warrant publication. For example, Paschalis et al.[35] describe a 78 yr old man who developed rapid mood oscillations, ranging from mania to depression. Each phase lasted approximately 24 h, and the cycles persisted for months. While depressed, he felt hopeless, worthless, and was inactive; while manic, he became jocular, overactive, and optimistic. The switch between the behavioral states always occurred during the daytime. However, the time of day the switch occurred varied in a predictable manner. Over 5–6 days, the switch time would be advanced by 1–2 h each cycle. Once the switch time was in early morning, the next switch time was advanced by 12–48 h, so that the subsequent switch occurred in late afternoon or evening.

C. Diaries

Often patients with recurring symptoms come to the attention of physicians when the patient and/or their family members keep a diary of their illness. For example, the letters of Vincent Van Gogh to his brother Theo[104] provide a diary of the episodic psychoses to which he was subject all his adult life and which informed his creative genius. The influence of an exogenous toxin, probably absinthe, may have modified the timing, as well as the content of his periodic psychoses.

Events documented in a diary are clearly of great significance to the author. Thus, it is surprising that so little has been written concerning the periodicity of pain. An exception is the study of Kaufmann et al.[105] on the timing of acute myocardial infarction pain. Nearly one-half (34/74) of the patients experienced their chest pain at extremes of the ACTH-cortisol excretion cycle, i.e., between 8 and 10 a.m. and between 8 and 10 p.m.

Lengthy diaries of recurring neurological and psychiatrical symptoms have been published: epilepsy,[27,42–45] headache,[47] and affective disorders.[10,34–36] Recently, these diaries have been subjected to time series analyses. For example, seizure diaries have been analyzed for evidence of an underlying deterministic mechanism with the aim of predicting the time of recurrence of the next seizure.[30,32–33]

Figure 1(a) shows a seizure diary and Fig. 1(b) a headache diary for two patients in our clinical practices. Although both patients felt that there was a definite periodic flavor to their illness, the time series are not clearly periodic. Indeed,

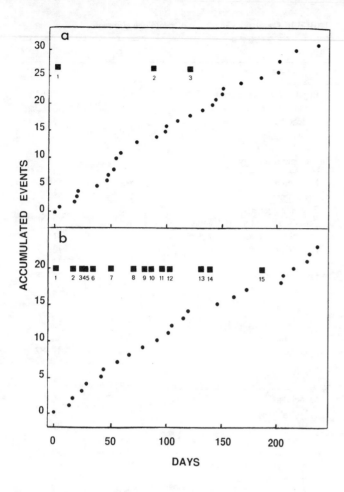

FIG. 1. Accumulated events (●) as a function of time for a (a) 17 yr old boy with seizures, and (b) a 46 yr old female with headaches. In (a) the events numbered 1 and 3 correspond to a change in medication and 2 to a headache. In (b) events 1, 8, 10, and 11 correspond to medication changes, 2, 6, 7, 9, 12, 13, and 15 to the onset of menses, and 3, 4, 5, and 14 to concurrent illness.

the approximate linearity of a plot of the accumulated number of events versus time is more suggestive of a random (Poisson) process.[27] However, over the course of the diary, both patients experienced concurrent illnesses, as well as changes in their medications. It is possible that these perturbations may obscure the periodic trends.

D. Institutionalized patients

Longitudinal studies of patients confined to institutions because of severe medical problems provide an excellent opportunity to study rhythmic phenomena. Since patients live in a controlled environment and concurrent events can be well documented, the response of the rhythm to exogenous perturbations can be recorded. For example, patients with epilepsy who were living on "epileptic communes" or "farms" at the turn of the century provide the best time series for seizure recurrence prior to the introduction of effective anticonvulsant medications.[42,44] With the development of modern medical therapies, studies of institutionalized patients have been largely limited to two patient groups: (1) severely mentally handicapped children, and (2) patients with psychiatric illness.

Stereotyped motor behaviors, such as rocking, head banging, arm flapping, and self-mutilation occur in severely mentally handicapped children.[59-64] The clinical significance of these behaviors, results from their interference with caretaker management to the loss of digits, and even blindness from self-mutilation. Recently, it has been observed that these motor behaviors recur with surprising regularity, with periods varying from 90 min to 8 h. Monthly and circaannual cycles have also been reported. In some children, the frequency and tempo of the stereotyped movements can be modified by playing strongly rhythmic marching music during the rocking episodes.[62]

Kleine–Levin syndrome, a recurrent disorder of unknown etiology occurring in adolescent boys, offers another fascinating glimpse into periodic behavioral phenomena.[39-41] Affected boys abruptly develop drowsiness, lethargy, confusion, and a craving for carbohydrates, sometimes accompanied by sexual preoccupations and inappropriate sexual behavior. Episodes last days to weeks and resolve spontaneously. Afterward, patients do not fully recall their behavior.

Perhaps the most exciting observations concerning a periodic disease have been made on patients with "rapid-cycling" manic-depressive illness.[10,31-37] Such patients oscillate between mania and depression with each phase lasting about 24 h. Recent interest has focused on the nature of the "switch" between the two behavioral states. Just before the switch patients may experience marked insomnia and decreased REM sleep, raising the possibility that brain monoamine metabolism may play a role in the switch process.

E. Time series

Thirty-six percent (36%) of the papers describing periodic diseases included a presentation of the raw time series. In 17%, only a statistical description of the observations (e.g., mean period, minimum/maximum interval) was presented. However, in 37% of the papers, no data were presented to either substantiate the recurring nature of the illness or describe its characteristics.

Raw time series data were typically presented for phenomena that recur rapidly (i.e., seconds) and that could be monitored with electrophysiological techniques. Examples include periodic phenomena in the electroencephalogram and a variety of neuro-ophthalmologic and movement disorders (Table II). In these cases, the time series were characteristically ≤1 minute, and were chosen to illustrate the phenomena under consideration. Notably, a number of raw time series lasting minutes to years for recurring diseases suitable for analyses have been published: epilepsy,[27,42-45] headache,[47] affective disorders,[10,34-36] Kleine–Levin syndrome,[39-41] and breathing patterns in patients with acute brain damage.[93]

Overnight video-EEG monitoring provides an excellent, but largely unexploited, opportunity to study sleep-related phenomena. An example is periodic leg movement during sleep, which consist of bursts of rhythmic leg movements occurring at multiple intervals throughout the night.[11] These movements show considerable night-to-night variations within the same subject.

F. Induced changes in periodic diseases

Qualitative changes in disease dynamics have been extensively described in patients with epilepsy and with sleep and affective disorders. These diseases are presently the best candidates for dynamic diseases of the nervous system.

Seizures can be induced in certain patients by a variety of stimuli, including hyperventilation and photic stimulation.[106] The period of the epileptic complexes in subacute sclerosing panencephalitis (SSPE) can be changed as body temperature is altered.[100] Attention and arousal also appear to play a role in modifying the frequency of epileptic spike-and-wave discharges.[107] When children with *petit mal* epilepsy became bored (for example, during inactivity), they had many more seizures than when their attention was engaged (for example, during IQ testing or a formal interview). Moreover, the frequency of epileptic discharges in the EEG during school exercises was approximately the same as during inactivity! These observations underscore the role of context in producing the variability in a periodic phenomena.

In patients with affective disorders, periods of mania and depression can be precipitated by, respectively, tricyclic antidepressants[108–110] and seasonal changes in ambient light levels.[10,111] The period of rapid-cycling manic-depressive illness can be changed by tricyclic antidepressants,[18,108–110] and in some patients the oscillation can be abolished with lithium. Stoddard *et al.*[112] describe a 39 yr old woman whose switch between mania and depression could be triggered by significant events in the patient's personal life, such as birthday, holidays, or therapy sessions with her husband.

G. Treatment strategies

When symptoms cause significant morbidity, it becomes necessary to develop a therapeutic strategy. Given that the underlying mechanism for a periodic disease is generally unknown, it would be anticipated that this can be a foreboding task. Nonetheless, patients and their physicians have often been able to arrive at effective treatments.

Several treatment strategies have emphasized the use of a discrete stimulus applied at a critical time. An example is the nonpharmacological treatment of patients with epilepsy. Caretakers of patients with epilepsy sometimes note that seizures can be aborted by startling the patient with a sudden noise or shaking. In the late 1960s, investigators developed an automated version of this strategy by constructing a special headset worn by the patient: one earphone monitored the EEG, and when a seizure was detected, triggered a loud noise in the contralateral ear.[113] By carefully tuning the intensity of the sound and its timing with respect to seizure onset, they were able to achieve seizure control in a number of otherwise difficult to manage patients with epilepsy. Unfortunately, this trial and error approach proved too time consuming for the method to be generally applicable. A more modern version of this approach is vagal stimulation.[114,115] Other examples include exposure to light to treat jet lag[111] and seasonal affective disorder.[10,111,116]

More commonly, the treatment of periodic disorders has focused on pharmacological strategies. From a dynamical disease standpoint, such approaches can be thought of as a "shotgun" method to alter control parameters. Examples include the use of lithium to dampen fluctuations in mood,[117] anticonvulsant medications to prevent seizures, melatonin to modify jet lag,[111] and the combination of thyroid hormone, benzodiazepines, and vitamin B12 to reset a free-running sleep wake cycle.[118] An example of a nonpharmacological approach to alter a control parameter is the addition of weights to a limb in a patient with cerebellar disease to decrease the oscillations of an intention tremor.[82]

IV. DISCUSSION

We have shown that there are at least 32 periodic diseases in psychiatry and neurology. These disorders arise at every level of the nervous system: muscle, nerve, spinal cord, brainstem, and cortex. Clinical experience suggests that patients with periodic recurrences in their symptoms can be especially refractory to treatment by traditional methods (for example, catamenial epilepsy[119]). It is possible that a careful study of disease dynamics might shed light onto the etiology of these disorders and how they can be best managed.

It is not unreasonable to hope that the recent mathematical advances into the nature of oscillatory processes might provide insights into the management of periodic diseases. For this to be fruitful, a necessary first step is that the time series be well enough described to permit analyses. A problem is that the clinical use of the term "periodic" differs from its mathematical meaning. Periodic diseases typically do not recur with clock-like regularity, but "every so often" or "every once in a while."

There are two possible explanations for the irregularity in the recurrence of symptoms and/or signs in periodic diseases. First, the periodicity of the disease may have been obscured by various randomly occurring endogenous and exogenous factors. Moreover, the behavioral and symptomatic measurements employed by physicians in the bedside assessment of a patient may be too crude to detect subclinical periodic oscillations. Second, it is possible that the disease process is inherently irregular. Time series methods to distinguish between these two possibilities are available.[120] However, these methods are currently of limited clinical value, since they require long time series that are impractical to obtain, particularly for those diseases in which the symptoms recur infrequently (e.g., monthly or yearly).

Social events and context can cause important perturbations in periodic phenomena in humans and animals. In a fascinating study of ten lizards housed in a group cage, Regal and Connolly[121] observed that the "omega lizard," at the bottom of the dominance hierarchy, desynchronized its sleep–wake-feeding rhythm from the other lizards in the cage, presumably as an adaptation to avoid aggression and conflict over food. Similar observations have been made in rats. Such perturbations are difficult to quantitate and are rarely described in clinical time series. This further underscores the difficulty in interpreting irregular time series.

An underlying mechanism for the recurrent diseases becomes conceptually plausible when a qualitative change in temporal pattern occurs in response to a therapeutic maneuver can be identified. Such changes have indeed been observed in a number of periodic diseases (see Sec. III D), and identify such diseases as dynamic diseases. Since a relatively short time series before and after the perturbation are all that is required to demonstrate a change in temporal pattern, it should be possible for physicians to readily identify such phenomena. Moreover, a control parameter, which potentially can be manipulated to therapeutic advantage, has necessarily been identified.

The temporal dimension of illness continues to receive little attention from physicians, whose major focus is the molecular pathophysiology and pharmacological treatment of disease. However, it is conceivable that the beneficial effects of a drug in the treatment of a periodic disease could be overlooked if proper attention is not given to details concerning, for example, the timing of drug administration.[105] In addition, it is possible that nonpharmacological therapeutic approaches may be as useful (as, for example, in the treatment of epilepsy). The challenge to the clinician will be to identify those patients in whom considerations of disease dynamics are necessary in order to formulate a treatment strategy.

ACKNOWLEDGMENTS

We gratefully acknowledge the invaluable assistance of the library staff at Hôtel Dieu Hospital. This work was supported by grants obtained from the National Institutes of Mental Health (NIMH) and the North Atlantic Treaty Organization (NATO).

[1] L. R. Silva, Y. Amital, and B. W. Connors, Science **251**, 432 (1991).
[2] R. Llinás, Science **242**, 1654 (1988).
[3] R. D. Traub, R. Miles, and R. K. S. Wong, Science **243**, 1319 (1989).
[4] J. C. Smith et al., Science **254**, 726 (1991).
[5] M. Von Krosigk, T. Bal, and D. A. McCormick, Science **261**, 361 (1993).
[6] M. Steraide, P. Gloor, R. R. Llinás, F. H. Lopes da Silva, and M.-M. Mesulam, Epilepsia **76**, 481 (1990).
[7] M. Steriade, D. A. McCormick, and T. J. Sejnowski, Science **262**, 679 (1993).
[8] C. A. Czeisler et al., Science **244**, 1328 (1989).
[9] D. D. Ginty, J. M. Kornhauser, M. A. Thompson, H. Bading, K. E. Mayo, J. S. Takahashi, and M. E. Greenberg, Science **260**, 238 (1993).
[10] T. A. Wehr and F. K. Goodwin, in Circadian Rhythms in Psychiatry (Boxwood, Pacific Grove, CA, 1983).
[11] S. Sheldon, J.-P. Spire, and H. Levy, Pediatric Sleep Medicine (Saunders, Philadelphia, 1992).
[12] E. Wylie in The Treatment of Epilepsy: Principles and Practice (Lea & Febinger, Philadelphia, 1993).
[13] M. C. Mackey and L. Glass, Science **197**, 287 (1977).
[14] L. Glass and M. C. Mackey, Ann. NY Acad. Sci. **316**, 214 (1979).
[15] U. an der Heiden and M. C. Mackey, J. Math. Biol. **16**, 75 (1982).
[16] M. C. Mackey and U. an der Heiden, Funkt. Biol. Med. **1**, 156 (1982).
[17] L. Rensing, U. an der Heiden, and M. C. Mackey, Temporal Disorder in Human Oscillatory Systems (Springer-Verlag, New York, 1987).
[18] M. C. Mackey and J. G. Milton, Ann. NY Acad. Sci. **504**, 16 (1987).
[19] L. Glass and M. C. Mackey, From Clocks to Chaos: The Rhythms of Life (Princeton University Press, Princeton, NJ, 1988).
[20] J. G. Milton et al., J. Theor. Biol. **138**, 129 (1989).
[21] J. G. Milton and M. C. Mackey, J. R. Colloid. Phys. London **23**, 236 (1989).
[22] J. G. Milton et al., Biomed. Biochim. Acta **49**, 697 (1990).
[23] M. C. Mackey and J. G. Milton, Comments Theor. Biol. **1**, 299
[24] L. Glass, Chaos **1**, 247 (1991).
[25] A. Asachenkov, G. Marchuk, R. Mohler, and S. Zuev, Disease Dynamics (Birhäuser, Boston, 1994).
[26] M. C. Mackey and U. an der Heiden, J. Math. Biol. **19**, 211 (1984).
[27] J. G. Milton et al., Epilepsia **28**, 471 (1987).
[28] J. G. Milton, S. A. Campbell, and J. Bélair, J. Biol. Sys. (in press).
[29] L. Glass, A. Beuter, and D. Larocque, Math. Biosci. **90**, 111 (1988).
[30] A. Longtin and J. G. Milton, Math. Biosci. **90**, 183 (1988).
[31] W. E. Bunney et al., Ann. Int. Med. **87**, 319 (1977).
[32] S. M. Hanna, F. A. Jenner, and L. P. Souster, Br. J. Psychiat. **149**, 229 (1986).
[33] D. J. King, S. A. M. Salem, and N. S. Meimary, Br. J. Psychiat. **135**, 190 (1979).
[34] G. Nikitopoulou and J. L. Crammer, Br. Med. J. **1**, 1311 (1976).
[35] C. Paschalis, A. Pavlou, and A. Papadimitriou, Br. J. Psychiat. **137**, 332 (1980).
[36] T. A. Wehr et al., Arch. Gen. Psychiat. **39**, 559 (1982).
[37] S. Zisook, J. Nerv. Ment. Dis. **176**, 53 (1988).
[38] K. Leonhard, J. Ment. Sci. **107**, 633 (1961).
[39] C. Billard et al., Arch. France Ped. **35**, 424 (1978).
[40] H. Garland, D. Sumner, and P. Fourman, Neurology **18**, 1161 (1965).
[41] M. Billiard, C. Guilleminault, and W. C. Dement, Neurology **25**, 436 (1975).
[42] R. Almqvist, Acta Psych. Neurol. Scand. (Suppl. 105) **30**, 1 (1955).
[43] G. W. Frank et al., Physica D **56**, 427 (1990).
[44] G. M. Griffiths and J. T. Fox, Lancet **409** (1938).
[45] L. Iasemidis et al., Epilepsy Res. **17**, 81 (1994).
[46] G. C. Manzoni et al., Eur. Neurol. **20**, 88 (1981).
[47] P. O. Osterman et al., Upsala J. Med. Sci. Suppl. **31**, 23 (1980).
[48] B. Weinshenker and G. Ebers, Can. J. Neurol. Sci. **14**, 255 (1987).
[49] B. Weinshenker et al., Brain **112**, 1419 (1989).
[50] R. W. Baloh and A. Winder, Neurology **41**, 429 (1991).
[51] W. DeCastro and J. Campbell, J. Am. Med. Assoc. **200**, 892 (1967).
[52] G. J. Hankey and S. S. Gubbay, Med. J. Austral. **150**, 277 (1989).
[53] R. H. Fox et al., Br. Med. J. **2**, 693 (1973).
[54] J. W. Lance, Ann. Neurol. **2**, 285 (1977).
[55] L. A. Mount and S. Reback, Arch. Neurol. Psychiat. **44**, 841 (1940).
[56] R. N. Richards and H. J. M. Barnett, Neurology **18**, 461 (1968).
[57] T. Johnson, Dan. Med. Bull. **28**, 1 (1981).
[58] R. B. Layzer, R. E. Lovelace, and L. P. Rowland, Arch. Neurol. **16**, 455 (1967).
[59] M. H. Lewis et al., Am. J. Mental Defic. **85**, 601 (1981).
[60] R. Brusca, Am. J. Mental Defic. **89**, 650 (1985).
[61] A. Meier-Koll and P. Pohl, Int. J. Chronobiol. **6**, 191 (1979).
[62] E. A. Stevens, Am. J. Mental Defic. **76**, 76 (1971).
[63] W. B. Quay, Chronobiologia **2**, 243 (1975).
[64] M. G. Wade, Am. J. Mental Defic. **78**, 262 (1973).
[65] N. R. Miller, in Walsh and Hoyt's Clinical Neuro-Ophthalmology (Williams & Wilkins, Baltimore, MD, 1985).
[66] H. Ishikawa, S. Ishikawa, and K. Mukuno, Neurology **43**, 1067 (1993).
[67] E. F. Masucci et al., Ann. Ophthalmol. **13**, 1123 (1981).
[68] R. W. Baloh, V. Honrubia, and H. R. Konrad, Brain **99**, 11 (1976).
[69] M. E. Norre and T. Puls, Acta Oto-Rhino-Laryngol. Belg. **35**, 198 (1981).
[70] P. Rudge and J. Leech, J. Neurol. Neurosurg. Psychiat. **39**, 314 (1976).
[71] B. T. Troost et al., Am. J. Ophthalmol. **91**, 8 (1981).
[72] M. Hallett and D. G. Cogan, Arch. Ophthalmol. **84**, 130 (1970).
[73] L. Stark, F. W. Campbell, and J. Atwood, Nature **182**, 857 (1958).
[74] S. D. Miller and H. S. Thompson, Br. J. Ophthalmol. **62**, 495 (1978).
[75] J. G. Milton et al., Am. J. Ophathalmol. **105**, 402 (1988).
[76] A. Longtin and J. G. Milton, Bull. Math. Biol. **51**, 605 (1989).
[77] A. Longtin and J. G. Milton, Biol. Cybern. **61**, 51 (1989).
[78] J. G. Milton and A. Longtin, Vision Res. **30**, 515 (1990).
[79] O. Lippold, Sci. Am. **224**, 65 (1971).
[80] W. C. Koller and N. Biary, Neurology **34**, 221 (1984).
[81] J. Bruce and C. McLellan, Lancet **1**, 1221 (1980).
[82] R. L. Hewer, R. Cooper, and M. H. Morgan, Brain **95**, 759 (1972).
[83] A. Beuter et al., Exp. Neurol. **110**, 228 (1990).
[84] A. Beuter and K. Vasilakos, Chaos **5**, 35 (1995).
[85] S. Toth, P. Zarand, and L. Lazar, Acta Neurochir. Suppl. **21**, 25 (1974).
[86] P. J. Wolf, Neurol. **215**, 39 (1977).
[87] W. A. Whitelaw and J-Ph. Derenne, Chaos **5**, 14 (1995).
[88] J. Lapresle, J. Neurol. **220**, 223 (1979).
[89] J. R. Keane, Neurology **34**, 251 (1984).
[90] R. R. Martin, L. J. Johnson, G. M. Siegel, and S. K. Haroldson, J. Speech Hear. Res. **28**, 487 (1985).
[91] J. Cambier et al., Rev. Neurol. (Paris) **139**, 531 (1983).

[92] R. D. Adams and M. Victor, *Principles of Neurology* (McGraw-Hill, Toronto, 1985).

[93] J. B. North and S. Jennett, Arch. Neurol. **31**, 338 (1974).

[94] F. Plum and J. B. Posner, *The Diagnosis of Stupor and Coma* (Davis, Philadelphia, 1980).

[95] A. C. Guyton, J. W. Crowell, and J. W. Moore, Am. J. Physiol. **187**, 395 (1956).

[96] E. Niedermeyer and L. da Silva, *Electroencephalography: Basic Principles, Clinical Applications and Related Fields* (Urban & Schwarzenberg, Baltimore, 1987).

[97] A. Janati, M. Z. Chesser, and M. M. Husain, Clin. Electroenceph. **17**, 36 (1986).

[98] G. G. Celesia, Electroenceph. Clin. Neurophysiol. **35**, 293 (1973).

[99] B. M. Evans, Electroenceph. Clin. Neurophysiol. **39**, 587 (1975).

[100] D. E. Farrell, A. Starr, and J. M. Freeman, Electroenceph. Clin. Neurophysiol. **30**, 415 (1971).

[101] P. Gloor, Ann. Neurol. **8**, 341 (1980).

[102] J. Kimura, *Electrodiagnosis in Diseases of Nerve and Muscle: Principles and Practice* (Davis, Philadelphia, 1983).

[103] D. Purves and B. Sakmann, J. Physiol. **239**, 125 (1974).

[104] R. R. Monroe, J. Nerv. Mental Disorders **166**, 480 (1978).

[105] M. W. Kaufman *et al.*, Psychosomatics **23**, 1109 (1982).

[106] R. B. Aird, Epilepsia **24**, 567 (1983).

[107] J. Guey *et al.*, Epilepsia **10**, 441 (1969).

[108] B. Lerer *et al.*, Br. J. Psychiat. **137**, 183 (1980).

[109] S. G. Siris, H. R. Chertoff, and J. M. Perel, Am. J. Psychiat. **136**, 341 (1979).

[110] T. A. Wehr and F. K. Goodwin, Arch. Gen. Psychiat. **36**, 555 (1979).

[111] A. J. Lewy and R. L. Sack, Proc. Soc. Exp. Biol. Med. **183**, 11 (1986).

[112] F. J. Stoddard, R. J. Post, and W. E. Bunney, Br. J. Psychiat. **130**, 72 (1977).

[113] F. M. Forster, *Reflex Epilepsy, Conditional Reflexes and Behavioural Treatment* (Thomas, Springfield, IL, 1975).

[114] A. R. M. Upton, Pacing Clin. Electrophysiol. **15**, 1543 (1992).

[115] B. J. Wilder, Epilepsia **31**, S1 (1990).

[116] A. Wirz-Justice, Prog. Drug Res. **31**, 383 (1987).

[117] Y. A. Rosier, P. Brousolle, and M. Fontany, Ann. Medico-Psychol. **132**, 389 (1974).

[118] B. Kamgar-Parsi, T. A. Wehr, and J. C. Gillin, Sleep **6**, 257 (1983).

[119] R. H. Mattson, J. M. Kamer, and J. A. Cramer, Epilepsia **22**, 242 (1981).

[120] D. Kaplan, Physica D **73**, 38 (1994).

[121] P. J. Regal and M. S. Connolly, Behavior **72**, 171 (1980).

Hiccups as a dynamical disease

W. A. Whitelaw
Department of Medicine, University of Calgary, 3330 Hospital Drive, NW, Calgary, Alberta T2N 2N1, Canada

J.-Ph. Derenne
Service de Pneumologie, Groupe Hospitalier Pitre-Salpétrière, Paris, France

J. Cabane
Service de Medicine Interne, Hoptial St. Antoine, Paris, France

(Received 20 June 1994; accepted for publication 21 September 1994)

I. INTRODUCTION

Everyone has had hiccups from time to time, either single ones or series (or bouts) of them, and knows tricks for putting an end to a bout. Hiccups can be observed in many mammalian species. In humans, they occur *in utero*, are common in babies, and decrease in frequency with age. Troublesome, prolonged, or repeated bouts are observed in connection with a wide range of diseases. In general, these can be classified as diseases of the stomach and esophagus, of the lungs and mediastinum or of the central nervous system, or as derangements of metabolism. There are no well-established animal models of hiccups produced experimentally.

A single hiccup is a coordinated movement involving contraction of many muscles. The glottis is closed actively, the soft palate rises, the diaphragm, inspiratory intercostal muscles, and neck accessory muscles of respiration all make a sudden violent contraction. Motor output to expiratory intercostal muscles is inhibited. There is a sudden sharp inspiratory rush of air that is interrupted by closure of the glottis to make the "hic" noise. Autonomic, parasympathetic discharge is thought to produce the bradycardia, contraction of tracheal smooth muscle and reverse peristalsis in the esophagus that are sometimes associated with hiccups.

The stereotyped motor pattern suggests strongly that hiccups are due to the activity of a central pattern generator (a neural network that can generate patterned behavior independently of peripheral feedback) somewhere in the nervous system. The activity is presumably suppressed most of the time, but can appear under the right circumstances. The purpose of such a pattern generator or of hiccups is unknown. What is known about a postulated hiccup generator comes from studying the behaviors of hiccups, and is rather scanty because hiccups do not usually threaten the health of a subject enough to justify complex or invasive investigations, and because bouts of hiccups are usually transient, tending to vanish just before the investigator gets the apparatus together. Most useful observations have been made on patients with chronic hiccups that recur in long bouts on and off over months or years. We have recently been able to study a series of these cases through a hiccup clinic in Paris that gathers referrals from a large population base and provides a systematic diagnosis and treatment service.

Hiccups are a dynamical disease in two senses: (1) Within one bout, individual hiccups have a rhythm of their own. (2) In chronic cases, bouts of hiccups of varying length come and go with varying intervals between them.

II. BEHAVIOR OF HICCUPS WITHIN A BOUT

The first good study (Newsom Davis)[1] not only described many details of the motor pattern of a hiccup, but showed in three patients that hiccups ran at a reasonably constant frequency, different for each subject, ranging from 13 to 30/min (Fig. 1). Hiccups were linked to respiration, with a strong tendency to occur in midinspiration (Fig. 2), and this tendency was enhanced when breathing was made more regular with the use of a metronome. When CO_2 (a stimulant to respiration) was given, hiccup frequency gradually declined, and sometimes the bout of hiccups would stop. The last observation was used to argue that hiccups are not generated by the network responsible for respiration, but by a separate one.

We studied the relationship between hiccup and heartbeat in ten subjects with chronic hiccups who had prolonged polygraphic recordings in a sleep laboratory. Monitoring included electroencephalograms, electromyograms, and electro-oculograms to determine sleep state. Respiration and hiccups were recorded by bands around the rib cage and abdomen. Hiccups could also be seen as bursts of electromyogram activity from electrodes placed on the anterior rib cage. The electrocardiogram was recorded separately, but showed as well on the rib cage electromyogram. Respiratory airflow was detected by a thermistor placed near the nose and mouth. A typical tracing of the band around the abdomen, the

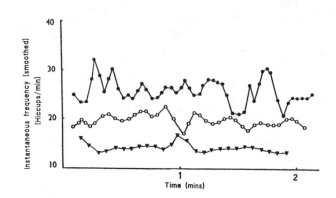

FIG. 1. Frequency of hiccups over time in three patients (from Newsom Davis).[1]

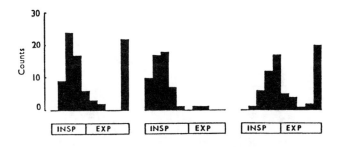

FIG. 2. Occurrence of hiccups in the respiratory cycle in three patients (from Newsom Davis).[1]

electrocardiogram, and the chest wall electromyogram is shown in Fig. 3. Paper speed is 15 mm/s and timing of events could be measured with an accuracy of 0.03 s. Recordings were made for one or two hours at a time, and contained from 1000 to 2000 hiccups. For analysis of hiccup/heartbeat relations, consecutive series of 100–150 hiccups were used.

Our observations have shown that the timing of hiccups is related to heartbeat, with a strong tendency in most patients to occur toward the end of systole (Fig. 4). Heart rhythm is generated by intrinsic pacemaker cells within the heart. The nervous system is able to accelerate and decelerate the heart rhythm generator, but cannot set off individual beats. Thus, there is no evident mechanism by which a hiccup generator in the nervous system could entrain heart rhythm. Instead, it is likely that heartbeat entrains hiccup rhythm. Numerous peripheral receptors, for blood pressure, ventricular tension, or atrial tension, for example, do send periodic discharges synchronous with heartbeat to the central nervous system, and these could conceivably entrain the periodic bursting of the hiccup generator.

We have also had the opportunity to explore the relation between respiration and hiccups in a patient who hiccupped while asleep and had central sleep apnea, a benign medical condition in which respiration becomes periodic, with long intervals of apnea (up to 40 s in this case) alternating with intervals of hyperpnea. In this patient, the hiccups continued during apneas, but their frequency would decline through

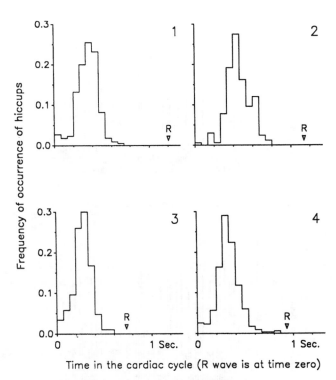

FIG. 4. Occurrence of hiccups in the cardiac cycle. Each histogram was constructed from observations on 100–150 consecutive hiccups from one subject. Data from four subjects are shown.

each apnea and then pick up again when breathing resumed (Fig. 5). The synchrony with respiration was 1:1 before the beginning of apneas, but when breathing resumed at the end of the apnea, hiccups would begin at 1:3 to respiration and change through 1:2 to 1:1 as hiccup frequency returned to its original level. The slowing of hiccups when breathing stops might well be explained by the blood carbon dioxide level, which rises during each apnea, and is known to be associated with a fall in hiccup frequency. A confounding factor is the sleep state, however, because this patient oscillated with each cycle between being awake through the interval when he was breathing to being asleep through the interval when he had

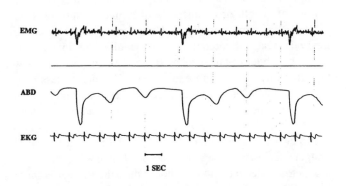

FIG. 3. Polygraph tracing. EMG: chest wall electromyogram. ABD: band around the abdomen. EKG: electrocardiogram. Large, sharp deflections on ABD, associated with large bursts on EMG are hiccups.

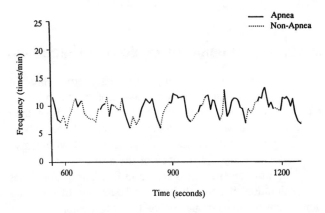

FIG. 5. Frequency of hiccups over time in a patient with recurrent apnea in sleep.

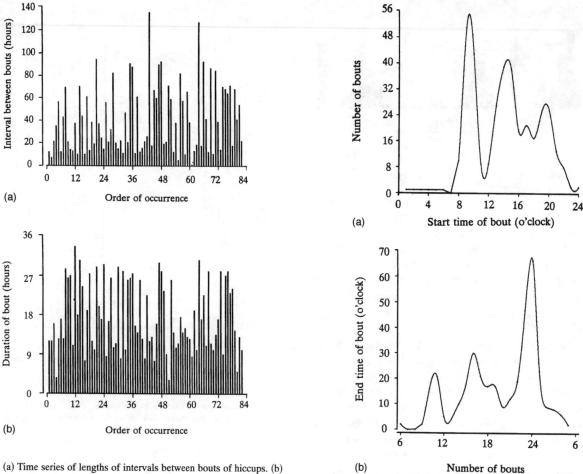

FIG. 6. (a) Time series of lengths of intervals between bouts of hiccups. (b) Time series of lengths of bouts of hiccups [the same database as (a)].

FIG. 7. (a) Distribution of times in the day when bouts of hiccups began in one subject. (b) Distribution of times in the day when bouts of hiccups ended in the same subject.

apnea. It is possible that sleep by itself changes the frequency of firing of the hiccup generator.

These data give a picture of three linked oscillators—a hiccup generator, the respiratory rhythm generator, and the heart. A hiccup integrate and fire model with input to the integrator from both the respiratory and cardiovascular systems, might be used to explain the timing of hiccups. Studies of hiccups, respiration and heartbeat over long periods could give insight into the behavior of the hiccup oscillator, and of the nature and strength of interactions with the other systems.

III. LONG TERM BEHAVIOR OF BOUTS OF HICCUPS

Among the hundred or so patients with chronic hiccups seen in Paris, there are a few who have kept exact continuous records over many months or years of when each of their recurrent bouts began, and when it ended. We have been analyzing these data in search of patterns that would give clues about the pathophysiology of the disorder.

Data from one patient is shown in Fig. 6 as a time series of the duration of intervals between bouts, and of the duration of bouts. Analysis has so far failed to demonstrate any clear pattern in these time series. Frequency plots of the number of bouts of hiccups beginning at each hour of the day

show several peaks that correspond to normal meal times of the patients [Fig. 7(a)]. Frequency plots of the number of bouts ending at each hour of the day show a strong tendency for bouts to end when the patient goes to sleep [Fig. 7(b)].

Frequency plots of the numbers of bouts of different durations [Fig. 8(a)], or the number of intervals of different durations [Fig. 8(b)] show that short bouts and short intervals are most common. The likelihood of the occurrence of bouts of a given length or of intervals of a given length falls off more or less exponentially with the length of the bouts or intervals. One interpretation of these plots for intervals is that once a bout of hiccups has stopped, the chance of a new bout starting in each subsequent hour is more or less constant. Similarly, the duration plots suggest that once a bout has started, the chance of its coming to an end in each subsequent hour is the same. The subject illustrated has a duration plot that seems to have a rapidly falling exponential at first, and a slowly falling one later on. This implies that there is a period after the end of a bout when the subject is more likely than at other times to start another bout.

The well-known ability to stop a bout of hiccups by means of maneuver (such as stimulating the back of the throat with a plastic catheter, or eating powdered sugar) that

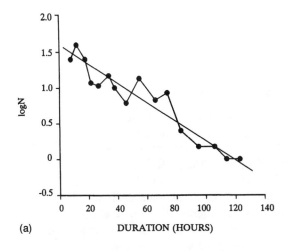

(a)

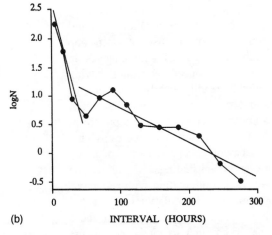

(b)

FIG. 8. (a) Frequency distribution of the lengths of bouts of hiccups. (b) Frequency distribution of lengths of intervals between bouts.

produce a brief discharge of sensory receptors in the pharynx, makes the point that the rhythmic activity of the hiccup generator can be permanently extinguished by a transient input. People with chronic hiccups often report that their hiccups are impossible to extinguish at the beginning of a bout, but the same maneuvers may be successful after a bout has been going on for a few hours or days.

Study of the patterns of the recurrence of hiccups and of the circumstances by which they can most successfully be extinguished may lead in the future to better hypotheses about the mechanism for generation and maintenance of this abnormal rhythmic behavior of the postulated hiccup generator.

APPENDIX: DATA SETS AVAILABLE

(1) We are beginning the collection and digitization of series of hiccups together with respiratory flow and volume and of heartbeat from subjects whose hiccups persist for hours. Typical series contain 1–2000 hiccups.

(2) We have digitized data sets of bouts of hiccups from diaries of four subjects with numbers of bouts: 364, 208, 119, and 84.

[1] J. Newsom Davis, "An experimental study of hiccup," Brain **93**, 851 (1970).

Dysrhythmias of the respiratory oscillator

David Paydarfar and Daniel M. Buerkel

Departments of Medicine and Biomedical Research, St. Elizabeth's Medical Center of Boston and Tufts University School of Medicine, Boston Massachusetts 02135

(Received 23 September 1994; accepted for publication 7 December 1994)

Breathing is regulated by a central neural oscillator that produces rhythmic output to the respiratory muscles. Pathological disturbances in rhythm (dysrhythmias) are observed in the breathing pattern of children and adults with neurological and cardiopulmonary diseases. The mechanisms responsible for genesis of respiratory dysrhythmias are poorly understood. The present studies take a novel approach to this problem. The basic postulate is that the rhythm of the respiratory oscillator can be altered by a variety of stimuli. When the oscillator recovers its rhythm after such perturbations, its phase may be reset relative to the original rhythm. The amount of phase resetting is dependent upon stimulus parameters and the level of respiratory drive. The long-range hypothesis is that respiratory dysrhythmias can be induced by stimuli that impinge upon or arise within the respiratory oscillator with certain combinations of strength and timing relative to the respiratory cycle. Animal studies were performed in anesthetized or decerebrate preparations. Neural respiratory rhythmicity is represented by phrenic nerve activity, allowing use of open-loop experimental conditions which avoid negative chemical feedback associated with changes in ventilation. In animal experiments, respiratory dysrhythmias can be induced by stimuli having specific combinations of strength and timing. Newborn animals readily exhibit spontaneous dysrhythmias which become more prominent at lower respiratory drives. In human subjects, swallowing was studied as a physiological perturbation of respiratory rhythm, causing a pattern of phase resetting that is characterized topologically as type 0. Computational studies of the Bonhoeffer–van der Pol (BvP) equations, whose qualitative behavior is representative of many excitable systems, supports a unified interpretation of these experimental findings. Rhythmicity is observed when the BvP model exhibits recurrent periods of excitation alternating with refractory periods. The same system can be perturbed to a state in which amplitude of oscillation is attenuated or abolished. We have characterized critical perturbations which induce transitions between these two states, giving rise to patterns of dysrhythmic activity that are similar to those seen in the experiments. We illustrate the importance of noise in initiation and termination of rhythm, comparable to normal respiratory rhythm intermixed with spontaneous dysrhythmias. In the BvP system the incidence and duration of dysrhythmia is shown to be strongly influenced by the level of noise. These studies should lead to greater understanding of rhythmicity and integrative responses of the respiratory control system, and provide insight into disturbances in control mechanisms that cause apnea and aspiration in clinical disease states. © *1995 American Institute of Physics.*

I. INTRODUCTION

Breathing is regulated by a central neural oscillator that produces rhythmic output to the respiratory muscles. Pathological disturbances in the rhythm of breathing can lead to prolonged apnea and severe hypoxemia. Respiratory recordings[1] of these potentially fatal episodes have shown that in some cases, most commonly in sleeping infants, the first sign of apnea is cessation of rhythmic contraction of the diaphragm without airway obstruction, suggesting that the disturbance is due to loss of rhythmicity of the brainstem respiratory oscillator. These dysrhythmias often arise unexpectedly, i.e., they are immediately preceded by a normal respiratory pattern and a normal metabolic profile. In some instances prolonged apneic pauses are associated with or triggered by brief physiological stimuli such as exposure to sound,[2,3] stimulation of the face,[4,5] oropharynx, or larynx,[6] and swallowing.[7] All infants are frequently exposed to these brief physiological stimuli, so the mechanism by which generally benign perturbations could on rare occasion cause prolonged apnea has remained a mystery.

Figure 1 shows an example[1] of prolonged non-obstructive expiratory apnea during sleep in a 30 month-old child. The respiratory pattern and oxygen saturation are normal during the first 40 s of the tracing followed by loss of chest wall movement and oxygen desaturation for nearly 1 min. During the apnea, there are no respiratory-related esophageal and gastric pressure changes, indicating lack of inspiratory effort, which would have been seen if the apnea was caused by acute airway obstruction. The large esophageal positive pressure wave near the onset and offset of the apnea was likely due to peristaltic activation of the esophagus several seconds after swallowing. The incidence of swallowing at the transitions between normal and abnormal respiratory rhythm has not been systematically examined. Otherwise, these tracings typify non-obstructive infant apnea syndrome.

A broad class of excitable systems can exhibit dysrhythmic behavior in response to perturbations that impinge upon the oscillation with specific combinations of strength and timing (critical stimuli).[8] A clock-pendulum system helps to

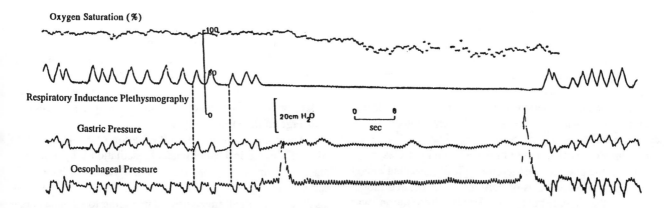

FIG. 1. Example of non-obstructive sleep apnea in a 30 month-old child. The normal respiratory pattern is interrupted by progressive oxygen desaturation and apnea lasting approximately 1 min. Absence of negative esophageal pressure waves during the apnea suggests lack of inspiratory effort. Note the large esophageal pressure waves at beginning and end of apnea, likely due to peristaltic esophageal activation related to swallowing. Adapted from S. P. Southall and D. G. Talbert, "Mechanisms for abnormal apnea of possible relevance to sudden infant death syndrome" Ann. NY Acad. Sci. **533**, p. 337, Fig. 6 (1988).

illustrate the phenomenon: counter striking the pendulum just as it passes to the bottom of its arc can stop the clock only if the strength of the impulse exactly opposes the momentum of the pendulum at that time. Other perturbations having strength or time of impact different from the critical impulse cause shifts in the phase the pendulum's rhythm of movement but do not stop the clock. Once stopped by a critical impulse, striking the pendulum with a second impulse, if strong enough, will reinitiate the normal operation of the clock.

In this paper, we review experimental work in animals[9-11] and humans[12] that characterizes the phase resetting properties of the mammalian respiratory oscillator. In adult animal experiments, respiratory dysrhythmias can be induced by stimuli having specific combinations of strength and timing. Newborn animals readily exhibit spontaneous dysrhythmias which become more prominent at lower respiratory drives. Computational studies of the Bonhoeffer–van der Pol (BvP) equations, whose qualitative behavior is representative of many excitable systems, support a unified interpretation of these experimental findings. Rhythmicity is observed when the BvP model exhibits recurrent periods of excitation alternating with refractory periods. The same system can be perturbed to a state in which amplitude of oscillation is attenuated or abolished. Critical perturbations induce transitions between these two states, giving rise to patterns of activity that are similar to those seen in the experiments. We illustrate the importance of noise in initiation and termination of rhythm, comparable to normal respiratory rhythm intermixed with spontaneous dysrhythmias. Our hypothesis on the dynamics of the respiratory oscillator can be further evaluated in neurophysiological experiments, and may have therapeutic implications for the treatment of respiratory dysrhythmias.

II. METHODS

Animal studies. These experiments in cats allowed for recording the rhythm of the respiratory oscillator in the absence of respiratory feedback mechanisms and influences from higher brain. Animals were anesthetized, mechanically ventilated through a tracheostomy, and paralyzed by neuromuscular blockade. In order to ablate feedback from lung and carotid body receptors, the vagosympathetic trunks and carotid sinus nerves were cut. A servo-ventilator was used to hold end-tidal P_{CO_2} within a narrow range (± 0.5 Torr) around any desired level.[13] Body core temperature was monitored and servo-controlled at 37 °C–38 °C by an electronic circuit and DC heating pad. Neural respiratory rhythm was recorded from the central end of a phrenic nerve; the electrical activity was half-wave rectified and integrated for each 100 ms period by means of an integrating digital voltmeter.[14] The onset of inspiration was designated by computer as the time when integrated phrenic activity increased to a level that was twice the baseline noise level. In order to study influences of neural maturation on dysrhythmias of the respiratory oscillator, experiments were performed in six newborn kittens (age 1–10 days), using a similar preparation. Anesthesia was achieved with intraperitoneal injection of sodium pentobarbital (30 mg/kg) in 2 kittens, a mixture of chloralose (40 mg/kg) and urethan (250 mg/kg) in 2 kittens. Because of the possibility that there are differential effects of anesthesia on the newborn vs adult respiratory oscillator, therefore leading to inconclusive results on the role of maturation, intercollicular decerebration followed by removal of inhaled ether was performed in 4 kittens. Decerebration in two kittens led to severe hypotension and no phrenic rhythm. In the remaining two, the preparation was viable throughout the study. There were no qualitative differences in the findings between anesthetized and decerebrate kittens.

In the adult animal studies, two series of experiments on respiratory phase resetting were performed, distinguished by the neural structure that was stimulated: superior laryngeal nerve (SLN)[9] or midbrain reticular formation.[10,11] Each stimulus throughout an experiment was preceded by 10 control breaths, during which end-tidal P_{CO_2} and neural respiratory rhythm remained constant (range: ± 0.5 Torr end-tidal P_{CO_2}; $\pm 5\%$ change in respiratory period). After each stimulus, an additional 4–15 breaths were recorded. Initially, a specific stimulus strength was selected and given at various times in the respiratory cycle. An attempt was made to give at least one stimulus in each 5% of the respiratory cycle. On completion of this set of runs, the stimulus strength was increased or decreased and the protocol was repeated. Stimulus strength was varied by changing the duration of the stimulus train, or by changing the frequency or intensity (current) of stimulation during a fixed interval.

Human studies. Relationships between the timing of respiration and swallowing (deglutition) were studied in 30 healthy subjects at rest.[12] Swallowing was evaluated by monitoring electrical activity of the submental muscles, pressure within the pharynx, and fluoroscopically detected movement of a swallowed bolus of barium and associated movements of the hyoid bone and larynx. Respiration was recorded by measurement of oro-nasal airflow through a pneumotachometer attached to a face mask, and chest wall movement using pressure tubing placed around the chest. Three types of deglutition were studied: injected bolus swallows, spontaneous swallows, and visually cued swallows of boluses previously placed in the mouth.

Computational studies. Fitzhugh[15] presented a generalization of the classic van der Pol "relaxation oscillator" equation which he called the Bonhoeffer–van der Pol (BvP) model:[16]

$$dx/dt = c \cdot (y + x - x^3/3 + z),$$

$$dy/dt = -(x - a + by)/c,$$

where

$$1 - 2b/3 < a < 1; \quad 0 < b < 1; \quad \text{and } b < c^2.$$

The model is a simple representative of a broad class of non-linear systems that exhibit excitability and oscillation. The phase plane of the BvP model, depicting the two variables of state (x,y), illustrates the various states of excitability to form a "physiological state diagram" which aids in illustrating the dynamics of excitability in familiar biological terms: resting, active, and refractory phases. We implemented the BvP model as follows. The solutions of the differential equations were estimated by computer, using the Runge–Kutta difference equation method ($\Delta t = 0.01$). Pseudorandom noise was incorporated into each iteration of x and y with a stochastic amplitude η. For example η of 0.01 means that a pseudorandom number between -0.005 and $+0.005$ was added to each iterative calculation of x and y. The noise amplitudes for x and y were independently generated. The effects of discrete perturbations on the model were studied by adding a fixed amount S_x and S_y to x and y, respectively, for a finite number of iterations. The strength of the perturbation is $|S| = (S_x^2 + S_y^2)^{1/2}$ and the direction of perturbation is $\tan^{-1} S_y/S_x$. In the present study, z was systematically varied, and $a = 0.7$, $b = 0.8$, $c = 3.0$.

Excitability of the BvP system was altered by changing the z value, which allowed for study of a broad range behavior.[15] In the noiseless Runge–Kutta approximations ($\Delta t = 0.01$) of the BvP equations, $z > -0.3356$ or $z < -1.4118$ results in a stable singular point and no spontaneous oscillation. A discrete perturbation can lead to a single regenerative cycle (action potential) but always results in trajectories that eventually lead back to the singular point. For $-0.3356 > z >$ -0.3452 or $-1.4023 > z > -1.4118$, the singular point is stable and trajectories within a circumscribed region (basin) converge to the singular point. However, trajectories outside the basin lead to sustained oscillatory behavior (attractor-cycles). Therefore, the approximated BvP equations can exhibit hard excitation.[17] For $-1.4023 < z < -0.3452$, the singular point is unstable and all trajectories eventually converge to the attractor-cycle.

The cubic term of the BvP equation of x was scaled to alter the numerical amplitude of oscillation[18] by replacing the $x^3/3$ term with $x^3/3d$; increasing d results in increase in amplitude. Unless stated otherwise, $d = 1$. In the non-oscillatory BvP (all trajectories converging to a stable singular point), increasing d can result in spontaneous oscillation (stable attractor-cycle with a stable or unstable singular point), similar to the effects of changing z. Changing z in the oscillatory BvP, however, can produce large shifts in the position of the singular point relative to the attractor-cycle, with little change in amplitude of oscillation.

The location of the singular point of the BvP equations was determined in two ways. First, we followed the classical approach of determining the singular point by solving for the intersection of the x and y nullclines ($dx/dt = 0$, $dy/dt = 0$). The second approach was by Runge–Kutta approximation of the BvP equations. For nonoscillatory solutions, the computations for any x,y initial condition eventually led to constant x and y values corresponding to the coordinate of the stable singular point. This approach was also applicable to the oscillatory BvP system with stable singular points by starting with x and y values located within the singular point's basin of attraction. We found that the two methods (analytic vs computational) resulted in very close concordance; the range of differences in coordinates for the singular point was within 0.001 for x and 0.015 for y. Localization of the singular point then allowed us to determine the distance from the singular point to the approximated attractor-cycle of the BvP equations, defining $\mathbf{D_{min}}$ as the distance from the singular point to the most proximate portion of the attractor-cycle. If the singular point was repelling, accurate localization of the singular point by Runge–Kutta computation was difficult. As an approximation, we used the topological method of Winfree[8] to find a critical perturbation of the approximated BvP oscillation. The x,y coordinates of the singular point were determined as the x,y value at which a phase singularity was observed, i.e., a singularity in the cophase vs old phase curves of phase resetting. The accuracy of this method is limited by the resolution of old phase, perturbation, and by the errors of Runge–Kutta approximation. Increased resolution can be achieved by using smaller Δt increments.

A. Definitions

Respiratory dysrhythmias. Expiratory apnea is identified when the chest wall and diaphragm are in the expiratory position longer than a normal expiratory period. Inspiratory apnea, also termed apneusis, is defined as tonic inspiratory activity, giving the appearance of "breath-holding." Respiratory rhythms are never exactly regular so designation of an expiratory or inspiratory period as prolonged should reflect normal variability of the respiratory cycle. In some respiratory recordings, there are low amplitude fluctuations in inspiratory or expiratory activity that are not normal and not completely arrhythmic. The distinction between normal rhythm and dysrhythmia is generally a clinical determination; the low amplitude fluctuations on the inspiratory or the expiratory side is still called apnea or apneusis because a clinically important parameter such as tissue oxygenation is compromised when the system develops such patterns.

Dysrhythmias were studied in the BvP equations with analogy to respiration as follows. BvP activity in $y(t)$ was depicted, and an activity threshold ($y = y_t$) was set which divided the observed phases into inspiratory-like activity and expiratory-like activity. Apneic-like dysrhythmia occurs if the activity remained below the activity threshold longer than the period of time expected for the unperturbed attractor-cycle below this threshold. Apneustic-like dysrhythmia was defined similarly for prolonged activity above the activity threshold. The time below the activity threshold is designated as T_b and time above as T_a, analogous to the expiratory and inspiratory periods, respectively.

In the noiseless BvP system, a state of permanent dysrhythmia is achieved when there is a stable singular point and x,y values are within the singular point's basin of attraction. We varied the position and size of the basin relative to the attractor-cycle by changing the equation parameters z and d. Transient dysrhythmia is observed if the x,y values are outside the basin, and divergence away from the vicinity of the basin to the attractor is slower than the expected period of the cycle. In the BvP system with an unstable ("repelling") singular point, the duration of dysrhythmia is similarly dependent upon the rate of divergence. This rate, and thence the duration of dysrhythmia, is influenced by all equation parameters.

Phases. The time from the onset of inspiration to the onset of a stimulus is defined as old phase (ϕ). Cophase (θ) is the time from the stimulus to the subsequent onsets of inspiration. The resulting times are expressed as normalized fractions, with the value of one being the average period of three control breaths prior to stimulation. Similar definitions are applied to phases of BvP oscillation, with old phase and cophase measured relative to onset of activity above y_t.

III. RESULTS

A. *In vivo* studies

Examples of respiratory perturbations and phase resetting of rhythm. Figure 2 illustrates different respiratory perturbations that cause transient alteration and phase resetting of respiratory rhythm. Figure 2(A) shows the effects of a 500 ms electrical stimulus (1 V, 0.1 ms pulses given at 100 Hz) of the superior laryngeal nerve (SLN)[9] in an anesthetized cat. SLN stimulation during the inspiratory phase inhibits inspiratory activity and shortens the duration of the inspiratory phase of rhythm. Expiratory stimuli cause prolongation of the expiratory phase, delaying the onsets of subsequent inspirations. Figure 2(B) shows the effects of stimulation (1 s duration, 10 Hz pulse frequency, 1 ms pulse duration, 600 μA mean current) of the midbrain reticular formation,[10]

A. CAT PHRENIC ACTIVITY - SLN STIM

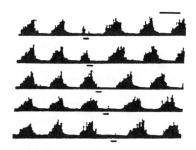

B. CAT PHRENIC ACTIVITY - MIDBRAIN STIM

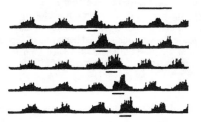

C. HUMAN AIRFLOW - SUBMENTAL EMG

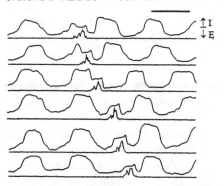

FIG. 2. Phase resetting of respiratory rhythm by strong superior laryngeal nerve (A) and midbrain reticular (B) stimulations in adult cats, and by swallowing in humans (C). In A and B, rhythm is half-wave rectified phrenic nerve activity. In (C) respiratory airflow is shown (↑ Inspiration; ↓ Expiration). Adapted from Refs. 9, 10, and 12, with permission from Am. J. Physiol. and J. Physiol. (London).

which causes marked inspiratory facilitation. These examples show that SLN and midbrain reticular stimuli have quite different immediate effects on respiratory rhythm. However, both cause a characteristic type of phase resetting of rhythm: the latency from the stimulus to onsets of subsequent breaths (cophases) are independent of the respiratory phase of stimulus onset (old phase). The tracings shown in Figs. 2(A) and 2(B) are examples of strong perturbation of respiratory rhythm in the absence of other respiratory feedback mechanisms and influences from higher brain. We also studied respiratory perturbations by swallowing in awake healthy humans,[12] shown in Fig. 2(C). Onset of swallowing, identified as the onset of submental electromyographic activity, is associated with inhibition of inspiratory airflow to a period of apnea, followed by expiration. The duration of expiration after swallowing is not the same in all runs: it is longest for swallows initiated at the transition between inspi-

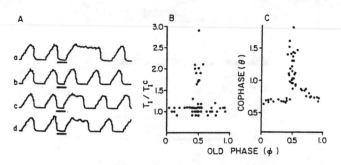

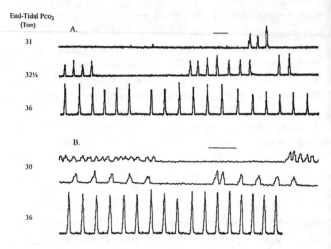

FIG. 3. Respiratory dysrhythmia evoked by critical midbrain reticular stimulus in a cat anesthetized with sodium pentobarbital. (A) The same stimulus given at approximately the same old phase [0.48±0.04 (SD)] had no effect on subsequent inspiratory duration (*run b*) or induced variable inspiratory prolongation (*runs a,c,d*). (B) Plot of inspiratory duration of first breath after stimulation normalized to control inspiratory durations before stimulation, vs old phase, showing the induced dysrhythmia appears only if the stimulus is given at a critical old phase. Reprinted from Ref. 10, with permission from Am. J. Physiol.

FIG. 4. Spontaneous dysrhythmias of newborn respiratory pattern in two kittens. Tracings are of integrated phrenic nerve activity at different levels of constant end-tidal P_{CO_2}. (A) 4-day old kitten anesthetized with sodium pentobarbital. Time bar: 3 s. (B) 2-day old kitten anesthetized with chloralose and urethan. Time bar: 3 s for top two tracings, 6 s for bottom tracing.

ration and expiration (I-E) and shortest for swallows initiated at the expiratory–inspiratory (E-I) transition. This pattern was found in all 30 subjects studied.

We have characterized the topological type of respiratory phase resetting by strong SLN and midbrain reticular stimuli, and by swallowing. Plots of cophase against old phase are suggestive of type 0 resetting, i.e., there is a net change of zero cycles of cophase as old phase varies through one full cycle.[9–12]

Stimulus-evoked dysrhythmias of the respiratory oscillator. In the animal experiments, we found that stimuli having strength less than that required to produce type 0 resetting, if properly timed, could cause dysrhythmic responses.[10] Such critical stimuli were identified by giving brief stimuli of constant strength at different times in the respiratory cycle as in Fig. 2, then reducing the strength of stimulation and repeating the protocol. We applied the topological search methodology of Winfree[8] to identify critical stimuli that cause the rhythm to be reset in a highly irregular fashion, thereby characterizing the respiratory oscillator's phase singularity. SLN stimuli of appropriate strength caused irregular phase resetting only if given at the E-I transition, whereas midbrain stimuli caused similar irregularities only if given at the I-E transition. In the majority of experiments, "highly irregular" meant that the normal rhythm resumed after an unpredictable latency after the stimulus, but never greater that a few seconds (i.e., one normal cycle period). However, in three cats studied with midbrain stimuli and anesthetized with pentobarbital sodium (instead of chloralose-urethan which was the usual anesthetic) critically timed midbrain reticular stimuli resulted in prolonged inspiratory activity of the breath following the stimulus. Figure 3(A) shows an example in one cat. The same stimulus (1 s duration, 20 Hz pulse frequency, 200 μA, 1 ms pulse duration) given at the same old phase had no effect on the subsequent inspiratory duration (*run b*) or resulted in variable inspiratory prolongation (*runs a,c,d*), lasting up to three times the inspiratory duration of the control breaths. Figure 3(B) (middle panel) shows a plot of the inspiratory duration of the first breath after stimulation, normalized to the mean inspiratory duration of five control

breaths, versus old phase. In twelve of the 55 runs in this cat, there was significant ($P<0.01$, unpaired Student's *t* test) prolongation of the inspiratory duration of the first breath after the stimulus. This prolonged response occurred only when the stimulus was given at an old phase of 0.48±0.04 (SD), which corresponds to stimuli initiated at the offset of inspiration. This plot therefore shows that post-stimulus prolongation of inspiratory activity occurred only when the stimulus was given at a specific time in the respiratory cycle. When the stimulus strength was increased to 50 Hz (other parameters unchanged) phase specific inspiratory prolongation did not occur, and strong (type 0) resetting similar to Fig. 2(B) was found.

Spontaneous dysrhythmias of the respiratory oscillator. In experiments in newborn kittens there were episodes of variable phrenic rhythm due to prolonged expiratory apnea. Figure 4 shows examples in two kittens, one anesthetized with chloralose and urethan [Fig. 4(A)], the other with sodium pentobarbital [Fig 4(B)]. Initially, the end-tidal P_{CO_2} was lowered to a level just below threshold of phrenic nerve activity, the apneic threshold. The ventilator's rate was then slowed to cause step increases in end-tidal P_{CO_2}; no further changes were made for at least 10 minutes, allowing for near-steady state phrenic recordings.

The two examples show that spontaneous apneas were more likely to appear, and were of greater duration, at respiratory drives that were near the threshold for rhythmicity compared to higher drives, readily demonstrated by changing end-tidal P_{CO_2} in a step-wise manner. Apnea was often immediately preceded and followed by apparently normal breaths. Figure 4(B) shows an example of low amplitude rapid phrenic rhythms that were sometimes seen just above apneic threshold.

B. Computational studies

Dysrhythmic behavior induced by critical perturbations. The approximated BvP equations exhibit sustained oscilla-

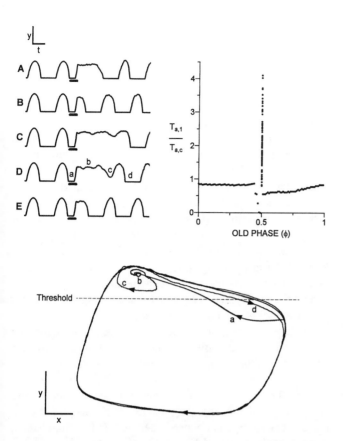

FIG. 5. Dysrhythmia induced by perturbation of computed BvP equations. Horizontal bars under rhythm tracings represent interval of perturbation. (A)–(E) Perturbations ($|S|$=0.06, direction 2.94 radians, duration 0.25) given at the same old phase (ϕ=0.5) cause highly variable resetting, sometimes delaying offset of T_a. Noise (η=0.05) is implemented at end of stimulation. Unit bars: y=1, t=5. Graph (top right) of first T_a after onset of stim, normalized to control T_a, vs old phase showing the dysrhythmic response only for perturbation at old phase of 0.5. Trajectories (bottom) before, during, and after perturbation for run D. Perturbation (a) caused displacement of the trajectory to a locus near the singular point (b), followed by spiral orbits (b,c) away from singular point toward attractor-cycle (d). Horizontal threshold: y_t=1.7. Unit bars: x=0.5, y=0.5.

tion over a range z values ($-0.3356 > z > -1.4118$). In order to find specific combinations of stimulus strength and stimulus timing that induce dysrhythmia, we applied the same topological search method that was used to find critical stimuli in the animal studies. We depict rhythm in $y(t)$ with activity threshold at y_t=1.7, and set $z=-1.34$ which places the singular point just below the maximum y value for the attractor. The system was perturbed with a critical stimulus ($|S|$ =0.06, direction 2.94 radians) lasting a finite fraction of the cycle (0.25). The direction of perturbation is oriented to facilitate y activity, analogous to the inspiratory-facilitatory effects of reticular stimuli. We found that strong perturbations cause patterns of resetting similar to those shown in Fig. 2. By systematically varying strength and timing of the stimulus, we found a unique stimulus which caused highly irregular resetting of the oscillator. Figure 5 shows five runs (A–E) of the simulated equations, with one full cycle before five perturbations having the same strength and old phase. These perturbations cause an unpredictable pattern of resetting, with some perturbations causing prolonged cessation of rhythmic activity, up to 4 times the duration of the positive

phase of the control cycles. Figure 5 (top right) shows a plot of first T_a after onset of stimulation, normalized to control T_a, versus old phase. The dysrhythmic response occurs only after perturbations given at an old phase of 0.5. In this example, the BvP equations were computed with pseudorandom noise added to each calculation. Without noise, each perturbation given at ϕ =0.5 would have resulted in the same response. The addition of noise leads to highly variable responses to this stimulus which perturbs the oscillator to a locus very close to its singular point. Figure 5 (bottom) shows the trajectories of the oscillator before, during, and after perturbation for the fourth run (D). The large closed-loop trajectory represents the stable attractor-cycle prior to perturbation. Perturbation (a) causes displacement of the attractor to a locus near the singular point (b). There are subsequent spiral orbits (b,c) away from the singular point leading back (d) to the stable attractor-cycle. In the example shown, the z-value ($=-1.34$) of the BvP equation was chosen to place the singular point on the "inspiratory" side of the attractor relative to the threshold y_t=1.7. The singular point in this example is unstable, i.e., trajectories arbitrarily close to the singular point diverge back towards the attractor-cycle. These critical stimuli cause responses of the model oscillator that are similar to the stimulus-evoked apneusis shown in Fig. 3. Fine adjustments of the stimulus direction was required to mimic the experimental results of dysrhythmia evoked at stimulus old phase of 0.5. However, the finding of a specific combination of stimulus strength and timing which induces dysrhythmic behavior is a general feature of attractor-cycle systems.[8] Changing the equation parameters and direction of perturbation alters the combination of stimulus strength and timing needed to induce dysrhythmia, and the duration of dysrhythmia (see Sec. II A).

Spontaneous dysrhythmias. Figure 6 illustrates this effect in the noisy BvP equations ($z=-0.34$, η =0.02), depicting $y(t)$ and x,y plots. The activity threshold (y_t) was set below the minimum $y(t)$ so that the entire range of cycling is seen. The conversion by increasing d of steady state to oscillation is not all-or-none. Figures 6(B) and 6(C) shows intermediate states in which variable periods of rhythmic activity are interrupted by variable periods of very low amplitude fluctuations. Figure 6(D) shows that increasing d further leads to relatively regular rhythm. The x,y trajectories in Figs. 6(B) and 6(C) show that the periods of dysrhythmia are associated with low amplitude orbits near the attractor-cycle orbit. These smaller orbits circumnavigate around the singular point of the system and at times there is true arrhythmia when the trajectory is so close to the singular point that the observed fluctuations are indistinguishable from noise. In the BvP system, patterns similar to Figs. 6(B) and 6(C) are readily generated if the singular point is close to the attractor-cycle and sufficient noise is added to the system. Figure 6 (bottom graph) shows that increasing d above 1 results in increases in D_{min} (calculated from the noiseless BvP system, see Sec. II). Below d=1 the singularity point is stable and there is no oscillation. One explanation for the prorhythmic effects of increasing d is that by increasing the distance from the singular point to the attractor, the noise is less likely to displace the trajectory off the attractor-cycle

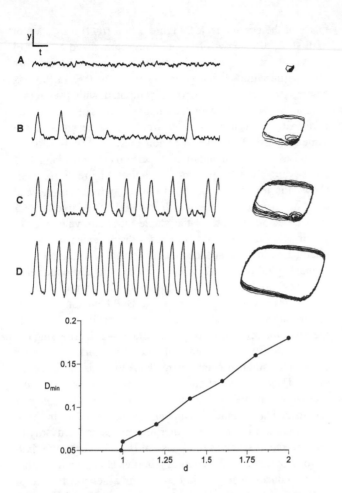

FIG. 6. Spontaneous dysrhythmia: effect of changing d. *Top*: $y(t)$ and x,y trajectories of the computed BvP equations ($z=-0.34$) with noise ($\eta=0.02$) for d value of 0.2 (*run A*), 0.5 (*run B*), 1.0 (*run C*), and 2.0 (*run D*). Increasing d results in conversion of the activity from continuous dysrhythmia (A) to episodic dysrhythmia [(B),(C)] and regular rhythm (D). Unit bars: $y=1$, $t=15$. *Bottom*: Plot of the distance from the singular point to the most proximate portion of the attractor-cycle (without noise) for values of d from 1 to 2. Lower values of d result in no spontaneous rhythm in noiseless system.

towards a dysrhythmic locus around or at the singular point. Another consideration is the stability of the singular point. Dysrhythmia is favored if there exists a basin within which trajectories converge to a singular point, allowing perturbations of sufficient strength to displace the trajectory off the attractor-cycle to this basin. On the other hand, dysrhythmia would be less prominent if the singular point is unstable. In this situation displacement off the attractor-cycle toward the singular point would always leads to trajectories that diverge away from the singular point back toward the attractor-cycle. However, the existence of a repelling (unstable) singular point does not preclude dysrhythmic behavior because trajectories near the singular point might take a long time (e.g., more than a "normal" cycle length) to return to the attractor-cycle. Noise or other perturbations can be prorhythmic. For example if the system is at the stable singular point, noise of sufficient magnitude can cause displacements outside the basin. In order to further characterize these relationships, we studied the effects of noise on BvP activities for different levels of excitability (z).

Figure 7 illustrates the remarkable influences of noise

(η) on rhythmicity of the BvP model. Noise can convert a non-oscillatory system to one that exhibits spontaneous cycles. In run A, there are no spontaneous oscillation ($z=-0.335$) and a steady state is reached, reflecting a stable singular point. Run B shows that addition of noise ($\eta=0.02$) causes the system to exhibit spontaneous regenerative cycles with spontaneous episodes of dysrhythmia.

In the oscillatory BvP system increasing noise leads to increases in the incidence and duration of dysrhythmia up to a critical level of noise. Further increases in noise above this critical level results in reduction in dysrhythmia. Runs C–G illustrate the critical effects of noise in the BvP oscillator with a stable singular point ($z=-0.3400$). A noise level of 0.001 results in permanent attenuation of rhythm; the tiny fluctuations reflect small orbits around the singular point. Runs H–J shows similar effects of noise even for the BvP oscillator with an unstable singular point ($z=-0.3450$), although the dysrhythmias are much less prolonged than those associated with a stable singular point.

Figure 8 shows the effects of changing noise on the cycle periods in the BvP oscillator with a stable singular point ($z=-0.340$), using 6 different noise levels. The histograms represent the distribution of times (T_b) spent below an activity threshold (y_t) midway between the maximum and minimum y value (transecting the attracter in half). For each noise level, computation proceeded for 75 000 time units, roughly equivalent to 5800 cycles of the noiseless rhythm (cycle period=13 time units) with the same parameters, and analogous to 6–8 hours of real breathing. The histograms show several features of the effects of noise on periodicity: (1) criticality, as illustrated in the shorter runs of Fig. 7; (2) skew distribution of the variability in T_b for a given noise level; (3) asymmetry of noise effects on T_b below and above the critical noise level, i.e., below the critical noise level, a small increase in noise causes transition of the pattern from very regular to highly dysrhythmic, whereas above the critical noise level, reduction in dysrhythmia by increases in noise are gradual rather than abrupt. Histograms of the times above the activity threshold (T_a) for the same set of runs show very little variability.

Let **max** T_b be the longest T_b of the run, analogous to the longest apnea of a continuous 6–8 hour respiratory tracing. Figure 9 shows the relationship between **max** T_b and noise level for different levels of excitability (z) including non-oscillatory [Fig. 9(A)], oscillatory with stable singular point [Figs. 9(B)–9(D)] and oscillatory with unstable singular point [Fig. 9(E)]. Criticality and asymmetry in the relationship between noise and **max** T_b are shown in these plots, similar to the full distribution of the T_b histograms. Another feature is noteworthy: the longest "apnea" is nearly the same at the highest noise levels for all plots. This underscores the finding that addition of noise to the non-oscillatory BvP system ($z>-0.3356$ or $z<-1.4118$) in sufficient amounts (0.05 or more in these examples) can produce an activity pattern that is indistinguishable from the pattern of the spontaneous oscillator in the presence of the same amount of noise.

In Fig. 10(A), we present the relationships among **max** T_b, noise and excitability for 1935 combinations of η (range 1.5×10^{-6} to 5×10^{-2}) and z (range -0.3331 to -0.3471).

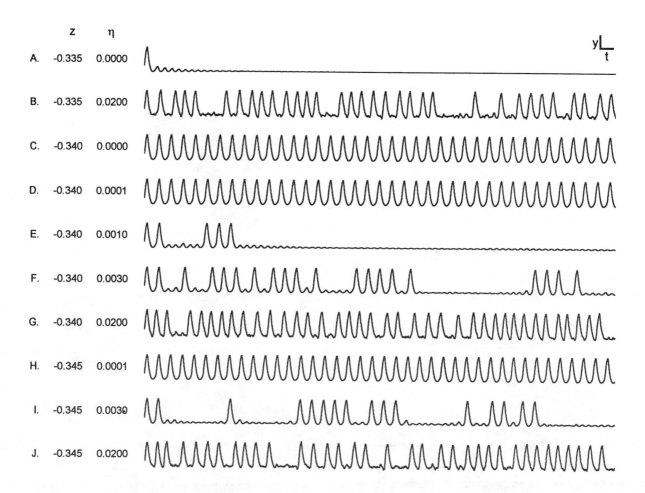

FIG. 7. Critical effects of noise (η) on rhythmicity of the BvP model. Noise converts non-oscillatory sytem to one that exhibits spontaneous cycles [(A), (B)]. The oscillatory system [(C)–(G), (H)–(J)] exhibits increased dysrhythmia with certain levels of noise further increases above this critical level results in decreased dysrhythmia. Unit bars: $y=1$, $t=15$.

The maximum T_b for each η, z combination is depicted as a shade of gray, with white being shortest (<50 time units, equivalent to approximately 5 cycles of oscillation) and black being longest ($>12\,000$ time units). For $z>-0.3356$ is no rhythmic activity up to a threshold of noise; increasing η above this threshold results in increased rhythmicity and progressive shortening of **max T_b**. For $z<-0.3356$ the plot

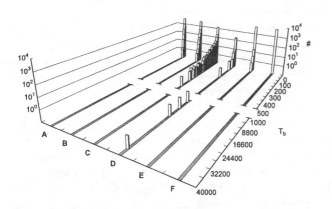

FIG. 8. Histograms of T_b for different amounts of noise in the BvP model ($z=-0.340$). Noise levels (η): (A) 0.05, (B) 0.02, (C) 0.003, (D) 0.001, (E) 0.0003, (F) 0.00006. The noiseless cycle has period=13, $T_a=4$, $T_b=9$.

shows an abrupt transition from eurhythmia to permanent dysrhythmia for intermediate noise levels and graded reductions in dysrhythmia with further increases in noise. The blending of gray tones across the top of the plot reflects the fact that in the presence of sufficient amounts of noise, the activity patterns of the BvP equations over a broad range of z values are indistinguishable and exhibit the same distribution of T_b values.

In Fig. 10(B), we have estimated the thresholds for initiation and termination of activitiy cycles of the BvP equations, computed for $t=75\,000$. The z domains are labeled to indicate noiseless BvP solutions with a stable singular point and no oscillation (I, $z>-0.3356$), stable singular point and attractor-cycle (II, $-0.3356>z>-0.3452$) and unstable singular point and attractor-cycle (III, $-0.3452>z>-1.4023$). Curve a is the threshold $\eta_a(z)$ below which activity cycles never take place if the equations are initially set at the singular point. Above this threshold, noise is of sufficient magnitude to eventually cause a large enough displacement away from the stable singular point to form a regenerative cycle. Below this threshold, noise results in small fluctuations of x,y activity around the singular point, i.e., dysrhythmia. Curve b is the threshold $\eta_b(z)$ below which oscillation is never interrupted by dysrhythmic activity because noise does not displace the activity cycles far enough away from the

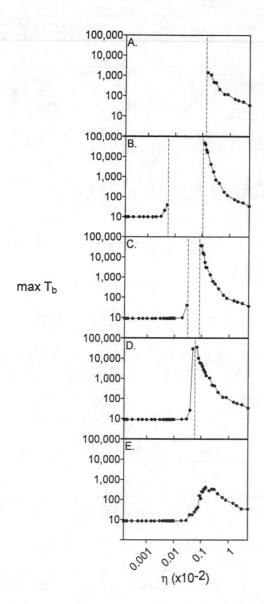

max T$_b$

FIG. 9. Relationship between **max T**$_b$ and η for five z values. (A) z = −0.3341, (B) z = −0.3364, (C) z = −0.3401, (D) z = −0.3421, (E) z = −0.3451. Vertical lines demarcate noise values for which there are no cycles of activity throughout the entire period of computation (t = 75 000).

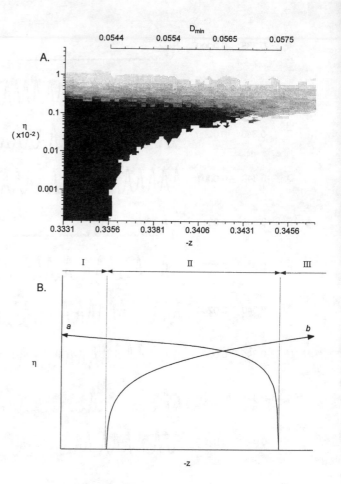

FIG. 10. Relationships among **max T**$_b$, noise (η) and excitability (z). (A) Gray-scale plot of **max T**$_b$ (t = 75 000) for 1935 combinations of η and z. Gray-scale white represents **max T**$_b$ < 50, Black is **max T**$_b$ > 12 000 units of time. Top scale shows **D**$_{min}$, defined as the distance from the singular point to the most proximate portion of the attractor-cycle. (B) Estimated threshold curves for noise levels η (z) that result in initiation and termination of BvP activity cycles. Curve a is threshold below which activity cycles never take place if the initial x,y values are at the singular point. Curve b is threshold below which oscillation is never interrupted by dysrhythmic activity. The scales for z and η are the same as in (A).

attractor-cycle. Permanent dysrhythmia of the oscillatory BvP is identified in the η,z domain only if two conditions are satisfied: noise is large enough to initiate dysrhythmia [$\eta > \eta_b(z)$] and too small to terminate dysrhythmia [$\eta < \eta_a(z)$].

IV. DISCUSSION

Irregularities in the pattern of breathing are most often pathological during sleep,[19] a time when respiratory drive is reduced. In adults, the most common form is obstructive apnea, due in part to sleep-induced reduction in inspiratory phasic and tonic activities of the upper airway muscles, allowing for them to occlude the airway. These muscle activities are sleep state dependent, so that once occlusion is initiated, arousal causes upper airway muscle activation thereby

relieving the obstruction. Recurrent cycles, not necessarily regular, of obstructive apnea terminated by arousal can take place throughout the night.

Another type of sleep apnea, most often seen in the infant, is sudden loss of phasic inspiratory effort,[1] suggesting that there is loss of rhythmicity of the brainstem respiratory controller. Identifiable neurological causes of recurrent non-obstructive infant apnea include focal cortical seizure activity[20] and posterior fossa lesions.[21] However, in current clinical practice most cases remain unexplained after an extensive evaluation.[1]

Apnea of central neural origin as a cause of sudden infant death syndrome (SIDS) has been speculated for a long time, but definitive evidence remains elusive. A number of neuropathological studies have shown brainstem abnormalities in some SIDS victims.[22] Specific findings include increases in dendritic spine density, delayed myelination and adrenergic alterations that are suggestive of brainstem immaturity. These abnormalities are not easily recognized on routine neuropathological examinations and even in the investigational studies there is overlap between the normal age matched population and SIDS victims. Direct investigation of apnea in SIDS has so far proven extraordinarily difficult because of the rarity of observing the life-threatening event under conditions of intensive monitoring. A recent prospective epidemiological study has found increased risk of SIDS in infants sleeping in the prone position.[23]

Our study on respiratory dysrhythmias should be viewed in this broader context of apnea and SIDS findings. The computational studies illustrate how an apparently normal respiratory pattern can be interrupted by apnea of the nonobstructive variety. These studies suggest that the apneic state can be induced by stimuli with specific combinations of strength and timing that impinge upon or arise within the respiratory oscillator. Dysrhythmias manifest as inspiratory apnea (apneusis) or expiratory apnea depending upon the dynamical structure of the respiratory oscillator: apneusis results when the singular point is situated near the inspiratory side of the attractor-cycle, whereas expiratory apnea occurs when the singular point happens to be below the inspiratory threshold. Small fluctuations in respiratory activity, clearly dysrhythmic but not arrhythmic, reflect small orbits expanding away from or contracting towards the singular point. Because we consider respiratory dysrhythmias as a disorder of state, a variety of parameter changes can result in the same pathological state, and there is no well-defined cutoff between "normal" and "abnormal." This may be relevant in the interpretation of clinical and pathological studies showing considerable overlap between "normal" infants and SIDS victims or those who are felt to be at high risk for SIDS.

A. Respiratory rhythm viewed as an attractor-cycle

Attractor-cycle oscillators have been the basis for many mathematical models of respiratory rhythm.[11,24–26] Experimental support for a respiratory attractor-cycle was published in the mid-1980s in which phase resetting of respiratory rhythm was studied by using respiratory perturbations with various combinations of stimulus strength and stimulus timing.[9–11] The data were analyzed using Winfree's definitions and topological classifications of phase resetting. The functional relationship of cophase was determined with respect to old phase and stimulus strength, defining the respiratory oscillator's resetting surface. The experimental data suggested that this surface is a helicoid that winds around a vertical axis and has contours of cophase that converge to this axis. Thus the axis represents a singularity in graphical terms. It is a phase singularity in dynamical terms because rhythmicity becomes more variable as stimuli are given closer to the point of convergence of the contours.

In the present investigation, we have developed the BvP metaphor to illustrate how attractor-cycle systems can exhibit the main features of dysrhythmia observed in the animal studies: (1) Critical stimuli, with only certain combinations of strength and timing, can induce dysrhythmias, and the stimuli that characterize the dysrhythmic response are intermediate in strength to stimuli that identify type 1 and type 0 resetting.[10] (2) As shown by Lumsden[27–29] spontaneous apneustic breaths are of varying duration and are often

immediately preceded and followed by apparently normal breaths. This same pattern is seen in the newborn animal except the dysrhythmic state is expiratory rather than inspiratory apnea. (3) Rapid low amplitude oscillations of phrenic activity during expiratory apnea can be seen in newborn animals (see Fig. 4). As illustrated by Euler,[30] apneustic neural inspiratory activity can also exhibit low amplitude oscillatory behavior having periodicity that is a fraction of the normal rhythm, approximately 1/3 in Euler's example.

The Bonhoeffer–van der Pol model of excitability was selected for study mainly because of its analytic simplicity and the broad range of excitable behaviors that it exhibits. The BvP singular point can be positioned off-center near one side of the attractor or the other (relative to an arbitrary threshold) by changing a single parameter (z). This proved convenient for illustrating dysrhythmic activity on either side of the cycle, analogous to inspiratory versus expiratory apnea. It is important to note that for a given z value, dysrhythmia occurs at or near a single state of activity. Indeed in respiratory recordings, spontaneous expiratory and inspiratory apneas rarely co-exist in the same experiment, supporting the idea of a unique singular point.

Other dynamical schemes have been proposed for the respiratory oscillator, notably integrate-and-fire and discrete models which have discontinuous dynamics. These models would be expected to exhibit discontinuities in phase resetting plots of cophase against old phase.[31] Indeed, some respiratory resetting plots appear discontinuous[9,32,33] and experimental limitations prevent finer resolution of the data in some experiments. Other experiments, particularly those with midbrain reticular stimulation,[10] show the full series of resetting plots with much greater resolution and the appearance of continuity. To our knowledge, the characteristics of respiratory dysrhythmia reviewed in the present study have not been demonstrated in integrate-and-fire or discrete models.

B. Importance of noise

The existence of stochastic processes over a broad time scale is a ubiquitous feature of neural systems,[34–36] demonstrated in experimental work that has identified irregular fluctuations in the activity of neural systems due to membrane, synaptic, and network properties. Noise has been proposed to have critical effects on neural sensory transduction[36] and phase locking of biological oscillators.[37]

In the present study, we have shown that stochastic fluctuations of the BvP system can lead to spontaneous dysrhythmias of varying durations. Our demonstration of critical levels of noise that are most pathological, i.e., produce the longest spontaneous dysrhythmias, can be viewed as noise levels in which stochastic combinations of strength and timing are most likely to perturb the trajectory away from the idealized attractor to the singular point or its dysrhythmic vicinity. If the level of noise is too large, stochastic fluctuations in state promote dispersion away from the singular point. Very small increases in noise can, for a certain range of excitability (z), cause a very dramatic transition in the activity pattern from highly regular rhythm to a permanent dysrhythmic state. Increases in noise above the critical level(s) lead to progressive reductions in dysrhythmic periods. In our computations, pseudorandom (deterministic) perturbations were uniformly distributed over a specified interval of amplitude and given for each iteration. We speculate that use of truly random perturbations with other distributions of amplitude and timing could shift the η,z domains of maximum dysrhythmia but criticality would still be found. Whether noise within or impinging upon the oscillator is deterministic or truly random has little bearing on the actual pathological state of dysrhythmia in the BvP system. More important is the distribution of amplitudes and timings of the fluctuations that perturb the oscillator.

The critical effects of noise on the initiation and termination of dysrhythmias are shown to be dependent on the level of excitability (z).The dysrhythmias are most prominent, i.e., are of greatest duration and initiated with smallest amplitudes of noise, for z values corresponding to a singular point situated closest to the attractor-cycle. In this regard, our findings are consistent with those of Kurrer and Schulten,[38] who studied the influence of Gaussian white noise on stability of the BvP oscillator, using statistical approximation methods. They concluded that noise normal to the attractor can have large effects on the trajectories and produce large shifts in the phase of the attractor-cycle ("quasistationary behavior"), whereas noise tangential to the attractor-cycle induces diffusion-like dispersion of trajectories. These shifts were most prominent for "critical" z values (i.e., close to values corresponding to a stable stationary point) and for portions of the attractor most proximate to the singular point.

C. Swallowing: A physiological perturbation of respiratory rhythm

The human studies have shown that in healthy subjects, swallowing causes phase resetting of respiratory rhythm with a pattern that we have characterized topologically as type 0. The latency from the swallow to the next breath (cophase) was largest for swallows initiated near the inspiratory–expiratory (I-E) transition, and smallest for swallows initiated near the expiratory–inspiratory (E-I) transition. We have related these respiratory phase effects with the timing of bolus flow through the pharynx during deglutition. The latency between departure of the bolus from the larynx to onset of next inspiration is also largest for I-E swallows and smallest for E-I. This finding raises the possibility that aspiration due to inspiration of swallowed material into the lung is most likely to occur for swallows initiated near the E-I transition, especially in pathological conditions that weaken the impact of swallowing on respiratory rhythm or slow the transport of the bolus through the pharynx.

In adults, aspiration normally causes rapid expiratory activation and coughing, aiding the expulsion of aspirated material from the airway. The infant, however, often lacks a vigorous cough reflex and can exhibit a different response to aspiration: prolonged apnea.[5] This response is thought to be due to stimulation by the aspirant of laryngeal and tracheal receptors that in turn causes reflex inhibition of respiration. Obstructive apnea due to laryngospasm, prolonged tonic closure of the vocal folds and cords, can also result from irritation of the laryngeal mucosa by the aspirant.

The phase of transition between expiration and inspiration was also shown in the animal studies to be the time at which irregular resetting was demonstrated with superior laryngeal nerve stimulation having critical strength, suggesting that this response represented the respiratory oscillator's phase singularity.

We propose that swallowing causes perturbations of the respiratory oscillator that are similar to strong SLN stimuli. Two forms of respiratory dysrhythmia could then result from conditions that weaken the normal (type 0) resetting effect of deglutition: apnea triggered by aspiration, or apnea due to perturbation off the respiratory attractor toward the singular point.

D. Prospects

What are the biological parameters that influence the frequency and duration of dysrhythmias of the respiratory oscillator? One factor that has already been implicated is respiratory drive which is reduced during sleep, a well known period of vulnerability for the infant. The preliminary experiments in newborn animals suggest that maturation of the neural circuits that make up the respiratory oscillator might have some bearing on the dynamical structure of the respiratory attractor and its singular point. In the BvP oscillator, dysrhythmia was readily induced by small perturbations if the basin of attraction to the singular point was large and the basin was near the attractor-cycle. Such might be the case in some infants. Neural maturation might result in migration of the singular point away from the attractor cycle and conversion of the singular point from one with a basin of attraction to a strongly repelling singular point, rendering the mature oscillator much less vulnerable. The spectrum of neural noise impacting on or arising within the newborn respiratory oscillator might be much closer to the critical domain for dysrhythmia.

Therapeutic interventions for infant apnea can be proposed based on the postulated effects of noise. If infant apnea is initiated by perturbation of the respiratory trajectory away from the respiratory attractor-cycle towards a singular point, then increasing the ambient level of noise impinging upon the respiratory oscillator could increase the likelihood of terminating the apneic episode. Noise therapy would therefore aim at shortening the duration of apnea analogous to the effects of noise on the BvP system for $\eta > \eta_a$ and $\eta > \eta_b$. On the other hand, lower levels of noise might be sufficient to trigger but not terminate apnea. Methods of introducing external noise to the respiratory control system include tactile vibration[39] and auditory stimulation,[2,3,40] both of which can cause perturbation of respiratory rhythm. The major challenge would be selecting the optimum stimulus frequencies and amplitudes that provide a therapeutic effect, i.e., reduction of respiratory dysrhythmia, without disrupting the sleep cycle.

ACKNOWLEDGMENTS

We thank J. A. Paydarfar for writing computer code, L. Glass for reviewing the manuscript, O. Piro and A. T. Winfree for direction to mathematical literature, and A. H. Ropper for administrative support. This work was funded in part by the Cecil B. Day Family and NIH Grant No. HL 49848-01. The animal studies were performed while D. Paydarfar was a Parker B. Francis Foundation Fellow in Pulmonary Research in the laboratory of F. L. Eldridge.

[1] D. P. Southall and D. G. Talbert, "Mechanisms for abnormal apnea of possible relevance to the sudden infant death syndrome," Ann. NY Acad. Sci. 533, 329–349 (1988).

[2] H.-J. Gerhart, H. Wagner, I. Thomschke, and B. Pasch, "Zur Beeinflussbarkeit der Atmung durch rhythmische akustische Reize," Z. Laryngol. Rhinol. Otol. 46, 235–247 (1967).

[3] T. G. Heron and R. Jacobs, "A physiological response of the neonate to auditory stimulation," Int. Aud. 7, 41–47 (1968).

[4] S. Wolf, "Sudden death and the oxygen conserving reflex," Am. Heart J. 71, 840–841 (1966).

[5] J. W. French, B. C. Morgan, and W. G. Guntheroth, "Infant monkeys–A model for crib death," Am. J. Dis. Child. 123, 480–484 (1972).

[6] S. E. Downing and J. C. Lee, "Laryngeal chemosensitivity: a possible mechanism for sudden infant death," Pediatrics 55, 640–649 (1975).

[7] S. L. Wilson, B. T. Thach, R. T. Brouillette, and Y. K. Abu-Osba, "Coordination of breathing and swallowing in human infants," J. Appl. Physiol. 50, 851–858 (1981). See p. 856.

[8] A. T. Winfree, The Geometry of Biological Time (Springer-Verlag, New York, 1980).

[9] D. Paydarfar, F. L. Eldridge, and J. P. Kiley, "Resetting of mammalian respiratory rhythm: existence of a phase singularity," Am. J. Physiol. 250, R721–R727 (1986).

[10] D. Paydarfar and F. L. Eldridge, "Phase resetting and dysrhythmic responses of the respiratory oscillator," Am. J. Physiol. 252, R55–R62 (1987).

[11] F. L. Eldridge, D. Paydarfar, P. G. Wagner, and R. T. Dowell, "Phase resetting of respiratory rhythm: effect of changing respiratory drive," Am. J. Physiol. 257, R271–R277 (1989).

[12] D. Paydarfar, R. J. Gilbert, C. Poppel, and P. Nassab, "Respiratory phase resetting and airflow changes induced by swallowing in humans," J. Physiol. (London), in press.

[13] D. M. Smith, R. R. Mercer, and F. L. Eldridge, "Servo control of end-tidal CO_2 in paralyzed animals," J. Appl. Physiol. 45, 133–136 (1978).

[14] F. L. Eldridge, "Relationship between respiratory nerve and muscle activity and muscle force output," J. Appl. Physiol. 39, 567–574 (1975).

[15] R. Fitzhugh, "Impulses and physiological states in theoretical models of nerve membrane," Biophys. J. 1, 445–466 (1961).

[16] Also called the Fitzhugh–Nagumo equations. See J. S. Nagumo, S. Arimoto, and S. Yoshizawa, "An active pulse transmission line simulating nerve axon," Proc. IRE 50, 2061–2070 (1962).

[17] Bifurcation analysis has led to the same conclusion. See K. P. Hadeler, U. An Der Heiden, and K. Schumacher, "Generation of nervous impulse and periodic oscillations," Biol. Cybernet. 23, 211–218 (1976); S. M. Baer, T. Erneux, and J. Rinzel, "The slow passage through a Hopf bifurcation: delay, memory effects, and resonance," SIAM J. Appl. Math. 49, 55–71, 1989.

[18] F. L. Eldridge (personal correspondence to D. Paydarfar, 1990). See also Ref. 11 for similar scaling factor for the van der Pol equation.

[19] D. Paydarfar and L. Castro, "Disorders of respiratory control," in Principles and Practice of Neurocritical Care, edited by D. F. Hanley, C. Borel, R. McPherson, W. Hacke, and G. Teasdale (Williams and Wilkins, Baltimore, in press).

[20] D. P. Southall, V. Stebbens, and N. Abraham, "Prolonged apnoea with severe arterial hypoxaemia resulting from complex partial seizures," Dev. Med. Child Neurol. 29, 784–804 (1987).

[21] J. E. Brazy, H. C. Kinney, and W. J. Oakes, "Central nervous system lesions causing apnea at birth," J. Pediatr. 111, 163–175 (1987).

[22] H. C. Kinney, J. J. Filiano, and R. M. Harper, "The neuropathology of the sudden infant death syndrome. A review," J. Neuropathol. Exp. Neurol. 51, 115–126 (1992).

[23] T. Dwyer, A.-L. B. Ponsonby, N. M. Newman, and L. E. Gibbons, "Prospective cohort study of prone sleeping position and sudden infant death syndrome," Lancet 337, 1244–1247 (1991).

[24] J. L. Feldman and J. D. Cowan, "Large-scale activity in neural nets II: A model for the brainstem respiratory oscillator," Biol. Cybern. 17, 39–51 (1975).

[25] S. M. Botros and E. N. Bruce, "Neural network implementation of a three-phase model of respiratory rhythm generation," Biol. Cybern. 63, 143–153 (1990).

[26] J. Lewis, L. Glass, M. Bachoo, and C. Polosa, "Phase resetting and fixed-delay stimulation of a simple model of respiratory rhythm generation," J. Theor. Biol. 159, 491–506 (1992).

[27] T. Lumsden, "Observations on the respiratory centers," J. Physiol. (London) 57, 354–367 (1923).

[28] T. Lumsden, "Observations on the respiratory centers in the cat," J. Physiol. (London) 57, 153–160 (1923).

[29] T. Lumsden, "The regulation of respiration. Part I," J. Physiol. (London) 58, 81–91 (1923).

[30] C. von Euler, "Brain stem mechanisms for generation and control of breathing pattern," in Handbook of Physiology. The Respiratory System II, edited by N. S. Cherniack and J. G. Widdicombe (American Physiological Society, Bethesda, MD, 1986), p. 43, Fig. 33.

[31] L. Glass and A. T. Winfree, "Discontinuities in phase-resetting experiments," Am. J. Physiol. 246, R251–R258 (1984).

[32] F. L. Eldridge and D. Paydarfar, "Phase resetting of respiratory rhythm studied in a model of a limit-cycle oscillator: influence of stochastic processes," in Respiratory Control, edited by G. D. Swanson, F. S. Grodins, and R. L. Hughson (Plenum, New York, 1989), pp. 379–388.

[33] J. Lewis, M. Bachoo, C. Polosa, and L. Glass, "The effects of superior laryngeal nerve stimulation on the respiratory rhythm: phase-resetting and aftereffects," Brain Res. 517, 44–50 (1989).

[34] G. P. Moore, D. H. Perkel, and J. P. Segundo, "Statistical analysis and functional interpretation of neuronal spike data," Annu. Rev. Physiol. 28, 493–522 (1966).

[35] L. J. Croner, K. Purpura, and E. Kaplan, "Response variability in retinal ganglion cells of primates," Proc. Natl. Acad. Sci. (USA) 90, 8128–8130 (1993).

[36] J. K. Douglass, L. Wilkens, E. Pantazelou, and F. Moss, "Noise enhancement of information transfer in crayfish mechanoreceptors by stochastic resonance," Nature 365, 337–340 (1993).

[37] L. Glass, C. Graves, G. A. Petrillo, and M. C. Mackey, "Unstable dynamics of a periodically driven oscillator in the presence of noise," J. Theor. Biol. 86, 455–475, 1980.

[38] C. Kurrer and K. Schulten, "Effect of noise and perturbations on limit cycle systems," Physica D 50, 311–320 (1991).

[39] R. Shannon, "Reflexes from respiratory muscles and costovertebral joints," in Handbook of Physiology. The Respiratory System II, edited by N. S. Cherniack and J. G. Widdicombe (American Physiological Society, Bethesda, MD, 1986), pp. 431–447.

[40] L. J. Bradford, "Respiratory Audiometry," in Physiological Measures of the Audio-Vestibular System, edited by L. J. Bradford (Academic, New York, 1975), pp. 249–317.

Nonlinear dynamics of the voice: Signal analysis and biomechanical modeling

Hanspeter Herzel
Institute of Theoretical Physics, Technical University, Hardenbergstrasse 36, D-10623 Berlin, Germany

David Berry and Ingo Titze
National Center for Voice and Speech, The University of Iowa, Iowa City, Iowa 52242

Ina Steinecke
Institute of Theoretical Physics, Humboldt University, Invalidenstrasse 110, D-10115 Berlin, Germany

(Received 17 May 1994; accepted for publication 8 August 1994)

Irregularities in voiced speech are often observed as a consequence of vocal fold lesions, paralyses, and other pathological conditions. Many of these instabilities are related to the intrinsic nonlinearities in the vibrations of the vocal folds. In this paper, bifurcations in voice signals are analyzed using narrow-band spectrograms. We study sustained phonation of patients with laryngeal paralysis and data from an excised larynx experiment. These spectrograms are compared with computer simulations of an asymmetric 2-mass model of the vocal folds. © 1995 American Institute of Physics.

I. INTRODUCTION

The vocal folds, together with glottal airflow, constitute a highly nonlinear self-oscillating system. According to the accepted myoelastic theory of voice production, the vocal folds are set into vibration by the combined effect of subglottal pressure, the viscoelastic properties of the folds, and the Bernoulli effect.[1,2] The effective length, mass, and tension of the vocal folds are determined by muscle action, and in this way the fundamental frequency ("pitch") and the waveform of the glottal pulses can be controlled. The vocal tract acts as a filter which transforms the primary signals into meaningful voiced speech.[3]

Normal sustained voiced sound appears to be nearly periodic, although small perturbations (on the order of a percent) are important for the naturalness of speech. Under certain circumstances, however, much larger irregularities are observed in vocalizations which are often associated with the term "roughness." In the phonetic literature phenomena such as "octave jumps," "biphonation" (two independent pitches), and "noise concentrations" have been reported for decades.[4,5] However, only within the past few years has it been suggested that these observations might be interpreted as period-doubling bifurcations, tori, and chaos, respectively,[6–10] It has been shown using Poincaré sections and estimations of attractor dimension and Lyapunov exponents that newborn cries[6] and vocal disorders[7–10] are intimately related to bifurcations and low-dimensional attractors. On the one hand, subharmonics and irregularities appear occasionally in normal vocalizations (newborn cries,[6] "vocal fry" phonation,[9] and speech[11]). On the other hand, vocal instabilities due to bifurcations are often symptomatic in voice pathology.[7–10] Laryngeal stroboscopy reveals that various voice disorders lead to irregular vibratory patterns of the vocal folds resulting in a rough voice quality.[12] The corresponding acoustic signals often show sudden jumps to subharmonic regimes (period-doubling or -tripling) and low-

frequency modulations (tori).[7,8,10] It is the aim of current research to understand the underlying physiological mechanisms of these bifurcations with the aid of high-speed films, excised larynx experiments,[13] and biomechanical modeling.[14,15]

In this paper we analyze voice signals with the aid of narrow-band spectrograms, allowing the detection of bifurcations in systems with slowly varying parameters.[4–6,16,17] Spectrograms are based on many subsequent short-time power spectra of overlapping segments. The spectral amplitude is encoded as a grey scale and, in this way, the (dis)appearance of spectral peaks due to bifurcations of the underlying dynamical system can be monitored. For example, period-doubling is reflected in additional peaks in the middle of the harmonics of the original pitch. Low-frequency modulations lead to sidebands of the main spectral peaks. An amplitude modulation with frequency f induces, e.g., peaks at $F_0 \pm f, 2F_0 \pm f,\dots$.

While normal phonation is characterized by synchronized motion of all vibratory modes of the vocal folds, various physiological mechanisms lead to the desynchronization of certain modes.[10] One source of instabilities is the tension imbalance of the left and right vocal fold which is relevant for unilateral laryngeal nerve paralyses. In these cases the rest position, the stiffness, and the effective mass of the affected fold may deviate drastically from normality. Often paralysis leads to turbulent fricative noise due to incomplete closure of the folds corresponding to a "breathy voice."[12] Frequently, subharmonics and low-frequency modulations have also been observed.[10,18–20] Here, the left–right asymmetry is presumably the origin of the instabilities.[15,18,21]

In the following sections we present left–right asymmetry from three perspectives. Spectrograms are presented from patients with unilateral paralyses, from excised larynx experiments with artificially induced asymmetry, and from

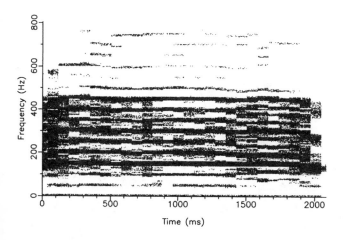

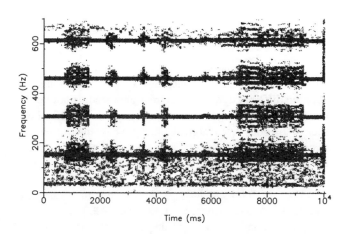

FIG. 1. Computer spectrogram of the vowel [i:] from a male patient with paralysis showing subharmonics. In order to get sufficient spectral resolution to resolve subharmonics and sidebands, segments of 4096 points (about 200 ms) have been used in all spectrograms. Higher frequencies have been boosted for a better visualization of harmonics.

FIG. 3. Spectrogram from an excised larynx experiment with asymmetric elongation of the folds. Around 1000 and 8000 ms episodes with low-frequency modulations of about 20 Hz can be seen.

simulations of an asymmetric 2-mass model of the vocal folds.

II. UNILATERAL LARYNGEAL NERVE PARALYSES

Figure 1 shows a spectrogram of a sustained vowel from a male patient with unilateral recurrent nerve paralysis. The fundamental frequency F_0 of about 150 Hz and its harmonics of 300 Hz and 450 Hz appear as dark horizontal lines. The audible rough voice quality results from the strong subharmonic components. Particularly, period-tripling, i.e. subharmonics at $\frac{1}{3}F_0, \frac{2}{3}F_0,...$ occur between 0 and 1500 ms. Moreover, around 1700 ms another subharmonic regime is found: there are subharmonics at one-fourth of the pitch F_0. Comparable transitions between subharmonic regimes will be discussed later in connection with our 2-mass model.

In Fig. 2 a sustained vowel of another male patient with recurrent nerve paralysis is shown. His voice is characterized by low-frequency modulations typically between 20 and 30 Hz. The modulations appear in the spectrogram as sidebands of the fundamental frequency (≈ 120 Hz) and its harmonics. These toroidal oscillations result in a very rough voice quality. Moreover, the voice sounds breathy due to turbulent air flow. In this case, two sources of hoarseness—complicated vibratory patterns of the folds and turbulence—superimpose on each other.

III. EXCISED LARYNX EXPERIMENTS

Experiments with human or animal larynges serve as a link between the human voice source *in vivo* and computer models.[1,18,22] They allow controlled and systematic parameter variations and easy observation of vibratory patterns.

We have examined three larynges from large (about 25 kg) mongrel dogs coming from coronary research units at The University of Iowa. The dissected larynges were mounted on an apparatus described in detail elsewhere.[13,22] Heated and humified air was supplied from below as the driving force of the oscillations. The device was attached to several micrometers to control the adduction and the elongation of the vocal folds. To facilitate observation of vocal fold movement, a strobe light with adjustable frequency was placed above the glottis. The data were recorded on a color video system and afterwards digitized with 16-bit resolution and a sampling rate of 20 kHz.

In our experiments instabilities have been studied for varying subglottal pressure and for asymmetric adduction and elongation of the vocal folds. 2-parameter bifurcation diagrams can be found elsewhere.[13] Here we only summarize briefly the various dynamic regimes which have been observed for overcritical asymmetry and pressure:

- Symmetric periodic phonation in head-like and chest-like registers;
- periodic vibrations of the lax fold only;
- subharmonics, modulations, and irregular vibrations with both folds involved;

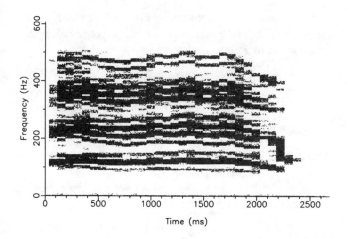

FIG. 2. Spectrogram (vowel [e:], recurrent nerve paralysis) displaying low-frequency modulations visible as sidebands.

- whistle-like sound;
- aphonia, i.e., vibrations ceased for very strong asymmetric tension.

Typically, the parameter ranges of these regimes overlap, i.e., hysteresis is observed. Sometimes spontaneous transitions between different dynamical regimes appeared without external parameter changes. The spectrogram in Fig. 3 shows such transitions from normal phonation to intermittent regimes with a low-frequency modulation of about 20 Hz, as evidenced by the spacing of the sidebands about the harmonics. The longest duration of low-frequency modulations occurs between 7000 and 9000 ms. An example of normal phonation is found between 5000 and 7000 ms. These modulations have been found due to lengthening of one of the folds. Note, that qualitatively comparable modulations appeared in the sustained vowel shown in Fig. 2.

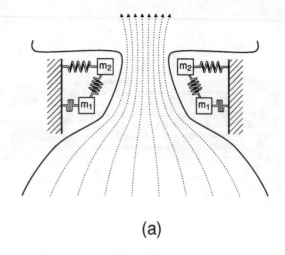

(a)

IV. TWO-MASS MODEL

Computer models of speech production are valuable to understand the basic mechanisms of normal and pathological phonation. There are conceptionally simple 2-mass models[9,15,18,21,23] and sophisticated continuum models simulating the viscoelastic equations.[2,8,14,24] In this section we discuss a simplified version of the intensively studied Ishizaka–Flanagan model.[23] For such relatively simple models extensive bifurcation analysis can be carried out.[9,15,25]

In our model, each fold is represented by two oscillators (defined by mass m, stiffness k, damping constant r) which are coupled by a spring with stiffness k_c (see Fig. 4). This realization enables the "vocal folds" to oscillate with a phase difference between the lower and the upper part. Another restoring force with stiffness c acts during collision of the left and the right vocal fold, i.e., if areas a_i become negative. We can describe the elongation of each of the four masses by Newton's law:

$$m_{i\alpha}\ddot{x}_{i\alpha}+r_{i\alpha}\dot{x}_{i\alpha}+k_{i\alpha}x_{i\alpha}+\Theta(-a_i)c_{i\alpha}\left(\frac{a_i}{2l}\right)+k_{c\alpha}(x_{i\alpha}-x_{j\alpha})$$

$$=F_i(x_{1l},x_{1r},x_{2l},x_{2r}), \tag{1}$$

$$a_{i\alpha}=a_{i0\alpha}+lx_{i\alpha},$$

$$a_i=a_{il}+a_{ir}, \tag{2}$$

with $a_{i0\alpha}$ the glottal rest area and l the length of the glottis

$$i,j=\begin{cases}1-\text{lower mass,}\\2-\text{upper mass;}\end{cases}$$

$$\alpha=\begin{cases}l-\text{left side,}\\r-\text{right side,}\end{cases}$$

where $F_i(x_{1l},x_{1r},x_{2l},x_{2r})$ is the force exerted by the pressure P_i on the corresponding part of the glottis,

$$F_i=ld_iP_i, \tag{3}$$

where d_i is the thickness of part i.

The air flow is considered to be laminar and is described by the Bernoulli equation (4). After passing the smallest gap

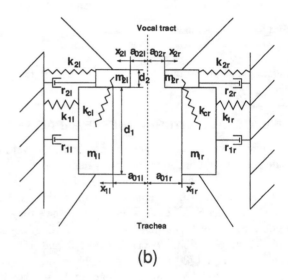

(b)

FIG. 4. (a) A cross section of the vocal folds with the airflow and 2-mass model superimposed. (b) A schematic of the asymmetric 2-mass model of vocal folds.

in the vertical direction with area $a_{\min}$, a jet is built up and the static pressure equals that of the supraglottal system which is set to zero.[2,15]

$$P_s=P_1+\frac{\rho}{2}\left(\frac{U}{a_1}\right)^2=\frac{\rho}{2}\left(\frac{U}{a_{\min}}\right)^2,$$

$$a_{\min}=\min(a_{1l},a_{2l})+\min(a_{1r},a_{2r}), \tag{4}$$

where P_s is the subglottal pressure, U the volume flow velocity, and ρ the density of air.

According to these assumptions we get the following pressure equations:

$$P_1=P_s\left[1-\Theta(a_{\min})\left(\frac{a_{\min}}{a_1}\right)^2\right]\Theta(a_1), \tag{5}$$

$$P_2=0, \tag{6}$$

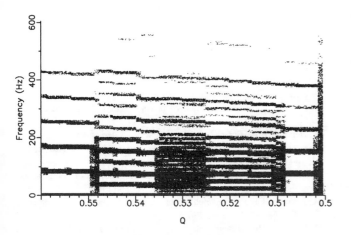

FIG. 5. Spectrogram from the asymmetric 2-mass model (calculated from the flow velocity U). The asymmetry parameter Q was reduced every 400 ms by 0.005 from 0.56 to 0.50. In this way jumps between different subharmonic regimes including period-doubling and -tripling are induced.

$$U = \sqrt{\frac{2P_s}{\rho}} a_{min}. \qquad (7)$$

It is emphasized that in this manner the upper masses are only driven by the lower ones. Our default parameter values representing a normal voice are given in the Appendix.

In the above model several aspects have been neglected: vertical motion, incompressibility, and nonlinear tissue properties of the folds. Moreover, the vocal fold vibrations were separated from the vocal tract by assuming constant pressures below and above the glottis. Nevertheless, several features of the human voice source such as the waveforms of glottal pulses and the phonation onset can be captured quite realistically.[9,15] However, we are aware that details such as localized lesions of the vocal folds cannot be treated by 2-mass models.

V. MODELING ASYMMETRY

In this section the effect of asymmetric mechanical properties of the folds is studied as a first approach to unilateral paralysis. Following earlier studies [15,18,21] we introduce an asymmetry parameter Q:

$$k_{ir} = Q k_{il},$$
$$m_{ir} = m_{il}/Q, \qquad (8)$$
$$0 < Q < 1.$$

In this way the eigenfrequency of the affected fold is reduced by the factor Q. Instabilities have been found for $Q < 0.6$ and subglottal pressure above $P_s = 0.013$.[15] Typically, at the borderline of normal phonation abrupt jumps to subharmonic regimes are observed.[15] Figure 5 shows a "spectral bifurcation diagram" for slowly decreasing Q. It can be seen that the pitch decreases with the ratio of the eigenfrequencies Q. Around $Q = 0.55$ subharmonics suddenly appear at one-half of the pitch. At $Q = 0.536$ another complicated subharmonic regime is reached. Inspection of the peaks of the elongations x_{1r} and x_{1l} [see Eq. (1)] reveals that during one cycle (about

5 times the original pitch period) five maxima of x_{1r} and eight maxima of x_{1l} occur, i.e., we can interpret this regime as a 5:8 resonance. From $Q = 0.525$ to 0.51 subharmonics of one-third of the original pitch ("period-tripling") dominate corresponding to a 3:5 resonance in the above sense. The sequence of decreasing ratios from 2:3 to 5:8 to 3:5 is reminiscent of "Arnold tongues" in bifurcation diagrams of coupled oscillators.

Our simulations show that for sufficiently large pressures, which couple the left and right folds, the detuning of the eigenfrequencies induces transitions to subharmonic regimes comparable to observations as in Fig. 1. Comprehensive bifurcation diagrams in the $P_s - Q$ parameter plane also reveal the appearance of toroidal and chaotic oscillations.[15]

Despite the qualitative resemblance of our simulations to observations, we have to keep in mind that a 2-mass model is only a crude approximation of the real vocal folds. However, in simulations of a three-dimensional model based on partial differential equations, similar bifurcations to subharmonic regimes and chaos have been found.[8,14] Moreover, the calculation of empirical orthogonal functions from the continuum model reveal that the dynamics is often governed by only a few dominant modes. This can be regarded as a justification to study specific aspects of vocal fold vibrations such as left–right asymmetry with appropriate low-order models.

VI. SUMMARY AND DISCUSSION

Analysis of acoustic signals from newborn cries,[6] voice disorders, and excised larynx studies reveals clear evidence of bifurcations and low-dimensional attractors.[6-10] Since vocal folds are vibrating rather fast compared to slowly varying parameters such as muscle tension and subglottal pressure, different dynamic regimes (normal phonation, subharmonics, modulations) can be characterized. Although the limited stationarity of such data allows no definite proof of chaos, nonlinear phenomena are plausible since the human voice source exhibits several essential nonlinearities:

- Nonlinear stress-strain characteristics of vocal fold tissue;[8,2]
- highly nonlinear relation between pressure and glottal area [cf. Eq. (5)];
- collision of the vocal folds;
- vortices and jet instabilities.

Simulations of the 2-mass model have shown that various bifurcations appear due to the desynchronization of the right and left fold for overcritical asymmetry. The corresponding instabilities are similar to observations of vocalizations of patients with unilateral paralysis. However, a more quantitative comparison would require the use of more sophisticated models and more detailed measurements of the biomechanical properties of vocal fold tissues, especially in the case of pathologies.

In forthcoming studies we plan to analyze the physiological mechanisms of vocal instabilities in detail using the continuum model,[8,14,2] excised larynx experiments, and high-speed films of vocal fold vibrations.

ACKNOWLEDGMENTS

Partial funding for this research was provided by the Deutsche Forschungsgemeinschaft and Grant No. P60 DC00976 from the National Institute of Deafness and Other Communication Disorders. We thank J. Wendler and M. Cebulla for providing data from patients with paralyses.

APPENDIX: PARAMETERS OF THE TWO-MASS MODEL

Following mostly Ishizaka and Flanagan we choose the following parameters to model a normal voice:

$$m_{1l} = m_{1r} = 0.125,$$

$$m_{2l} = m_{2r} = 0.025,$$

$$k_{1l} = k_{1r} = 0.08,$$

$$k_{2l} = k_{2r} = 0.008,$$

$$k_{cl} = k_{cr} = 0.025,$$

$$c_{1l} = c_{1r} = 3k_1,$$

$$c_{2l} = c_{2r} = 3k_2,$$

$$r_{1l} = r_{1r} = 0.02,$$

$$r_{2l} = r_{2r} = 0.02,$$

$$d_1 = 0.25, \qquad a_{01} = a_{01l} + a_{01r} = 0.05,$$

$$d_2 = 0.05, \qquad a_{02} = a_{02l} + a_{02r} = 0.05,$$

$$P_s = 0.008 \qquad (\approx 8\text{cm H}_2\text{O}),$$

$$\rho = 0.00113.$$

All units are given in cm, g, ms, and their corresponding combinations.

[1] J. van den Berg, "Myoelastic-aerodynamic theory of voice production," J. Speech Hearing Res. 1, 227–244 (1958).

[2] I. R. Titze and F. Alipour-Haghighi, "Myoelastic aerodynamic theory of phonation" (in preparation).

[3] G. Fant, Acoustic Theory of Speech Production (Mouton, The Hague, 1960).

[4] J. Lind (editor), Newborn Infant Cry (Almquist and Wiksells Boktrycken, Uppsala, 1965).

[5] A. W. Kelman, "Vibratory pattern of the vocal folds," Folia Phoniat. 33, 73–99 (1981).

[6] W. Mende, H. Herzel, and K. Wermke, "Bifurcations and chaos in newborn cries," Phys. Lett. A 145, 418–424 (1990).

[7] H. Herzel and J. Wendler, "Evidence of chaos in phonatory samples," in EUROSPEECH (ESCA, Genova, 1991), pp.263–266.

[8] I. R. Titze, R. Baken, and H. Herzel, "Evidence of chaos in vocal fold vibration," in Vocal Fold Physiology: Frontiers in Basic Science, edited by I. R. Titze (Singular Publishing Group, San Diego, 1993), pp.143–188.

[9] H. Herzel, "Bifurcations and chaos in voice signals," Appl. Mech. Rev. 46, 399–413 (1993).

[10] H. Herzel, D. A. Berry, I. R. Titze, and M. Saleh, "Analysis of vocal disorders with methods from nonlinear dynamics," J. Speech Hearing Res. 37, 1008–1019 (1994).

[11] L. Dolansky and P. Tjernlund, "On certain irregularities of voiced-speech waveforms," IEEE Trans. Audio AU-16, 51–56 (1968).

[12] M. Hirano, "Objective evaluation of the human voice: clinical aspects," Folia Phoniat. 41, 89–144 (1989).

[13] D. Berry, H. Herzel, and I. R. Titze, "Bifurcations in excised larynx experiments due to asymmetric vocal folds" (in preparation).

[14] B. A. Berry, H. Herzel, I. R. Titze, and K. Krischer, "Interpretation of biomechanical simulations of normal and chaotic vocal fold oscillations with empirical eigenfunctions," J. Acoust. Soc. Am. 95, 3595–3604 (1994).

[15] I. Steinecke and H. Herzel, "Bifurcations in an asymmetric vocal fold model," J. Acoust. Soc. Am. (in press).

[16] W. Lauterborn and E. Cramer, "Subharmonic routes to chaos observed in acoustics," Phys. Rev. Lett. 47, 1445–1448 (1981).

[17] M. A. Liauw, K. Koblitz, N. I. Jaeger, and P. Plath, "Periodic perturbation of a drifting heterogeneous catalytic system," J. Phys. Chem. 97, 11724–11730 (1993).

[18] K. Ishizaka and N. Isshiki, "Computer simulation of pathological vocal-cord vibrations," J. Acoust. Soc. Am. 60, 1194–1198 (1976).

[19] B. Hammarberg, B. Fritzell, J. Gauffin, and J. Sundberg, "Acoustic and perceptual analysis of vocal dysfunction," J. Phonetics 14, 533–547 (1986).

[20] M. Ptok, G. Sesterhenn, and R. Arold, "Bewertung der laryngealen Klanggeneration mit der FFT-Analyse der glottischen Impedanz bei Patienten mit Rekurrensparese," Folia Phoniat. 45, 182–197 (1993).

[21] M. E. Smith, G. S. Berke, B. R. Gerrat, and J. Kreimann, " Laryngeal paralyses: theoretical considerations and effects on laryngeal vibration," J. Speech Hearing Res. 35, 545–554 (1992).

[22] T. Baer, "Investigation of the phonatory mechanism, " ASHA Rep. 11, 38–47 (1981).

[23] K. Ishizaka and J. L. Flanagan, "Synthesis of voiced sounds from a two-mass model of the vocal cords," Bell Syst. Technol. J. 51, 1233–1268 (1972).

[24] I. R. Titze and D. T. Talkin, "A theoretical study of the effects of various laryngeal configurations on the acoustics of phonation," J. Acoust. Soc. Am. 66, 60–74 (1979).

[25] H. Herzel, I. Steinecke, W. Mende, and K. Wermke, "Chaos and bifurcations during voiced speech," in Complexity, Chaos and Biological Evolution, edited by E. Mosekilde and L. Mosekilde (Plenum, New York, 1991), pp. 41–50.

Tremor: Is Parkinson's disease a dynamical disease?

Anne Beuter[a)]

Laboratoire de Neurocinétique (N-8280), Université du Québec à Montréal, CP 8888, SUC. A, H3C 3P8 Montréal, Canada

Konstantinon Vasilakos[a)]

Department of Physiology, McGill University, 3655 Drummond Street, Montréal H3G 1Y6, Canada

(Received 2 June 1994; accepted for publication 2 August 1994)

Experimental evidence has shown a plethora of short-term fluctuations in patients with Parkinson's disease. We investigate these transitory events using the concept of dynamical disease. Several examples of short-term fluctuations in tremor are analyzed, and in two cases, other systemic variables (i.e., respiration and blood pressure) are examined as well. A model for tremor, based on negative feedback with delays is proposed, and the transient events are simulated. The theoretical implications of the model suggest that interactions between the central and peripheral loops, as well as interactions between the control loops and other systemic signals, can give rise to transitory events in tremor, both in the pathological and in the normal case. © *1995 American Institute of Physics.*

I. INTRODUCTION

There are numerous oscillatory phenomena in motor control that occur regularly or irregularly, both in health and disease. For example, myoclonus is an intermittent muscle jerking, irregular or rhythmic, arising in the central nervous system,[1] chorea corresponds to sudden bursts of activity occurring in antagonist muscles,[2] and finally, clonus is composed of rhythmical muscle contractions evoked by active or passive stretch of a joint.[3] The qualitative changes occurring in regular and irregular oscillatory phenomena have been described by the concept of dynamical disease. For Mackey and Glass, a dynamical disease is defined as an intact physiological control system operating in a range of control parameters that leads to abnormal dynamics.[4,5] Later, Mackey and Milton indicated that the signature of a dynamical disease is a change in the qualitative dynamics of some observable nature as one or more parameters are varied. Thus, dynamical diseases tend to exhibit transient behaviors, and the severity of their symptoms varies over time.[6] These qualitative changes or transitions correspond mathematically to bifurcations in the relevant nonlinear equations describing the physiological system.

Parkinson's disease (PD) is a chronic progressive neurodegenerative disorder characterized by tremor, rigidity, and bradykinesia that affects mainly dopamine neurotransmission in the basal ganglia.[7] PD is a complex multisystem disease characterized by a great variability, both between individuals and within individuals throughout the course of the illness. Mackey and Milton describe three main characteristics of dynamical diseases.[6] These characteristics are observed in PD. Namely, (1) the appearance of a regular oscillation in a physiological control system not normally characterized by rhythmic processes, such as the appearance of cogwheeling, a rhythmic resistance in a mobilized joint at a frequency of about 6 Hz; another example is the appearance of a resting tremor, where normally only a physiological tremor is present; (2) the disappearance of a rhythmical process, such as the progressive loss of oscillation in the swinging arms during locomotion; another example is freezing, which is a disturbance of voluntary repetitive movements (walking, writing, or speech) in one part of the body; and (3) the development of a new periodicity in an already periodic process, such as the increase in amplitude and decrease in frequency noted in a resting tremor; another example is the marked fluctuations in motor functioning ("yoyoing").

There are additional experimental or clinical observations that make PD a good candidate for being a dynamical disease:

(1) PD symptoms are reversible. Symptons appear when 80%–90% of the dopaminergic neurons of the substantia nigra are destroyed and can be reversed through replacement of striatal dopamine. However, an accidental overdose of dopamine causes hyperkinetic symptoms in patients normally described to have hypokinetic disorders.[8] Visual or auditory stimuli can also overcome freezing episodes.[8]

(2) Clamping of movement and tremor frequencies. In normal subjects, the frequency of movements can be modulated voluntarily throughout the performance range. However, in PD, tapping and tremor are slowed down. In addition, at higher frequencies tapping is clamped to a fixed frequency that seems to corresponds to tremor frequency.[9] This hastening phenomena may suggest that tremor acts as an attractor for frequencies close to its range.[9]

(3) Thalamic stimulation can diminish resting tremor. Thalamic stimulation of the ventral intermediate nucleus at a frequency above 100 Hz suppresses Parkinsonian tremor. Tremor suppression is also accompanied by depressed activity medially and paramedially in the rostral cerebellum, and suggests that resting tremor suppression is associated with a decrease in synaptic activity in the cerebellum.[10] In addition, resetting of a tremor using sensory stimulation at various phases of the tremor cycle is rarely seen in PD tremor, suggesting that sensory involvement is limited in PD.[11]

(4) Pathological tremor can be simulated. The occurrence of pathological-like oscillations in the hand of a normal subject simulating pathological tremor induced without

[a)]Also at the Centre for Nonlinear Dynamics in Physiology and Medicine, McGill University.

the use of drugs or accidental CNS lesions provides a good example of the fuzzy distinction between normality and pathology.[12] In addition, paired discharges (two discharges) of the same motor unit with a short interval are associated with larger tremor amplitude in PD, or in control subjects receiving intramuscular microstimulation. Until recently, they were believed to be restricted to pathological tremor, but now it is known that they can also be produced by normal subjects mimicking tremor.[13]

Finally, recent work by Gantert, Honerkamp, and Timmer has suggested that Parkinsonian tremor is a nonlinear, deterministic, and even chaotic process, and physiological tremor is a linear stochastic process.[14] However, these results still have to be confirmed by using a variety of experimental results, as it is known that the symptoms of PD are highly variable.

Now that some indication that PD might be a dynamical disease has been presented, it is interesting to explore more precisely one of the symptoms (i.e., a resting tremor) and analyze the rich dynamics underlying this manifestation of the disease.

Fluctuations in tremor are commonly observed in patients with PD and follow three different time scales:[15] long-term fluctuations with improvement or deterioration over a few days, medium-term fluctuations with variations over several hours, and short-term fluctuations with variations occurring over seconds or minutes. Since they are seen in the untreated disease, short duration fluctuations are felt to be mainly due to the disease itself, while the other two (medium and long term) are believed to be caused by the treatment. In this paper, the origin of these short-term fluctuations is explored using a dynamical systems approach. Previous research on resting tremor has focused mainly on the neurological aspects. In the present study, we hypothesize that changes in tremor correspond to changes in some critical parameter(s) in the equations governing the system. Following Marsden's elegant study in 1969 correlating tremor and ballistocardiac impulse,[16] we also hypothesize that these changes may be associated with changes in other physiological systems. Subsequently, in several subjects we have recorded respiration, blood pressure, and electrocardiogram simultaneously with tremor.

II. METHODOLOGY AND RESULTS

Tremor is an involuntary movement characterized by rhythmic oscillations of a part of the body.[3] In PD, the resting tremor or "pill rolling" has a frequency around 4–5 Hz, and static tremor observed during a maintained posture may also be present. Clonus and cogwheeling, when present, have frequencies around 6–6.5 Hz. Finally, patients with PD, like all subjects, display physiological tremor, although this tremor being of very low amplitude cannot always be recognized against the background of tremor at rest. In normal subjects, physiological tremor in an extended hand generates frequencies up to 15 Hz.[17]

Typically in our experiments, we record tremor at rest while the subject sits comfortably in a chair and relaxes with closed eyes. The forearms are resting on foam padded supports, and the wrists and hands hang freely over the edge of

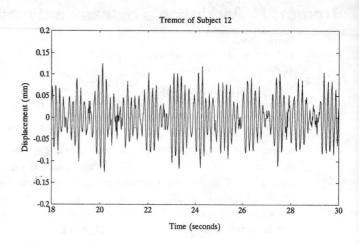

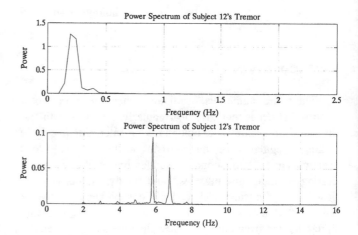

FIG. 1. Data and power spectrum of subject 12's resting tremor; note the "bursting" every second or so and the presence of two peaks in the spectrum indicative of the beat phenomenon. The power spectrum is displayed in two segments; one containing power below 2 Hz and the other containing power between 2 and 16 Hz.

the supports. A resting tremor is recorded using position laser systems (Matsushita), with the laser sensor positioned at 7.5 cm from the tip of the index finger. The laser accurately records position (resolution 35 μm), providing for a higher resolution of low-frequency components.[18] In some subjects, heart rate and respiration are also recorded using a infant respiration/heart rate monitor (Aequitron Medical) measuring electrical activity of the chest, and blood pressure is recorded with a CBM 3000 system (Colin) using pressure sensors at the wrist. Each test lasts 5 min.

Figure 1 presents data recorded from subject #12, a 60 yr old right-handed patient with an akinetic form of PD, stage III.[19] As the subject's breathing created significant lateral movement in the resting hand, the data is presented with frequencies below 1.5 Hz filtered out. One can see that the time series contains a "burst" of activity every second or so (Fig. 1). The subject is fully relaxed, and although muscle activity is not measured, flexor and extensor muscles assumably have almost no EMG discharge.[20] Tremor, however, is present and appears to be subjected to mechanical disturbances, e.g., ballistocardiac impulse, respiration. These mechanical disturbances may have (through the skin of the fin-

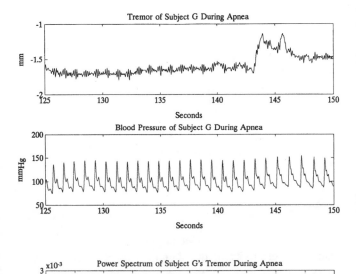

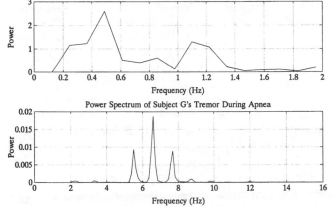

FIG. 2. Resting tremor, blood pressure, and power spectrum of tremor of control subject G during an apnea. Note the correlation of the "bursts" with the systolic upstroke of the blood pressure. The spectrum contains a structure indicative of amplitude modulation (see the text). The power spectrum is displayed in two segments: one containing power below 2 Hz and the other containing power between 2 and 16 Hz.

ger) profound effects on the discharges of the motoneuron (MN) supplying the hand.[20] The power spectrum of subject 12's entire run is also displayed in Fig. 1. The spectrum was computed by averaging two 2048 point segments of data. Notice the two sharp peaks, one at approximately 6 Hz, the other at approximately 7 Hz, other smaller peaks appear at approximately 3, 4, 5, and 8 Hz. As the peaks are evenly spaced (every one Hz), it would seem likely that they are harmonics, despite the difficulty in ascertaining which peak is the main frequency. It is well known that a "bursting" pattern may be produced by the beat phenomenon that occurs when two independent oscillations appear with frequencies in close proximity. The spectra of other trials with subject 12 (not shown) contain a different structure. These spectra have one main peak, and equally spaced sidebands radiating out from this peak.

Figure 2 shows the tremor and blood pressure of control subject G, recorded while the subject performed an apnea. Note how the tremor "bursts" with each systolic upstroke of the blood pressure. Some variance of tremor is to be expected from blood pressure, as the ballistocardiac component

of tremor has been estimated to be about 10%.[21] As well, the constant oscillation of blood pressure in the finger might induce resonance of the finger. We tested this hypothesis by perturbing the hand mechanically at 1.2 Hz while recording tremor, and found that such direct mechanical stimulation led to a different power spectrum (not shown). Subsequently, we infer that the mechanical properties of the system create unavoidable instabilities that probably interact with peripheral (and perhaps central) reflex mechanisms. No special contribution of the Central Nervous System (CNS) is required during resting tremor, at least under normal circumstances. Thus, the variation of blood pressure, with each cardiac cycle, may drive this instability and influence tremor amplitude.

Figure 2 also contains the power spectrum of subject G's tremor during the apnea, again calculated by averaging two 2048 point segments. Here we see a main peak at approximately 6.5 Hz, with two equally spaced sidebands. Other smaller (seemingly equally spaced) peaks appear as well throughout the spectrum. As manipulations with trigonometric identities will indicate, the power spectrum of an amplitude modulated signal will contain such a structure,[22] in accord with our hypothesis that blood pressure is modulating tremor amplitude in some indirect fashion.

Fluctuations in tremor of a different time scale are presented in Fig. 3 (subject H). Three basic factors may be responsible for these fluctuations, including the stage of the disease, changes in the environment (mood, fatigue, degree of motor effort), and drug therapy. Subject H is a 63 yr old man who is a stage IV on the Hoehn and Yahr scale. The respiration rate of this subject was recorded by measuring chest impedance. As the subject breathes, the physical properties of the chest, and subsequently the impedance, changes. Note how the subject's respiration rate changes around 195 s. Soon after, the amplitude of the tremor drops dramatically. Then, around 210 s, the subject's breathing returns to the previous rate, and later, the amplitude of the tremor rises. The power spectrum, calculated by averaging four 2048 point segments, exhibits a single peak just under 4 Hz, in accord with typical results for patients with PD. Further examples of such correlations between changes in respiration and tremor amplitude were recorded on this subject (not shown), which suggest somehow a link, at least in this subject, between tremor fluctuations and other physiological variables, such as breathing or blood pressure.

III. MODELING

It is safe to say that the neuromuscular system at rest contains feedback mechanisms and that time delays play an important role in these mechanisms. It has also been suggested that physiological systems are noisy.[23] Furthermore, as traces from subject G and H have indicated, other physiological variables (i.e., blood pressure and respiration) interact with the system affecting the output.

As Llinas suggested ten years ago,[24] we should abandon the question of a centrally versus peripherally generated tremor. Instead we should look at tremor as the result of central and peripheral factors interacting dynamically according to the state of health (or disease), supraspinal influ-

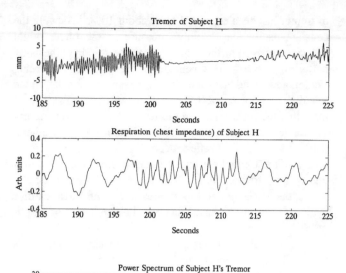

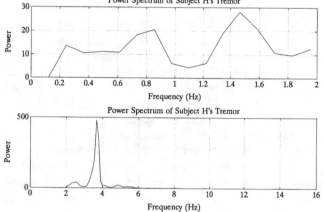

FIG. 3. Resting tremor, respiration, and power spectrum of tremor of subject H. Note the correlation between the change in respiration rate and the amplitude of tremor. The power spectrum is displayed in two segments: one containing power below 2 Hz and the other containing power between 2 and 16 Hz.

ences (such as vision), circulating catecholamines, posture, muscle tone, etc. Therefore we decided to explore the coupling between central and peripheral oscillations with a simple model describing the fluctuations.

The model itself is based on the work of Glass and Malta.[25] Their work was primarily interested in the interaction of multiple feedback loops, but we limit ourselves to studying just two: the central loop (x_c) and the peripheral loop (x_p). The variable of primary interest P is the limb (finger in our case) position. It is given by

$$P = \frac{wt_c \cdot x_c + wt_p \cdot x_p}{wt_c + wt_p},$$

where x_c and x_p are the intended finger position of the central and peripheral loops, respectively, while wt_c and wt_p are weights determining each loop's (central and peripheral) actual contribution to the final finger position. The individual loops are controlled by the feedback:

$$\frac{dx_i}{dt} = S_i(X_i) - x_i, \quad i = c, p,$$

where

$$X_i = \alpha P(t - \tau_i) + (1 - \alpha) x_i(t - \tau_i), \quad 0 \leqslant \alpha \leqslant 1.$$

Here $S_i(X_i)$ is a nonlinear function that depends on both the finger position (P), and the loop itself (x_c or x_p) at a time $t - \tau_i$ in the past. Given the finite conduction velocity in the nervous system, the presence of delays in the equation fits quite naturally. As the human body is intent on maintaining homeostasis, the existence of the damping term, $-x_i$, is completely in accord. As well, physiological systems generally operate using negative feedback, and thus we choose $S_i(X_i)$ to be monotonically decreasing, and use the negative hyperbolic tangent function;

$$S_i(X_i) = -g_i \cdot \tanh(s_i \cdot X_i),$$

where g_i and s_i are parameters governing, respectively, the gain and sensitivity of the sigmoidal function, S_i. Preliminary work has indicated that the results are not dependent on the choice of function for S_i provided that the function is monotonically decreasing. The hyperbolic tangent function has been used previously to model finger position,[26,27] although for a motor task involving visual feedback.

Biological considerations lead us to believe that the central loop would, when acting, have a greater impact on the system,[28] while the peripheral loop would be much more sensitive and responsible for minor corrections.[28] Subsequently, in all simulations studied, we set g_c to 1000, s_c to 0.1, g_p to 100, and s_p to 1. As a bifurcation occurs in an isolated loop when $g \cdot s \cdot \tau > \pi/2$, the stability of each loop is identical with the same delays, while the dynamics do vary. Delays were chosen in the range of reported values for central and peripheral neural transmission; between 50 and 120 ms for the central loop and between 20 and 50 ms for the peripheral loop.[29]

The parameters in the two loops were set so that the central loop would react more vigorously to large changes, whereas the peripheral loop would be much more sensitive to small variations, as it is well known that the gain in exteroceptors and proprioceptors is very high. Meanwhile, each loop's weight will determine which loop dominates in controlling finger position and contributing to tremor. Thus, changes in relative weights and which loop is favored will prove to be the deciding factor on the dynamics of the model. As much as possible, we have kept the weight on the peripheral loop ten times larger than the weight on the central loop. In this way, although the peripheral loop initially seems favored with the higher weight, the gain in the central loop is ten times higher than in the peripheral loop; consequently, the two loops actually have the same relative contributions.

The model proves to have robust dynamics. Once the steady state becomes unstable, periodic dynamics are exhibited. Interestingly, for most sets of parameters, a narrow range of α can be found over which quasiperiodic or periodic behavior with long periods can be found. The role of α in the model is in determining to what degree each loop is controlled by its own activity or by the position of the limb. As α increases, the model becomes more dependent on the limb position; as α decreases, each loop becomes more reactive to its own activity. The physiological reasoning behind the level

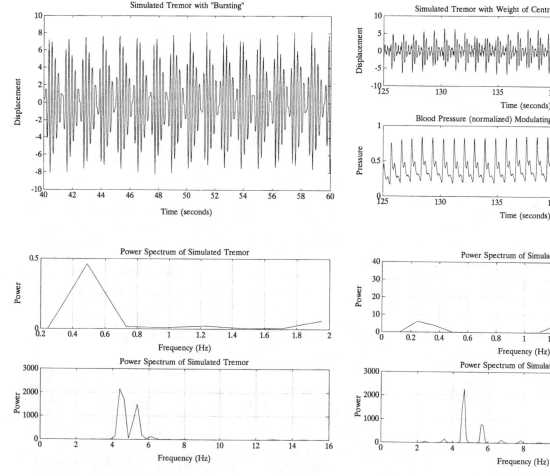

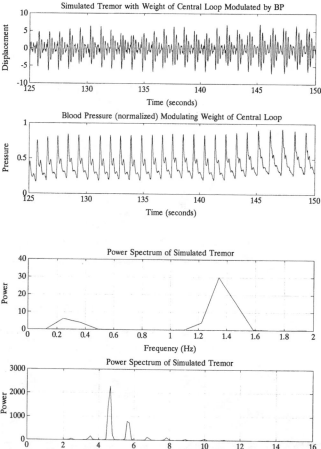

FIG. 4. Simulation with parameters τ_p=48 ms, τ_c=60 ms, g_p=100, g_c=1000, s_p=1, s_c=0.1, wt_p=10, wt_c=1, α=0.15, step size=0.004, and initial offset for all $t \leqslant 0$=0.4. Note the "bursting" behavior of the simulation and the presence of two peaks in the power spectrum indicative of the beat phenomenon. The power spectrum is displayed in two segments: one containing power below 2 Hz and the other containing power between 2 and 16 Hz.

FIG. 5. Simulation with parameters τ_p=24 ms, τ_c=60 ms, g_p=100, g_c=1000, s_p=1, s_c=0.1, wt_p=3.144 [10·mean(bp)], wt_c=bp, α=0.65, step size=0.004, and initial offset for all $t \leqslant 0$=0.4. Normalized blood pressure used at wt_c in the simulation and the power spectrum appears below the data. Results quite similar to Fig. 2 are evident, with a power spectrum indicative of amplitude modulation (see the text). The power spectrum is displayed in two segments: one containing power below 2 Hz and the other containing power between 2 and 16 Hz.

of α is less than clear. In the first simulation, we display (Fig. 4), an α was chosen, such that long period (or quasiperiodic) behavior was present. For the two other simulations (Figs. 5 and 6), α was set to 0.65. Similar dynamics were seen in these two simulations with different α's, gains, delays, weights, and sensitivities.

Since the model contains delays, integration of the equations (analytically or numerically) requires initial conditions for all times up to the largest delay in the past. Numerically we set an offset of 0.4 for all $t<0$, providing an unstable initial condition. All simulations were integrated using a fourth-order Runge–Kutta method with a time step of 0.004.

Figure 4 displays a simulation with the delays in the peripheral and central loop of 48 and 60 ms, respectively, w_p=10, w_c=1, and α equal to 0.15. The results are quite startling, showing a modulation in the amplitude of the oscillations quite akin to what was seen in subject G (Fig. 2) and in subject 12 (Fig. 1). The power spectrum of the run, computed by averaging four 2048 point segments, appears below the data. Note the presence of two large peaks at ap-

proximately 4.5 and 5.5 Hz, and a third smaller peak just over 6 Hz. This spectrum proves to be quite similar to the spectrum seen in subject 12 (Fig. 1). A peak three orders of magnitude smaller than the main peak appears at 0.5 Hz; careful scrutiny has indicated that this peak is most likely a numerical artifact. Again, the spectrum indicates the existence of the beat phenomenon, which seems natural as the model is constructed from two equations oscillating at different frequencies. Initial work done with this equation indicated extensive quasiperiodic activity,[25] while the slight up/down warbling of the simulation and the third, albeit small, peak indicate the possible existence of a three-torus.

Unfortunately, as would be expected from the presence of a three-torus, these dynamics occur for only a narrow range of parameter values. Furthermore, the correlation between blood pressure and the "bursting" is quite apparent in subject G (Fig. 2). The appearance of the three peak structure in the power spectra, indicative of amplitude modulation,

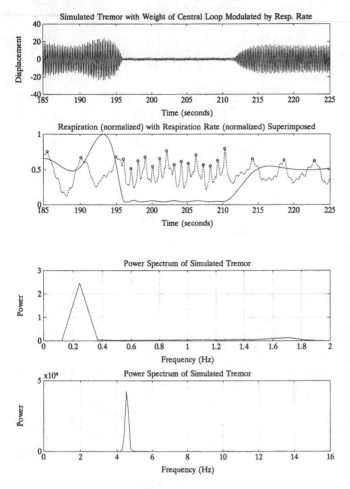

FIG. 6. Simulation with parameters $\tau_p=24$ ms, $\tau_c=60$ ms, $g_p=100$, $g_c=1000$, $s_p=1$, $s_c=0.1$, $wt_p=1$, $wt_c=$rr (respiration rate), $\alpha=0.65$, step size=0.004, and initial offset for all $t\leqslant 0=0.4$. Normalized respiration (dashed), normalized calculated respiration rate (solid), times of inspiration (circles) and power spectrum appear below the simulation. Note the similarity between the results and Fig. 3. The power spectrum is displayed in two segments: one containing power below 2 Hz and the other containing power between 2 and 16 Hz.

suggests that somehow blood pressure should be incorporated in the model in a modulating role.

Subsequently, we took subject G's blood pressure (bp), normalized the scaling to [0,1], and used the trace itself as one of the parameters. Figure 5 shows a run using $\tau_p=24$ ms, $\tau_c=60$ ms, $\alpha=0.65$, $wt_p=3.114$ [10·mean(bp)], and $wt_c=$bp. With g_c ten times higher than g_p, the activity of the central loop is significantly higher than the peripheral one. Variations in either weight (central or peripheral) would then lead to modulations in the oscillation size. The results displayed in Fig. 5 clearly show an increase in the amplitude of the oscillation with each systolic upstroke, which bears strong resemblance with those of Fig. 2 (subject G). The power spectra, computed by averaging two 2048 point segments, show the presence of a main peak around 4.5 Hz, as well as a second large peak just under 6 Hz. Several smaller equally spaced peaks also appear between 1 and 12 Hz. As well, a peak exists around 1.3 Hz, which may result from the input of real blood pressure as the main peak of the power

spectrum of the blood pressure (not shown) is at 1.3 Hz. The two large peaks initially indicate a beat phenomenon, but the existence of equally spaced smaller sidebands do arise from amplitude modulation. Furthermore, if the fluctuations are not independent of the system, the sidebands will be asymmetric, and may appear similar to the results of the beat phenomenon.[22] As the model is nonlinear, the effect of changes in weights is highly dependent on the physical state of the model. Subsequently, the amplitude modulations arising from the variations in blood pressure (and hence wt_c) are not independent, and clearly demonstrate the misleading results of spectral analysis of amplitude modulation.

The modulation of the weights by blood pressure is a natural way of linking the model to a systemic variable. With each stroke of the heart, the structures in the periphery will be perturbed. Subsequently, the activity of the periphery is bound to change with each cardiac cycle. These changes will undoubtedly lead to a shift in the balance of which loop dominates the control of the finger. Although in the simulations the weight of the central loop is modulated, the real issue is the ratio between the weights of the two loops; we could have easily fixed the central weight and modulated the peripheral loop weight instead.

To mimic the results seen in subject H (Fig. 3), the subject's respiration record was normalized to the scale [0,1]. The peaks of the trace, giving the times of inspiration, were then found, and the time between peaks was calculated. A cubic spline was then fitted to these times to give an approximate respiration rate (rr) given as the time between inspirations. This rate was then normalized to the scale [0,1]. Figure 6 displays the results of a run using rr to modulate the weights instead of blood pressure. The delays used were again 24 and 60 ms, while the weights of the peripheral and central loops were set to 1 and rr, respectively; α was set to 0.65. Here we see that as the respiration rate changes, the amplitude of the oscillations rises and falls. Indeed this simulation is quite similar to what is seen in the pathological case (Fig. 3), where the tremor amplitude suddenly increased or decreased with respiration rate. The power spectrum, computed by averaging four 2048 point segments appears below the data. Presence of a single peak at just over 4 Hz is consistent with the example of tremor amplitude modulation on this time scale (Fig. 3).

Linking the weights to the respiration rate is a more tenuous hypothesis. The motivation for this undertaking were the results seen in subject H (Fig. 3). As several examples of a change in tremor corresponding to a change in respiration rate were recorded (only one was shown), we investigated the correlation between tremor amplitude and respiration rate, hypothesizing that some critical parameter must be changing. The most obvious place to initiate the search was the modulation in the weights. The results were encouraging, although the change in tremor amplitude was significantly smaller in the simulations. In addition, in the simulation the change in tremor amplitude follows immediately after the change in respiration rate, whereas in the experimental trace, there is a lag of several seconds. As only correlation is implied by the several examples of this phenomenon, we may be hasty in our approach of using respiration rate to vary the weight of the central loop. In subject H, the lag of several seconds implies that either the change in respiration rate led to a change in one (or more) significant physiological variable(s), which, in turn, led to a change in tremor amplitude, or that something else changed in the system, causing both the respiration rate and the tremor amplitude to change.

IV. DISCUSSION AND CONCLUSION

Having seen several examples of short-term fluctuations in physiological and pathological tremor, we have modeled the observed results from the perspective of dynamical systems. We modeled short-term fluctuations in finger tremor using a linked pair of delay differential equations. The variations in tremor were provided by both a narrow range of parameter values and by the inclusion of a second signal into the framework of the model. The results in both the time domain and the frequency domain proved to be quite similar to our experimental results.

Variation of tremor over a one second period was demonstrated in both a patient with PD and in a control subject. We duplicated these short fluctuations in two methods, one involving the beat phenomenon, and the second involving amplitude modulation. The beat phenomenon gives us an easy handle on the system; simply two oscillations are occurring, perhaps one central and one peripheral, which results in the "bursting," which is seen. But, the possibility of amplitude modulation also proves tempting. According to Gresty and Buckwell,[22] amplitude modulation will lead to characteristic sidebands appearing equally spaced on each side of the main peak in the power spectrum. Moreover, if the fluctuations in amplitude are not independent of the system, then the sidebands will be asymmetric, and it may prove difficult to discern this phenomenon from the beat phenomenon. Still, the model gives us insight on what may be happening in the system. In the future, it will be interesting to pursue this investigation, and to discover under which situations the beat phenomenon occurs, and under which amplitude modulation exists.

The simulation presented in Fig. 6 demonstrates how longer (several seconds) fluctuations may arise. Of course, the lag present in the experimental data indicates that our correlation between respiratory rate and tremor amplitude is too simplistic. The results still highlight an extremely important point; they demonstrate a working example of the principal idea of the concept of dynamical disease. Simply, the change in one parameter has led to the disappearance and appearance of a symptom in a pathological range. The possibility exists to accurately delineate which parameters are changing, to determine which physiological processes these parameters represent, and to modify and control the pathology through these parameters.

The difficulty, of course, is to work backward from observing the oscillations to inferring the appropriate underlying dynamics. If we are successful, it will become possible to develop therapeutic strategies to reposition the system (mechanically, electrically, or pharmacologically) in a range of parameter space associated with "healthy" dynamical behavior. So, what makes PD a dynamical disease is not just the presence of multiple oscillatory phenomena or even their in-

teractions, it is really the possibility that coupling between these different rhythms is changing over time in ways that we do not understand yet. Pathological tremor in PD is probably expressed because of a dynamic shift in the functional organization of neuronal circuits or a modification of basic electrophysiological properties of cells in some nuclei; not just damage to a specific site. We must not forget that the patient suffers from functional abnormalities and not from anatomical problems.[24]

ACKNOWLEDGMENTS

The authors would like to acknowledge their collaborators Leon Glass (McGill University), Jacques Bélair (Université de Montréal), and Daniel Kaplan (McGill University).

[1] C. D. Marsden, M. Hallett, and S. Fahn, in *Movement Disorders*, edited by C. D. Marsden and S. Fahn (Butterworths, London, 1981), pp. 196–248.

[2] J. W. Lance and J. G. McLeod, *A Physiological Approach to Clinical Neurology*, 3rd ed. (Butterworths, London, 1981).

[3] L. J. Findley, M. A. Gresty, and G. M. Halmagyi, "Tremor, the cogwheel phenomenon and clonus in Parkinson's disease," J. Neurol. Neurosurg. Psych. **44**, 534–546 (1981).

[4] M. C. Mackey and L. Glass, "Oscillation and chaos in physiological control systems," Sciences **197**, 287–289 (1977).

[5] L. Glass and M. C. Mackey, "Pathological conditions resulting from instabilities in physiological control systems," Ann. NY Acad. Sci. **316**, 214–235 (1979).

[6] M. C. Mackey and J. G. Milton, "Dynamical diseases," Ann. NY Acad. Sci. **504**, 16–32 (1987).

[7] J. G. Nutt, "Therapy of Parkinson's disease," Neurosci. Fact **3**, 85–86 (1992).

[8] G. E. Alexander, M. D. Crutcher, and M. R. DeLong, "Basal ganglia-thalamocortical circuits: Parallel substrates for motor, oculomotor, 'prefrontal' and 'limbic' functions," Prog. Brain Res. **85**, 119–146 (1990).

[9] H. H. Freund and H. Hefter, "The role of basal ganglia in rhythmic movement," in *Parkinson's Disease From Basic Research to Treatment*, Advances in Neurology, edited by H. Narabayashi, T. Nagatsu, N. Yanagisawa, and Y. Mizuno (Raven, New York, 1993), Vol. 60, pp. 88–92.

[10] M.-P. Deiber, P. Pollak, R. Passingham, P. Landais, C. Gervason, L. Cinotti, K. Friston, R. Frackowiak, F. Mauguiere, and A. L. Benabid, "Thalamic stimulation and suppression of Parkinsonian tremor," Brain **116**, 267–279 (1993).

[11] R. B. Stein, R. G. Lee, and T. R. Nichols, "Modifications of ongoing tremors and locomotion by sensory feedback," in *Contemporary Clinical Neurophysiology*, EEG Suppl. 34, edited by W. A. Cobb and H. W. Duijn (Elsevier, Amsterdam, 1978), pp. 511–519.

[12] R. N. Stiles, "Frequency and displacement amplitude relations for normal hand tremor," J. Appl. Physiol. **40**, 44–54 (1976).

[13] J. M. Elek, R. Dengler, A. Konstanzer, S. Hesse, and W. Wolf, "Mechanical implications of paired motor unit discharges in pathological and voluntary tremor," Electroencephal. Cin. Neurophysiol. **81**, 279–283 (1991).

[14] C. Gantert, J. Honerkamp, and J. Timmer, "Analyzing the dynamics of hand tremor time series," Biol. Cybernet. **66**, 479–484 (1992).

[15] C. D. Marsden, J. D. Parkes, and N. Quinn, "Fluctuations of disability in Parkinson's disease—clinical aspect," in *Movement Disorders*, Butterworths International Medical Reviews of Neurology, edtied by C. D. Marsden and S. Fahn (Buttersworths, London, 1982), Vol. 7, pp. 96–121.

[16] C. D. Marsden, J. C. Meadows, G. W. Lange, and R. S. Watson, "The role of the ballistocardiac impulse in the genesis of physiological tremor," Brain **92**, 647–662 (1969).

[17] A. M. Halliday and J. W. T. Redfearn, "An analysis of the frequencies of finger tremor in healthy subjects," J. Physiol. **134**, 660–611 (1956).

[18] A. Beuter, A. de Geoffroy, and P. Cordo, "The measurement of tremor using simple laser systems," J. Neurosci. Methods **53**, 47–54 (1994).

[19] M. M. Hoen and M. D. Yahr, "Parkinsonism: Onset, progression and mortality," Neurology **17**, 427–442 (1967).

[20] M. Lakie E. G. Walsh, and G. W. Wright, "Passive mechanical properties of the wrist and physiological tremor," J. Neurol. Neurosurg. Psych. **49**, 669–676 (1986).

[21] C. D. Marsden, "Origins of normal and pathological tremor," in *Move-*

ment Disorders: Tremor, edited by L. J. Findley and R. Capildeo (Butterworths, London, 1984), pp. 37–83.

[22] M. Gresty and D. Buckwell, "Spectral analysis of tremor: Understanding the results," J. Neurol. Neurosurg. Psych. **53**, 976–981 (1990).

[23] C. A. Bloxham, D. J. Dick, and M. Moore, "Reaction times and attention in Parkinson's disease," J. Neurol. Neurosurg. Psych. **50**, 1178–1183 (1987).

[24] R. R. Llinas, "Possible role of tremor in the organisation of the nervous system," in Ref. 21, pp. 475–477.

[25] L. Glass and C. P. Malta, "Chaos in multi-looped negative feedback systems," J. Theor. Biol. **145**, 217–223 (1990).

[26] K. Vasilakos and A. Beuter, "Effect of noise on a delayed visual feedback system," J. Theor. Biol. **165**, 389–407 (1993).

[27] A. Beuter, J. Belair, and C. Labrie, "Feedback and delays in neurological disease: A modeling study using dynamical systems," Bull. Math. Biol. **55**, 525–541 (1993).

[28] I. Fukumoto, "Computer simulation of Parkinsonian tremor," J. Biomed. Eng. **8**, 49–55 (1986).

[29] H. S. Milner-Brown, R. B. Stein, and R. G. Lee, "'Synchronization of human motor units: Possible roles of exercise and supraspinal reflexes," Electroencephal. Clin. Neurophysiol. **38**, 245–254 (1975).

The dynamical structure of tremor in tardive dyskinesia

K. M. Newell and F. Gao
The Pennsylvania State University, University Park, Pennsylvania 16802

R. L. Sprague
University of Illinois at Urbana—Champaign, Champaign, Illinois 61820

(Received 26 May 1994; accepted for publication 22 August 1994)

The movement disorder syndrome of tardive dyskinesia arises as a consequence of prolonged regimens of neuroleptic medication, and is characterized, although not exclusively, by jerky and sometimes rhythmical stereotypical motions in a wide range of muscle systems. It is well established that the degree and variability of tremor in tardive dyskinesia is greater than that in normal age-matched subjects. The findings from the current experiment show that the dimension of the tardive dyskinetic finger tremor time series is systematically lower than that evident in normal finger tremor. Furthermore, the variability of finger motion in both groups is inversely related to the dimension of the respective attractor dynamic. The neuroleptic medication appears to constrain the degrees of freedom regulated in organization of the motor system. © *1995 American Institute of Physics.*

I. INTRODUCTION

Tardive dyskinesia is the movement disorder syndrome that arises from prolonged intake of neuroleptic medication (American Psychiatric Association, 1992; Jeste and Wyatt, 1982), and has a high prevalence in schizophrenic and mentally retarded populations (Kalachnik, 1984; Khot *et al.*, 1992), particularly in institutionalized individuals. A hallmark characteristic of tardive dyskinesia is the production of jerky and sometimes rhythmical stereotypic motions in the peripheral effector systems, including tongue, lips, jaws, hands, fingers, legs, ankles, and toes. Tremor has been proposed as a useful task to examine the dynamical properties of tardive dyskinesia (Alpert, Diamond, and Friedhoff, 1976; Sprague and Newell, 1987).

Tremor can be observed in normal healthy individuals (Elble and Koller, 1990) and persons suffering from various disease states (Findley and Capildeo, 1984). To the eye of an observer, tremor is apparent in a variety of body segments of tardive dyskinetic individuals (Hansen, Glazer, and Moore, 1986), but there have been only a few direct measurements of the tremor dynamic (Caligiuri and Lohr, 1990; van Emmerik, Sprague, and Newell, 1993; Hansen *et al.*, 1986; Rondot and Bathien, 1986; Stacy and Jankovic, 1992; Tyron and Pologe, 1987). Most of these analyses have focused on the time and frequency domain of the finger accelerometer signal. The general finding is that the degree and variability of tremor is greater in tardive dyskinetic than normal subjects, and that there is a shift to a lower and more broadband finger frequency in tardive dyskinesia.

A recent study from our research program examined the dimensionality of whole-body postural tremor as an approach to understanding if the structure of the tremor dynamic is different in tardive dyskinesia, in addition to its degree of motion and modal frequency characteristics (Newell, van Emmerik, Lee, and Sprague, 1993). Tardive dyskinetic subjects were split into two groups, based upon whether to the eye of observers the structure of the center of pressure time series appeared random or rhythmical. The center of pressure is the position on the surface of support of the global ground reaction force. All trials of the normal group were judged by the eye of an observer to have an unstructured center of pressure pattern. The dimensionality of the center of pressure dynamic was lower in the rhythmical tardive dyskinetic group ($D=1.30$), than the random tardive dyskinetic group ($D=1.75$), and the normal group ($D=2.20$). These dimension estimates of the center of pressure are in the range of others reported for posture (Myklebust and Myklebust, 1989). This postural study showed that the dimensionality measure could distinguish between the tardive dyskinetic and normal groups, and that the dimension was inversely related to the variability of the motion of the center of pressure. Also of interest was the result that the dimensionality measure could distinguish differences in the structural properties of the center of pressure pattern that were indistinguishable to the eye of the observer. This later finding has interesting implications for the possibility of using dynamic measures as part of the diagnostic protocol for tardive dyskinesia.

In this paper, we report a study of the dimensionality of the finger tremor of tardive dyskinetic and normal adult subjects. Our focus is the use of the dimensionality estimate as a discriminator between population groups, rather than the determination of a strange attractor *per se* in the tremor time series. Finger tremor was examined in the postural tasks of both the left and right index fingers considered alone, and in a task where both fingers were held simultaneously in a posture. Given the above findings on postural tremor, one might anticipate that the dimension of the finger tremor of the tardive dyskinetic group would be lower than that of the normal group. The finger effector unit is also of relatively low mass in contrast to the other biokinematic linkages, and is therefore, likely to be influenced by the reactive force motions of the other larger mass body parts. This relative mass factor could contribute to creating a higher-dimensional estimate in finger tremor than that found for the whole body posture. A final feature of interest was whether the variability of the finger tremor motion was inversely related to the dimension estimate.

II. METHOD

A. Subjects

The tardive dyskinetic subjects were 16 developmentally disabled adults who ranged in age from 23 to 60 years. The exact medication history of the tardive dyskinetic group was not known, but all subjects had been on neuroleptic medication for some years, were diagnosed as tardive dyskinetic by supervising medical personnel, and displayed stereotypes normally associated with tardive dyskinesia. The subjects also scored above the cutoff for a diagnosis of tardive dyskinesia on the DISCUS dyskinesia identification scheme (Sprague and Kalachnik, 1991). There were also 16 normal health age-matched adult subjects that acted as a control group. The age of the control group ranged from 24 to 59 years, and each subject was age matched (±6 months) to an individual from the tardive dyskinetic group.

B. Apparatus

The acceleration of each finger was measured with a Coulbourn T45-10 accelerometer. The T45-10 is a one-axial miniature solid state piezoresistive accelerometer with a full-scale direct current (DC) frequency response up to 500 Hz. The accelerometers used for the right and left fingers were factory calibrated and provided with an individual sensitivity level (mV/g). To obtain absolute acceleration levels, we zero balanced the accelerometer in the DC mode in a vertical position on a level surface. The signal from the accelerometer was amplified through a Coulbourn transducer coupler (S72-25) with an excitation voltage of 5 V. The hardware factory standard sensitivity of the accelerometer is 1 mV/V/g. The standard output noise of the accelerometer is uV p-p.

The amplified accelerometer data were collected on a PC through a 12-bit analog-to-digital converter and stored on magnetic tape for further processing. The acceleration signals were collected with a sampling frequency of 200 Hz. This sample frequency was considered adequate to avoid aliasing of the signal.

C. Procedures

The procedure for testing the finger tremor was the same for both the tardive dyskinetic group and the normal group. Subjects were tested individually in a quiet testing room. The subject sat in a chair and rested both arms on a rigidly fixed table. Accelerometers were attached (taped) to the tip (nail) of the index finger of both the left and right hands. In all conditions the subjects were asked to make a fist with their hand, rest the hand on the table, and outstretch the index finger so that it was still and parallel to the table. In one condition, the acceleration of the left index finger was measured while it was stretched out, and the right index finger rested on the table. In the second condition the reverse occurred with the right index finger stretched out and the left index finger resting on the table. In the third condition, both

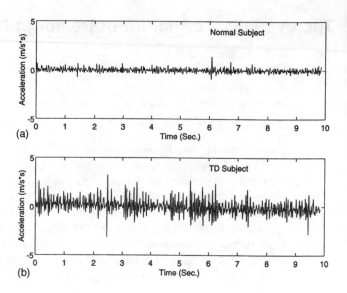

FIG. 1. Example acceleration time series from the two groups: (a) normal group; (b) tardive dyskinetic group.

fingers were stretched out and the acceleration of both fingers was recorded simultaneously. There were two trials that were blocked at each finger condition. Each trial was of ten seconds duration.

D. Data analyses

All analyses were conducted on the raw data. The basic analyses examined the mean and standard deviation of the acceleration signal as a function of finger condition and trial. Dimensionality analysis was performed on the acceleration time series of each trial. The dimension was calculated by using the correlation dimension algorithm, as proposed by Grassberger and Procaccia (1983). The derivation of the correlation dimension requires resconstruction of the original state space that generated the acceleration dynamic. These higher-dimensional state spaces were constructed by time lagging the originial acceleration time series (e.g., Packard et al., 1980). A criterion for choosing the appropriate time delay is maximal independence of the original and delayed signals. This was obtained by using the mutual information technique, as introduced by Fraser and Swinney (1986). From these time-lagged series, higher-dimensional state spaces were reconstructed, in which the number of added delay series is an indication of the "embedding dimension" of the state space. By adding additional embedding dimensions, the dimension of the attractor can be determined. In the present experiment we calculated the correlation dimension of the center of pressure on the basis of iterations up to 25 embedding dimensions by which point the dimensionality estimate had saturated. Surrogate data analyses were run as checks on the structure of the time-series data (Theiler et al., 1992).

III. RESULTS

Representative finger acceleration data for normal and tardive dyskinetic trials are shown in Fig. 1. In general, and as reflected in the example trials shown in Fig. 1, there was

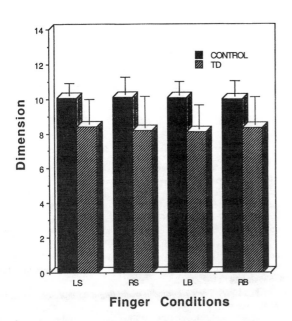

FIG. 2. Average dimension and standard deviation as a function of group and finger condition.

TABLE I. Correlations of dimension and the standard deviation of acceleration as a function of group and finger condition.

| | Finger condition | | | |
| | Alone | | Together | |
Group	left	right	left	right
Control	−0.44	−0.39	−0.34	−0.43
Tardive dyskinesia	−0.30	−0.80	−0.58	−0.56

more acceleration activity in the tardive dyskinetic group than the normal group, as reflected in the standard deviation of the acceleration signal, $F(1,28)=9.07$, $p<0.01$. These findings are consistent with those previously published from time domain analyses of the tremor of tardive dyskinesia.

Of more interest here are the estimates of dimension for the two groups as a function of finger condition and trial. Figure 2 shows the mean and standard deviation of dimension for the two groups as a function of the finger conditions (averaged over the two trials). An analysis of variance confirmed that, on average, the dimensionality of the normal group was higher than that of the tardive dyskinetic group, $F(1,28)=37.54$, $p<0.01$. There was no effect for either finger condition, $F(3,84)<1$, or trial, $F(1,28)<1$. None of the interactions were significant (all p's>0.05).

The dimensionality analysis was repeated on surrogate data of the original data set (Theiler $et\ al.$, 1992). For surrogate analysis, we took 25% of the finger tremor trials and transformed the raw data by randomly shuffling the acceleration values prior to recalculating the dimension estimate. With this strategy, the estimate of dimensionality never saturated over the 25 embedding dimensions and the average calculated dimension on the 25th embedding dimension for all trials was significantly larger than that derived from the original data set, $t(15)=7.75$, $p<0.05$.

The correlation between dimension and the variability of the acceleration signal was calculated within a group for each trial and finger condition. Table I shows the correlations averaged over trials as a function of the group and finger condition. All the correlations between dimension and acceleration variability were negative and statistically significant (p's<0.05). There was also a trend for the correlations to be higher in the tardive dyskinetic group than the normal control group, suggesting a stronger relation between dimension and variability in the tardive dyskinetic group.

It is difficult to obtain long duration time samples of the tremor time series in tardive dyskinetic subjects due to their inability to stay still or persevere at an experimental protocol. To examine if this limitation provides a significant influence to the estimate of the dimension, three normal subjects were tested in the same protocol as outlined above on 60 s trials. The dimension was calculated over the first 10, 20, 30, 40, 50, and 60 s of the trial. The dimension estimate was essentially uninfluenced by trial duration and the means for each of the subjects over each of the time sample calculations were between 10–11. These numbers are consistent with those reported earlier for the normal subjects in the 10 s trials. These tests provide an indication that the high dimension estimates in the main protocol are not driven significantly by the short duration trials.

IV. DISCUSSION

The data presented here provide additional evidence that the structure of the tremor dynamic is different between normal healthy adult individuals and age-matched tardive dyskinetic subjects. The dimension of the finger tremor time series was lower in the tardive dyskinesia group than the normal group. This finding was evident across both individual and combined finger tremor conditions, and is consistent with data reported previously for whole-body postural tremor (Newell $et\ al.$, 1993).

It appears that one consequence of the prolonged medication is the overconstraint on the degrees of freedom regulated in the motor system (Newell and McDonald, in press). This overconstraint is inversely related to the variability of the finger motion, as revealed by the correlational analysis of dimension and the standard deviation of the acceleration signal. The relation between dimensionality and variability is higher in the lower dimension attractor of the tardive dyskinetic group. The dimension of the time series does not fully predict its variability, but it apparently accounts for a significant portion of the acceleration variance. It would be useful to examine the change of the dimension and variability estimates over both drug addiction and withdrawal regimens. These kinds of tests are particularly necessary to determine if dynamic analyses, such as dimension, are useful (more sensitive) than traditional acceleration measures in a clinical setting.

The absolute estimates of the dimension of the finger acceleration signal are relatively high, and higher than those reported for whole-body postural motion (Newell $et\ al.$, 1993). These values could be due to the artifact of noise introduced into the experimental setup, the technique used for dimensionality estimates, or because they are a natural reflection of the actual organization of the motor system in solving the finger tremor task. The techniques for data collection used here were standard for postural finger tremor, and the signal to noise ratio was acceptably high. There are a number of limitations to current methods of estimating dimension in biological data (Rapp, Albano, and Mees, 1988; Theiler *et al.*, 1992), but under a number of approaches to measuring the dimension in the current data, the estimate is always essentially in the range reported, and the direction and statistical effect of the group difference always remains. Thus, the artifacts of experimental noise and the influence of the dimension measurement technique could contribute to the overall absolute estimate of dimension reported, but it seems doubtful that these extraneous contributions account for the majority of the variance to either the high numbers for dimension or in the relative group difference.

A postural finger tremor task is often considered as if it is a one degree of freedom motion, but this is not the case. All the degrees of freedom of the body are being coordinated and controlled in the attempt to minimize the degree of motion and the variability of the fingertip. It is worth noting that even the index finger has four degrees of freedom in joint space, without considering the potential contribution of other biokinematic linkages to the coordination problem. Furthermore, the mass of the index finger is relatively low in contrast to its connected other body parts, which increases the probability of reactive forces from the other relatively larger mass effector units, influencing the motion, and hence the dimensionality of the finger. Thus, the relatively high estimate of dimensionality may be due to the many degrees of freedom regulated in the commonly defined "simple" finger tremor task, with a skilled tremor performance actually having more independent degrees of freedom regulated than a nonskilled (Arutyunyan, Gurfinkel, and Mirskii, 1968, 1969; Bernstein, 1967; Newell and McDonald, 1994), or drug influenced performance. More direct tests of this degrees of freedom hypothesis for movement disorders need to be conducted. It should also be noted that the dimension analysis reveals that the variation in the normal finger acceleration signal is not without structure, and thus it is not entirely a reflection of noise—as it is often characterized (cf. Elble and Koller, 1990; Findley and Capildeo, 1984).

In summary, tardive dyskinesia finger tremor appears to exhibit a lower dimension than that of normal subjects in the organization of postural dynamics. The finger tremor findings reported here are consistent with this emerging theoretical position of the influence of neuroleptic medication on the degrees of freedom regulated in the coordination of posture (Newell, in press), although clearly more work is required that examines the postural dynamics over the *change* of the neuroleptic medication. Dynamical analysis could prove a useful diagnostic tool in the evaluation of tardive dyskinesia and the regulation of neuroleptic medication regimens.

ACKNOWLEDGMENTS

The preparation of this paper was supported by NIH Grant No. PHS 1 R01 HD21212 awarded to K. M. Newell. This project was completed with the assistance of many staff and clients at Lanterman Developmental Center, Pomona, CA. In particular, we would like to thank Dr. Donald Dean for his cooperation and interest in the project. Requests for reprints should be addressed to K. M. Newell, The Pennsylvania State University, 109 White Building, University Park, PA 16802.

Alpert, M., Diamond, F., and Friedhoff, A. J. (**1976**). "Tremorgraphic studies in tardive dyskinesia," Psychopharmacol. Bull. **12**, 5–7.

American Psychiatric Association Task Force on Tardive Dyskinesia (**1992**). "Tardive dyskinesia: A task force report of the American Psychiatric Association," Washington, DC (American Psychiatric Association).

Arutyunyan, G. H., Gurfinkel, V. S., and Mirskii, M. L. (**1968**). "Investigation of aiming at a target," Biophysics **13**, 536–538.

Arutyunyan, G. H., Gurfinkel, V. S., and Mirskii, M. L. (**1969**). "Organization of movements on execution by man of an exact postural task," Biophysics **14**, 1162–1167.

Bernstein, N. (**1967**). *The Co-ordination and Regulation of Movements* (Pergamon, Oxford).

Caligiuri, M., and Lohr, J. B. (**1990**). "Fine force instability: A quantitative measure of neuroleptic-induced dyskinesia in the hand," J. Neuropsychol. **2**, 395–398.

Elble, R. J., and Koller, W. C. (**1990**). *Tremor* (The Johns Hopkins University Press, Baltimore).

van Emmerik, R. E. A., Sprague, R. L., and Newell, K. M. (**1993**). "Finger tremor and tardive dyskinesia," Exp. Clin. Psychopharmacol. **1**, 259–268.

Findley, L. J., and Capildeo, R. (**1984**). *Movement Disorders: Tremor* (Oxford University Press, New York).

Fraser, A. M., and Swinney, H. L. (**1986**). "Independent coordinates for strange attractors from mutual information," Phys. Rev. A **33**, 1134–1140.

Grassberger, P., and Procaccia, I. (**1983**). "Measuring the strangeness of strange attractors," Physica D **9**, 189–208.

Hansen, T. E., Glazer, W. M., and Moore, D. C. (**1986**). "Tremor and tardive dyskinesia," J. Clin. Psychol. **47**, 461–464.

Jeste, D. V., and Wyatt, R. J. (**1982**). *Understanding and Treating Tardive Dyskinesia* (Guildford, New York).

Kalachnik, J. E. (**1984**). "Tardive dyskinesia and the mentally retarded: A review," in *Advances in Mental Retardation and Developmental Disabilities*, edited by S. B. Bruening (JAI, Greenwich, CT), Vol. 2, pp. 329–356.

Khot, V. Egan, M. F., Hyde, T. M., and Wyatt, R. J. (**1992**). "Neuroleptics and classic tardive dyskinesia," in *Drug-induced Movement Disorders*, edited by A. E. Lang and W. J. Weiner (Futura, Mt. Kisco, NY), pp. 121–166.

May, P. R. A. (**1987**). "Measurement of extrapyramidal symptoms and involuntary movement by electronic instruments," Psychopharmacol. Bull. **23**, 187–188.

Mayer-Kress, G. (**1986**). *Dimensions and Entropies in Chaotic Systems* (Springer-Verlag, New York).

Myklebust, J. B., and Myklebust, B. M. (**1989**). "Fractals in kinesiology," Abstract No. 243.2 at the Society for Neuroscience Meeting.

Nan, X., and Jinghua, X. (**1988**). "The fractal dimension of EEG as a physical measure of conscious human brain activities," Bull. Math. Biol. **50**, 559–565.

Newell, K. M. (in press). "The dynamics of tardive dyskinesia," in *Stereotypes: Brain–Behavior Relationships*, edited by R. L. Sprague and K. M. Newell (American Psychological Association, Washington, DC).

Newell, K. M., and McDonald, P. V. (**1994**). "Learning to coordinate redundant biomechanical degrees of freedom," in *Interlimb Coordination: Neural, Dynamical, and Cognitive Constraints*, edited by S. Swinnen, H. Heuer, J. Massion, and P. Casaer (Academic, New York), pp. 515–536.

Newell, K. M., van Emmerik, R. E. A., Lee, D., and Sprague, R. L. (**1993**). "On postural stability and variability," Gait Posture **4**, 225–230.

Packard, N. H., Crutchfield, J. P., Farmer, J. D., and Shaw, R. S. (**1980**). "Geometry from a time series," Phys. Rev. Lett. **45**, 712–716.

Rapp, P. E., Albano, A. M., and Mees, A. I. (**1988**). "Calculation of correlation dimension from experimental data: Progress and problems," in *Dynamic Patterns in Complex Systems*, edited by J. A. S. Kelso, A. J.

Mandel, and M. F. Schlesinger (World Scientific, Singapore), pp. 191–205.

Rondot, P., and Bathien, N. (**1986**). "Movement disorders in patients with coexistent neuroleptic-induced tremor and tardive dyskinesia: EMG and pharmacological study, in *Advances in Neurology*, edited by M. D. Yahr and K. J. Bergmann (Raven, New York), Vol. 45, pp. 361–366.

Sprague, R. L., and Kalachnik, J. E. (**1991**). "Reliability, validity, and a total score cutoff for the Dyskinesia Identification System: Condensed User Scale (DISCUS) with mentally ill and mentally retarded populations," Psychopharmacol. Bull. **27**, 51–58.

Sprague, R. L., and Newell, K. M. (**1987**). "Toward a movement control perspective of tardive dyskinesia," in *Psychopharmacology: The Third Generation of Progress*, edited by H. Y. Meltzer (Raven, New York).

Stacy, M., and Jankovic, J. (**1992**). "Tardive tremor," Movement Disorders **7**, 53–57.

Theiler, J., Galdrikian, B., Longtin, A., Eubank, S., and Farmer, J. D. (**1992**). "Using surrogate data to detect nonlinearity in time series," in *Nonlinear Modelling and Forecasting: SFI Studies in the Sciences of Complexity*, edited by M. Casdalgi and S. Eubank, Proceedings of Colloquium XII (Addison–Wesley, Reading, MA).

Tyron, W. W., and Pologe, B. (**1987**). "Accelerometric assessment of tardive dyskinesia," Am. J. Psychol. **144**, 1584–1587.

Tremor classification and tremor time series analysis

Günther Deuschl and Michael Lauk
Department of Neurology, University of Freiburg/Breisgau, Germany

Jens Timmer
Department of Physics, University of Freiburg/Breisgau, Germany

(Received 2 June 1994; accepted for publication 22 August 1994)

The separation between physiologic tremor (PT) in normal subjects and the pathological tremors of essential tremor (ET) or Parkinson's disease (PD) was investigated on the basis of monoaxial accelerometric recordings of 35 s hand tremor epochs. Frequency and amplitude were insufficient to separate between these conditions, except for the trivial distinction between normal and pathologic tremors that is already defined on the basis of amplitude. We found that waveform analysis revealed highly significant differences between normal and pathologic tremors, and, more importantly, among different forms of pathologic tremors. We found in our group of 25 patients with PT and 15 with ET a reasonable distinction with the third momentum and the time reversal invariance. A nearly complete distinction between these two conditions on the basis of the asymmetric decay of the autocorrelation function. We conclude that time series analysis can probably be developed into a powerful tool for the objective analysis of tremors. © *1995 American Institute of Physics.*

I. INTRODUCTION

Tremor with a small amplitude is accompanying normal posture and movement and is called physiologic tremor. It has been claimed that its function is to keep the motor system in an oscillating state in order to gate the timing of motor events.[1] The strongest evidence for this hypothesis comes from experiments demonstrating that voluntary movements start usually at the peak momentum of physiologic tremor.[2]

Movement disorders with involuntary, rhythmic oscillating movements of one or more functional regions of the body are commonly labeled as pathologic tremors. The distinction between pathologic and physiologic tremor is mainly on the basis of amplitude and frequency. The physiologic basis of pathologic tremors is far from being understood,[3] and it is likely that different mechanisms are mediating the various tremors seen in clinical neurology. A first mechanism is the mechanical oscillations of the hand/muscle system. A second mechanism may be upregulated or abnormal reflexes of the central nervous system maintaining abnormal oscillations. Third, central pacemakers may play an important role in pacing the motor output at a certain frequency. In a particular patient these mechanisms are probably interacting rather than excluding each other.

The distinction of the different tremors is based on some traditional clinical criteria, which reflect more than a century of clinical experience. The criteria are first the frequency of tremors separating into low-, middle-, and high-frequency tremors. Second, the motor task during which the tremor is manifesting is taken into account. It is separated into tremors during rest, posture or goal-directed movements. Finally, additional anamnestic data or clinical findings like symptoms of akinesia or rigidity in Parkinson's disease or a family history for tremor are helpful to separate the conditions.[3–6] These criteria are mostly good enough to separate the conditions. However, especially in the beginning of the diseases, significant errors may occur. For the two most frequent

pathologic tremors, Parkinson's disease and essential tremor, it has been estimated[7] that up to 20% are misdiagnosed during the first years of the disease.

Thus, objective measures and schemes of classification are wanted to overcome the diagnostic problems. Another reason to look for such quantitative measures is related to underlying mechanisms: Once objective criteria can be established, it can be expected that these differences may reflect meaningful physiologic differences, and may prompt new hypotheses, which can be tested with appropriate physiologic investigations. Our previous work[8,9] has shown that nonlinear deterministic models do only describe a small percentage of the real tremor curves and, therefore, the present approach was developed. We present evidence that tests analyzing the waveform characteristics of the accelerometer series of tremor are able to separate different forms of tremor.

II. SUBJECTS AND METHODS

A. Subjects

Fifty-two normal subjects with a mean age of 51 years (range: 22–83 yr), 62 patients with Parkinson's disease (mean age: 65, range: 35–84), and 42 patients with essential tremor (mean age: 57, range 22–87) underwent a standardized procedure of tremor recording. The diagnosis was made on the basis of clinical criteria. Any doubt or uncertainty with the diagnosis was an exclusion criterion.

B. Recording

The subjects were seated in a comfortable chair with both forearms supported by comfortable armmolds. A monoaxial accelerometer (50 mV/gravity) was fixed 9 cm distal to the ulnar epicondylus at the right hand. No movement was possible between the accelerometer and the finger. The subjects were asked to keep the hand outstretched. The accelerometer signals were digitized (300 Hz with a 12-bit resolution) and epochs of 10 240 data points corresponding to a time period of 35 s were stored on a computer for further analysis.[8,9]

C. Basic data analysis

The time series underwent Fourier analysis and appropriate smoothing was performed according to a frequency and amplitude-dependent algorithm.[9] The peak frequency of each spectrum and the total power between 1 and 30 Hz was determined.

D. Further data analysis

Additional tests were limited to unselected subgroups of 50 normal subjects; 25 patients with Parkinson's disease and 15 patients with essential tremor.

To exclude amplitude information, all the time series were normalized to have a variance of unity. The mean was set to zero. Three different mathematical transformations were applied, and specific numbers for each time series were extracted, which have been later used as classificators for the different time series.

Third momentum: The third momentum was calculated. Each point of the time series was taken at the third power, and all the obtained data points were added and divided by their number. This number was taken as the classificator.

Time reversal invariance: Second, a test was developed that is quantifying the invariance of the time series to reversal of the time direction ("time reversal invariance").[10] The difference of the conditional expectations forward and backward, was defined by

$$D_1 = E(x(t+\tau)|x(t)=y) - E(x(t-\tau)|x(t)=y),$$

$$D_1 = D_1(\tau, y).$$

Thus, the time reversal is a function of the lag τ and the value y,

$$D_2(\tau) = \int D_1(\tau, y)^2 \, dy,$$

where $D_2(\tau)$ is a measure of the mean deviation of the conditional expectations, $D_m = \max D_2(\tau)$, and D_m characterizes the maximal deviation of the conditional expectations.

The basic idea behind this test is that linear stochastic time series are invariant under time reversal, but nonlinear might not. This feature might, therefore, separate on the one hand tremors exhibiting nonlinear behavior from linear stochastic waveforms and on the other hand tremors showing different types of nonlinear behavior.

Asymmetric decay of the autocorrelation function: The autocorrelation function AF(h) of a linear damped oscillator with a frequency ω shows a typical (exponential) decay,

$$AF(h) = \cos \omega h \exp(-|h|/\tau),$$

with the decay time τ.

In the case of linear damped oscillations, the absolute values of the extrema of the autocorrelation function form a monotonous decreasing series. In the case of nonlinear oscillations, especially in a skewed time series, the absolute value of a minimum can be less than the next maximum [Figs. 4(A) and 4(B)]. Thus, we used the difference (diff_{1-2}) be-

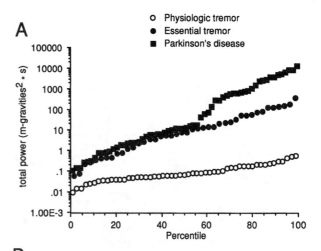

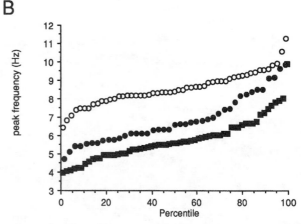

FIG. 1. Tremor amplitude (A) and frequency (B) in subjects with physiologic tremor, essential tremor, and Parkinson's disease. The data are displayed as cumulative percentage plots, indicating which percentage of each category of subjects exhibits the parameter under investigation above or below a certain value.

tween the absolute value of the first and the second extremum as a classification number for the time series.[10] In other words, this test is also testing asymmetries of the tremor curves.

III. RESULTS

Two questions are of interest for the present study. The first is whether the criteria defined with this approach separate between normal and pathologic tremors, and the second if they separate among the different pathologic tremors.

The amplitudes and frequencies of the controls and patients are displayed in Fig. 1. In this, as well as in all the other figures, the cumulative probability is compared for normals (PT), patients with essential tremor (ET), and patients with Parkinson's disease (PD), which allow us to decide if a criterium separates between the different groups. By definition, the patients amplitude [Fig. 1(A)] is larger than the one of the normals, except for those patients displaying only minimal tremor amplitudes during the postural task being investigated in this study or those with unilateral pathologic tremors at the healthy hand. Generally, this criterium separated 80% of the patients from the controls. The situation is

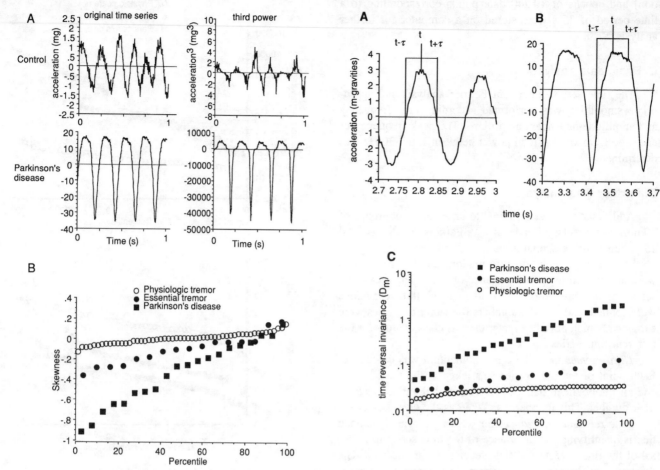

FIG. 2. Calculation of the third power of a time series illustrated for a physiologic tremor and tremor in Parkinson's disease (A). It is evident that asymmetries of the amplitude are accentuated by this test. (B) shows the cumulative percentage plot for the three tremor categories. The distinction between normal and pathologic tremor is reasonable, but between essential tremor and Parkinson's disease, the distinction is poor.

FIG. 3. Time reversal invariance as a test to separate different tremors. (A) and (B) are showing two tremor cycles with the values that are observed and calculated. Completely symmetric waveforms would show identical values for $(t+\tau)$ and $(t-\tau)$. The waveform in (A) shows a pretty good symmetry, whereas the one in (B) does not. Asymmetries of the waveform, as seen in (B), will give higher values when entering the mathematical equations of the time reversal (see Sec. II D) as the values for curves like in (A). This feature shows higher values for the patients with Parkinson's disease than for the normal subjects and the patients with essential tremor (C).

even worse when looking at the frequencies [Fig. 1(B)]. Only about 50% of the patients with ET and 70% of the patients with PD have a lower frequency than 6 Hz, which we found to be the lowest value of the normal controls. The discrimination between the two pathologic tremors is poor.

The further mathematic tests developed in this paper are dealing with the waveforms, rather than with frequency and amplitude characteristics of the tremors.

The most simple approach was to calculate the third power of every point of the time series. This is shown in Fig. 2(A) for a time series of subjects with PT and PD, respectively. It is evident that this test is separating only 30% of the ET and 70% of the PD patients from PT [Fig. 2(B)], and that the separation between ET and PD is less than 50%.

The time reversal invariance is explained in Figs. 3(A) and 3(B) (see also Sec. II D). The critical feature is the asymmetry of the waveform with respect to the inversion of time. Figure 3(C) shows the resulting discrimination. The distinction between PT and ET is poor, but ET and PD are separated already at a percentage of 75%.

The decay of the autocorrelation function may express

the asymmetries of a tremor time series. The feature that we calculated is simply the difference between the absolute values of the first and the second extremum of the autocorrelation function, as shown in Figs. 4(A) and 4(B). Figure 4(C) shows the resulting discrimination. This test does not separate between PT and ET, but it is almost separating 95% of the ET from PD for the analyzed cases.

IV. DISCUSSION

The use of a time series analysis for the distinction of different tremors is a new field of application for these mathematical tools, and has been used, hitherto, only in limited number of studies.[10-12] Nevertheless, this first approach already shows a number of features that could eventually be used in future experiments.

The basic idea of our application of time series analysis is to extract features from the time series that reflect the different dynamical properties of the various types of tremor.

The message of the present paper is that the three major groups of tremor assessed with the present study differ in

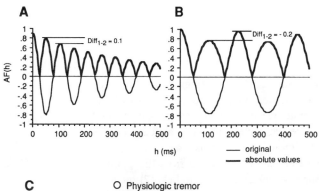

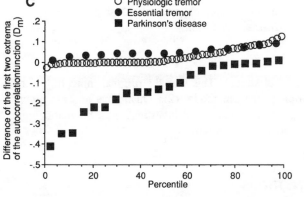

FIG. 4. Asymmetries of the autocorrelation function as a test for differences between time series. The first few cycles of two typical autocorrelation functions of a normal subject (A) and a patient with Parkinson's disease (B) are shown as thin lines. The thick lines display their absolute values. The maxima form a monoton decreasing series in the normal subject, whereas they show alternating high and low values in the patient. The absolute values of the first two extrema are subtracted (D_{1-2}) and taken as a classification value. This is displayed for all the subjects in (C). The patients with Parkinson's disease have smaller values than the normals and essential tremor subjects.

various dimensions from each other: For the separation of pathologic and normal tremor, the amplitude will be sufficient in most cases. The separation among different pathologic tremors, however, is not possible, on the basis of frequency or amplitude criteria of tremors. In this case, the waveforms seem to be helpful to separate the different pathologic conditions. The applied classificators are relatively simple and straightforward tools for assessing asymmetry of time series. This is the result of our recent approaches to classify tremor with different tests. Tests for linearity were helpful in separating physiologic and pathologic tremors,[12] as well as measures of the third moments and the peakedness.[10] The tests being able to separate between PD and ET tremor curves seem all to reflect asymmetries of the tremor curves: For the third momentum, this is mostly the asymmetry of the time series, with respect to a change of the

sign of each value of the time series. For the time reversal invariance, this is the asymmetry with respect to a change of the direction of time, and for the decay of the autocorrelation function both asymmetries play a role.

The tests operating in the time domain proved to be helpful especially for the distinction between ET and PD. This is the most relevant clinical question, as the separation of these two tremors may be difficult in a particular patient. The result of a nearly complete separation of a PD tremor time series from ET is surprising, and may be due to the selection of typical examples. It obviously requires further confirmation in a larger prospective series of patients.

At present, it seems interesting that it is possible to make reasonably good judgements about diagnostic categories of tremor on the basis of 35 s records of the waveform. This is hope toward an identification of the features that experienced movement disorder clinicians use to subclassify tremors just by looking at the trembling extremity. It is most likely the nonlinear behavior of the rhythmic hand movement that is causing both the clinical impression of Parkinson-like trembling and the quantitative features separating PD tremor from the other ones tested with the present series. This will be investigated with EMG/tremor correlation's in a larger group of patients in the future.

ACKNOWLEDGMENT

The work was supported by the Deutsche Forschungsgemeinschaft (SFB 325).

[1] A. T. Winfree, *The Geometry of Biological Time* (Springer-Verlag, New York, 1980).

[2] D. Goodman and J. A. Kelso, "Exploring the functional significance of physiological tremor: A biospectroscopic approach," Exp. Brain Res. **49**, 419–431 (1983).

[3] R. J. Elble and W. C. Koller, *Tremor* (The Johns Hopkins University Press, Baltimore, 1990).

[4] G. Deuschl, "Tremor–Aktueller Stand in Forschung und Klinik," in *Jahrbuch der Neurologie 1994/95*, edited C. E. Elger and R. Dengler (Biermann-Verlag, Zülpich, 1994).

[5] L. J. Findley and R. Capildeo, *Movement Disorders: Tremor* (MacMillan, London, 1984).

[6] W. C. Koller, K. Busenbark, C. Gray, R. S. Hassanein, and R. Dubinsky, "Classification of essential tremor," Clinical Neuropharmacol. **15**, 81–87 (1992).

[7] L. J. Findley and W. C. Koller, "Essential tremor: a review," Neurology **37**, 1194–1197 (1987).

[8] G. Deuschl, H. Blumberg, and C. H. Lücking, "Tremor in reflex sympathetic dystrophy," Arch. Neurol. **48**, 1247–1252 (1991).

[9] J. Timmer, M. Lauk, and G. Deuschl, "Quantitative analysis of tremor time series" (in preparation).

[10] J. Timmer, C. Gantert, G. Deuschl, and J. Honerkamp, "Characteristics of hand tremor time series," Biol. Cybernet. **70**, 75–80 (1993).

[11] G. Mayer-Kress, F. E. Yates, L. Benton, M. Keidel, W. Tirsch, S. J. Pöppl and K. Geist, "Dimensional analysis of nonlinear oscillations in brain, heart and muscle," Math. Biosci. **90**, 155–182 (1988).

[12] C. Gantert, J. Honerkamp, nd J. Timmer, "Analyzing the dynamics of hand tremor time series," Biol. Cybernet. **66**, 479–484 (1992).

Variations on tremor parameters

A. Boose, Ch. Jentgens, S. Spieker, and J. Dichgans
University of Tübingen, Department of Neurology, Hoppe-Seyler-Str. 3, 72076 Tübingen, Germany

(Received 25 May 1994; accepted for publication 22 August 1994)

This paper describes our analysis procedure for long-term tremor EMG recordings, as well as three examples of applications. The description of the method focuses on how characteristics of the tremor (e.g. frequency, intensity, agonist–antagonist interaction) can be defined and calculated based on surface EMG data. The resulting quantitative characteristics are called "tremor parameters." We discuss sinusoidally modulated, band-limited white noise as a model for pathological tremor-EMG, and show how the basic parameters can be extracted from this class of signals. The method is then applied to (1) estimate tremor severity in clinical studies, (2) quantify agonist–antagonist interaction, and (3) investigate the variations of the tremor parameters using simple methods from time-series analysis. © *1995 American Institute of Physics.*

I. INTRODUCTION

Tremor is a potentially disabling sign that appears in several neurological diseases including Parkinson's disease and essential tremor. It is defined as involuntary, roughly periodic oscillation of a limb, the head or any other part of the body. For more than a century instrumental methods have been used to precisely quantify tremor, both for pathophysiological and pharmacological studies and to monitor patient therapy. Instrumental methods can also be used in diagnosis, to distinguish between clinically similar diseases.

The methods used range from a 19th-Century technique, where a tambour was applied to the limb under study, transferring its displacement to a mechanical lever which wrote a permanent record on a smoked rotating drum,[1] to the use of modern laser equipment.[2] Other approaches include accelerometry with piezoresistive devices, displacement transducers using potentiometers, force transducers, and the recording of muscle activity via EMG.

Usually these techniques are applied in the laboratory for recording durations not longer than several minutes. When used in this manner, they share the weakness that they do not take into account the variability of tremor, making use of only a short portion of a strongly varying time-series. We have therefore developed a *long-term* recording method where the EMGs of wrist extensors and flexors are recorded by a portable tape recorder for up to 24 hours. As most pathological tremors are markedly influenced by anxiety, our method has the additional advantage that patients are free to move in their everyday environment and maintain their daily activities, giving us access to the tremor as it is in the absence of physicians and exciting laboratory equipment. One reason for using EMG rather than e.g. accelerometry is that the inconvenience to the patient is minimal, as nothing has to be attached to the hands and the recording equipment can be hidden under a shirt or a jacket. Another advantage is that the EMG is a direct measure of the pathological muscle activity.

In this paper we first describe our recording method and the model "sinusoidally modulated band-limited white noise" which is the basis for the definition of our "tremor parameters." We then give three examples of applications: (1) The use of long-term averages of the tremor parameters

in clinical studies. This was the original motivation for developing the method. (2) Quantification of agonist–antagonist interaction. (3) Investigation of fluctuations in the properties of the tremor.

II. METHODS

A. Band-limited white noise: A model for surface EMG

The surface EMG signal is the sum of many action potentials which travel along the muscle fibers. As in most cases the action potentials occur independently, the resulting signal is approximately normally distributed (central limit theorem). Because of the frequency content of the single action potentials and the low-pass filtering effect of skin and fat tissues normal surface EMGs are confined to a frequency range of approximately 50 to 300 Hz. One can therefore model raw EMG as band-limited white noise.[3–5]

B. Demodulation: Estimation of the variance

The information about the state of activity of the muscle must be encoded in the only parameter that this model allows for, the variance or the standard deviation of the EMG. Different terms have been used in the literature, contraction level or activity level being two of them. So we have

$$x(t) = c(t) \cdot n(t) , \qquad (1)$$

where $x(t)$ is the EMG signal, $n(t)$ is band-limited white noise with unit variance and $c(t)$ the contraction level. The muscle force is an increasing function of $c(t)$. Countless attempts have been made to determine this force-EMG relationship, the majority favoring a nonlinear relationship. In order to determine the contraction level $c(t)$ for a given EMG recording—i.e. to *demodulate* it—let us assume that c varies slowly compared to the noise, so that it may be estimated from an approximately stationary interval. Assume further that we have N independent samples $x_i, i=1,..,N$ from such an interval, then the maximum-likelihood-estimate is[4]

$$\hat{c} = \left(\frac{1}{N} \sum_{i=1}^{N} x_i^2 \right)^{1/2}. \tag{2}$$

Note that the independence of the samples is violated if the sampling rate is too high. In practical terms, sampling faster than 500 Hz will not increase the quality of the estimate. Sampling with a lower rate will usually lead to an increase in the variance of the estimate, because the duration of the stationary intervals is limited. However, lower sampling rates do not affect the expectation of this estimate.

Most commonly the demodulation of surface EMG is accomplished by first rectifying and then smoothing the signal. Although this procedure has the advantage of being the simplest one, the estimate has a higher variance than the estimate (2), which has been shown to be optimal in this respect.[4]

C. Sinusoidally modulated white noise: A model for *tremor* EMG

If we now assume sinusoidal modulation[5]

$$x(t) = n(t) \cdot (1 + M \sin(2\pi f t)), \tag{3}$$

the power-spectrum of the demodulated signal can be calculated.[5] It consists of three components: First, there is a nearly constant component resulting from the noise. Second, we find delta peaks at the modulation frequency as the rectification or squaring introduces a periodically fluctuating mean. In general, if the modulating function is not perfectly sinusoidal or if rectification is used instead of squaring, one should also expect harmonic peaks at integer multiples of this frequency. Third, there is a delta peak at zero frequency because the mean of the signal is not zero. The ratio of the power in the peak at the modulating frequency and the power per unit frequency contained in the noise is called "signal-to-noise ratio." This quantity, which can be estimated directly from the estimate of the spectrum,[3] is monotonically (roughly quadratically) related to the modulation depth M.

D. Recording method

The recording procedure has been described by Bacher *et al.*[3] Briefly, the EMG signal is recorded with surface electrodes placed over the extensor carpi radialis and flexor carpi ulnaris muscles of both forearms. We use a portable (walkman-sized) analog tape recorder with a maximum recording duration of 24 hours. The frequency is limited to $\leqslant 100$ Hz because of the tape velocity. We therefore sample the signal at 200 Hz. This may appear to be relatively low, but this limitation affects only the variance, not the expectation of the contraction level estimate. Afterwards we store the data on a PC where low-frequency motion artifacts are detected and removed.

E. Tremor parameters

The tremor parameters are the parameters that emerge from this model of tremor-EMG. We extract them on the basis of a spectral analysis of 15-second intervals, that are assumed to be approximately stationary. The analysis is per-

formed by standard techniques (see e.g. Bendat and Piersol[6]) on contiguous (nonoverlapping) intervals. For the present data we analyzed 10 hours of the waking time as most pathological tremors vanish during sleep. The **tremor frequency** is the frequency of the modulating sine wave. It is estimated by looking for the highest peak in the estimate of the spectrum. The **signal-to-noise ratio** (SNR) is defined above. It can be used as a measure of tremor intensity. A decision, whether there is **tremor** or not, can be considered as third tremor parameter: If the SNR is small (we use a cutoff of 4.0), or the frequency is not in a reasonable range for tremor, this indicates that the model is not adequate for the data. We assume that in these intervals there was no tremor present. Thus the parameter "tremor" can take two values: Yes and No, or 1 and 0, respectively. It therefore has to be either smoothed or averaged, yielding a local or a global estimate, respectively, of the "tremor occurrence rate."

F. Cross-spectral analysis

Additional tremor parameters that describe agonist-antagonist interaction can be derived using cross-spectral analysis: For two stochastic processes $x(t)$ and $y(t)$ with Fourier transforms $X(f)$ and $Y(f)$ the power spectral densities are

$$G_{xx}(f) = \frac{2}{T} E[X^*(f)X(f)],$$

$$G_{yy}(f) = \frac{2}{T} E[Y^*(f)Y(f)], \tag{4}$$

and the cross-spectral density function of x and y is given by

$$G_{xy}(f) = \frac{2}{T} E[X^*(f)Y(f)]. \tag{5}$$

This complex quantity is common in linear systems analysis where it is used to describe the transmission characteristics between an input signal $x(t)$ and the corresponding output $y(t)$. The phase of $G_{xy}(f)$ is called phase spectrum and denoted $\theta_{xy}(f)$. It can be thought of as phase lag between the individual frequency components of x and y.

In addition to the phase we are interested in the *coherency spectrum* $\gamma_{xy}^2(f)$, which is defined as

$$\gamma_{xy}^2(f) = \frac{|G_{xy}(f)|^2}{G_{xx}(f)G_{yy}(f)}. \tag{6}$$

This coherency function measures the extent to which $y(t)$ may be predicted from $x(t)$ by an optimum linear least squares relationship.[6] It can be thought of as a conventional linear correlation coefficient for each frequency component.

Assuming that the cross-spectrum is estimated by averaging n_d independent pieces of data, then the variance of the estimate of the phase spectrum is[6]

$$\text{var}(\hat{\theta}_{xy}(f)) = \frac{1 - \gamma_{xy}^2(f)}{2 n_d \gamma_{xy}^2(f)}. \tag{7}$$

In order to apply this to the problem of agonist-antagonist interaction we calculate the cross-spectra of the demodulated extensor and flexor signals. If there is tremor in

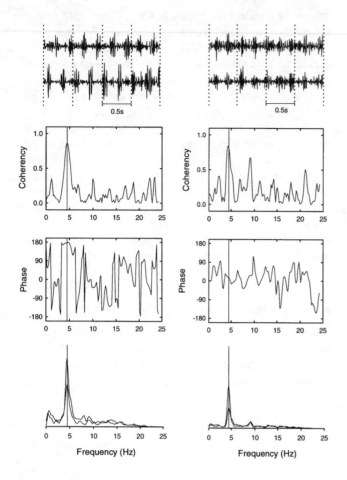

CHAOS, Vol. 5, No. 1, 1995

III. LONG-TERM AVERAGES AS TOOLS FOR CLINICAL STUDIES

The basic idea of our method is that the tremor occurrence rate and the averages of frequency and intensity (SNR) are better suited for clinical studies than frequency and amplitude values obtained from short measurements. This issue has been quantitatively investigated.

In a repeated measurements study we have shown the reliability of these quantities. Twelve patients with essential tremor and 13 Parkinsonian patients were recorded on three consecutive days. The intraclass correlation coefficients are excellent for each of the parameters.[7] Corresponding results concerning short-term mesurements are not known in the literature.

From this clinical point of view, "tremor" is the most important parameter, as the "tremor occurrence rate," i.e. the percentage of intervals that contain tremor is well correlated with the patients subjective impression of tremor severity.[8]

With the percentage of tremor and the average SNR as test quantities we performed an open study of the tremorlytic activity of budipine, an NMDA-antagonist that is believed to relieve Parkinsonian tremor. Most patients in our study showed a marked reduction in both the average SNR and the percentage of intervals that contain tremor.[9] This study is currently being repeated in a double-blind, multicentric fashion.

IV. AGONIST–ANTAGONIST INTERACTION

Pathological tremors are characterized not only by their frequency and intensity, but also by the interaction of antagonistic muscles that are involved in the tremor. In Parkinsonian tremor extensors and flexors usually are activated alternatingly, whereas in essential tremor simultaneous contraction is more common. Some patients with essential tremor, however, show the alternating pattern, and it is controversial, whether essential tremor can be subdivided by this criterion.[10–12]

We have derived a quantitative expression for these "alternating" versus "simultaneous" behaviors using cross-spectral analysis.[13] With this approach we were able to contribute new information to this discussion. It is not only possible to check, whether a patient changes patterns at some time of the day, we can also quantitatively assess which patterns occur how often.

In Fig. 2 phase values of two patients with essential tremor are shown. The first patient shows both the alternating and the simultaneous patterns. The dynamics seems to consist of a discrete background process, which switches between the patterns and noisy fluctuations in the phase values. The second patient shows no significant amount of alternating activity, but mostly simultaneous activity and some activity at −50 degrees. In both panels one observes some points loosely scattered over the whole phase range. These can easily be explained, as the tails of the phase distributions are "wrapped" around the circle, so that, given a certain interaction pattern there is a nonzero probability for any of the "false" phase values to be obtained.

FIG. 1. Cross-spectral analysis procedure illustrated for two intervals from one recording of a patient with essential tremor. Left column: An interval where alternating activity occurs. Right column: Simultaneous contraction. Top row: Raw-EMG of extensor (upper trace) and flexor. Second row: Coherency spectra. Third row: Phase spectra. Bottom row: Autospectra. The vertical line indicates the tremor frequency, where the phase is read from the phase spectrum. On the left, the coherency is higher than 0.6 and the phase is near 180°, indicating significantly alternating activity, which is in accordance with the visual impression. On the right the coherency is also sufficient, and now the phase value is near 0°, indicating simultaneous contraction, again in accordance with the visual impression. The autospectra and the coherency spectra show a harmonic peak at roughly 8 Hz.

one of the signals, the tremor frequency is determined and the coherency at this frequency is evaluated. If the coherency lies below a certain limit, it is likely that the two signals are sufficiently uncorrelated to make the phase conceptually meaningless. In addition, the random error of the phase will increase with falling coherency according to (7). In our experimental setup we chose a lower bound of 0.6 for the coherency, corresponding to a standard deviation of roughly 20 degrees.

If the coherency is higher than this value, the phase is a valid indicator of the temporal relationship of extensor and flexor bursts; e.g. a value near +/−180° indicates alternating activity and a value near zero indicates simultaneous contraction. This is exemplified in Fig. 1, where we compare two intervals from one long-term recording of a patient with essential tremor.

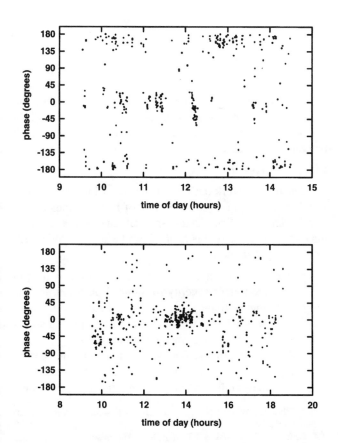

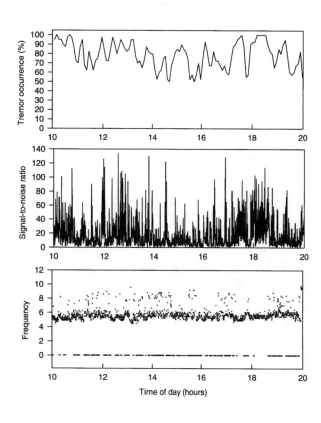

FIG. 2. Phase values of two patients with essential tremor. The patient above shows both the alternating and the simultaneous patterns, the other patient shows simultaneous activity and some activity near −50°.

FIG. 3. Tremor parameter time series from a patient with Parkinson's disease. Top panel: The parameter "Tremor" averaged over 10-minute intervals that overlap 5 minutes. Middle panel: SNR values of all intervals. Bottom panel: Frequency values of the intervals where tremor was detected. In the other intervals the frequency has been set to zero.

An important conclusion can be drawn from the results in Figs. 1 and 2: If different interaction modes occur in the same patient—a result which is in agreement with earlier observations based on short recordings[1,14,15]—then essential tremor cannot be subdivided into two groups by this criterion.

V. VARIATIONS OF TREMOR PARAMETERS

Although the long-term recording method was originally designed to obtain more reliable quantities by averaging the tremor parameters, we now use its unique potential for revealing their time-dependence. All patients with Parkinsonian tremor (PT) or essential tremor (ET) show a marked variability in all of the tremor parameters, particularly in "tremor" and in "SNR." Even in patients with only 10% total occurrence of tremor there are 10-minute intervals where 70% of the 15-second intervals contain tremor. Figure 3 shows examples of time-series plots of the tremor parameters. The time series of "tremor" was averaged over 10-minute intervals that overlapped 5 minutes. In this patient the parameter "frequency" fluctuates around 5–6 Hz, but sometimes we observe a frequency near 8 Hz.

This section will concentrate on the parameter "tremor," which is clinically most important. The plots in Fig. 4 show different phenomena we observed in analyzing recordings from 13 patients with PT and 12 patients with ET.

In Parkinsonian patients with little tremor the tremor activity appears to be grouped. Especially in the early afternoon, but also in the morning and in the evening, there are peaks in the "tremor occurrence rate" [cf. Fig. 4(A)]. In Parkinsonian patients with more severe tremor as well as in ET patients this grouping does not appear.

In both patient groups (in 8 patients with PT and in 10 with ET) there are longer periods (15 minutes to 1.5 hours) where there is no tremor present. [cf. Fig. 4(B)]. The average duration of these intervals is 30 minutes in ET and 45 minutes in PT. Some of the recordings show a prominent periodic behavior [cf. Fig. 4(C)]. However, these oscillations were not reproduced in repeated recordings of the same patient.

In 4 patients with PT and in 5 patients with ET we observed a slow, steady increase or decrease in tremor occurrence, lasting for more than three hours [cf. Figs. 4(D) and 4(E)]. Sudden changes, i.e. immediate transitions from phases with much tremor to phases with few tremor or vice versa can also be observed [cf. Figs. 4(D) and 4(E)]. Generally, the time series look "noisy" and their spectra appear to be very broadband, indicating that the parameters fluctuate on many different time scales.

From the variability of the present data we can again conclude that extracting tremor parameters from short-term measurements is likely to give random results. The peaks in the tremor occurrence in PT patients with mild tremor are

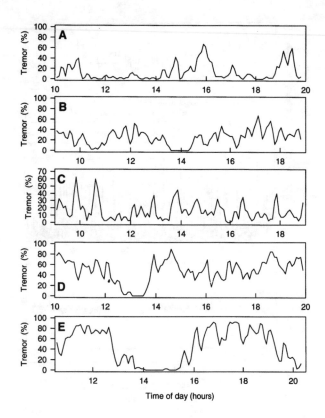

FIG. 4. The parameter "Tremor" averaged over 10-minute intervals that overlap 5 min. (A) This patient shows three peaks of tremor activity, which were reproducible in repeated recordings. (B) This patient shows a period without tremor near 2 p.m. (C) In this recording there seems to be periodic activity at roughly 1/hour. (D) This is an example of a slow, gradual decrease in tremor occurrence from 80% at 10 a.m. to zero at 1 p.m. Then a sudden jump back to 80% occurs. (E) This patient shows a downwards jump as well as a slow increase and a slow decrease in the evening.

probably related to resting phases. From clinical observation it is known, that PT is in most cases a "resting tremor," suppressed by voluntary muscle activity. This corresponds well to our observation that in the periods with more tremor there are fewer motion artifacts. In a minority of patients with PT, however, a "postural tremor," which appears during voluntary activity, occurs in addition to the resting tremor. This is the most probable explanation for the "frequency" behavior in Fig. 3: In those periods where the patient maintains a posture, the postural tremor—which has a higher frequency—appears, but the resting tremor at 5–6 Hz is suppressed.

The periods without tremor in ET can be explained as resting phases, because ET is known to be a postural tremor. Correspondingly, we observe fewer motion artifacts in these time intervals. In PT, phases without tremor might be due either to increased voluntary activity or to sleep.

Because in our setup the patients are free to live in their usual surroundings, there are many factors that can influence the tremor. From clinical observation we know, for example, that mental excitement can increase tremor amplitude by almost an order of magnitude. On the other hand, postural

tremors in particular are very sensitive to changes in hand position. These and similar effects may account for many of the peaks and dips we observed.

Thus, although we are still far from completely understanding the dynamics of tremor, our method seems to be an important contribution to this end: It is the first method that provides a quantitative view of the diurnal variations of the characteristics of human hand tremor, and this view seems to be consistent with what we know from clinical experience.

VI. CONCLUSION

The present work outlines the basics of long-term tremor EMG recording, gives an overview of how "tremor parameters" can be defined using spectral analysis, and shows three examples where this method can be applied giving new insights about tremor.

- Averaged tremor parameters can be used to reliably estimate tremor severity for clinical purposes.
- Defining a tremor parameter "phase" from cross-spectral analysis, we obtain a new approach to the problem of agonist–antagonist interaction.
- An analysis of the fluctuations in the tremor parameters reveals a very complex behavior, that is, insofar it is analyzable, consistent with clinical observation.

[1] R. J. Elble and W. C. Koller, *Tremor* (Johns Hopkins University Press, Baltimore, 1990)
[2] A. Beuter and K. Vasilakos, "Tremor: Is Parkinson's disease a dynamical disease," Chaos **5**, 35–42 (1995).
[3] M. Bacher, E. Scholz, and H. C. Diener, 24-hour continuous tremor quantification based on EMG recording," Electroencephalogr. Clin. Neurophysiol. **72**, 176–183 (1989).
[4] N. Hogan and R. W. Mann, "Myoelectric signal processing: Optimal estimation applied to EMG: Part I, derivation," IEEE Trans. Biomed. Eng. **27**, 382–395 (1980).
[5] H. L. Journée, "Demodulation of amplitude modulated noise: A mathematical evaluation of a demodulator for pathological tremor EMG's," IEEE Trans. Biomed. Eng. **30**, 304–308 (1983).
[6] J. S. Bendat and A. G. Piersol, *Random Data: Analysis and Measurement Procedures* (Wiley, New York, 1986).
[7] S. Spieker, C. Jentgens, A. Boose, and J. Dichgans, "Reliability and specifity of long-term tremor recordings," New Trends Clin. Neuropharmacol. **VIII**, 140 (1994).
[8] A. Boose, S. Spieker, Ch. Jentgens, T. Klockgether, E. Scholz, and J. Dichgans, "Assessing tremor severity with long-term tremor recordings," J. Neurol. Neurosurg. Psychiatry **57**, 397 (1994).
[9] S. Spieker, E. Scholz, M. Bacher, and J. Dichgans, "Long-term measurement of tremor," edited by A. D. Korczyn, P. H. Kraus, and H. Przuntek, in *Instrumental Methods and Scoring in Diagnosis and Quantification of Extrapyramidal Disorders* (Springer-Verlag, Berlin, 1994).
[10] G. Deuschl, C. H. Lücking, and E. Schenk, "Essential tremor: Electrophysiological and pharmacological evidence for a subdivision," J. Neurol. Neurosurg. Psychiatry **50**, 1435–1441 (1987).
[11] A. F. Sabra and M. Hallett, "Action tremor with alternating activity in antagonist muscles," Neurology **34**, 151–156 (1984).
[12] W. C. Koller, K. Busenbark, C. Gray, R. S. Hassanein, and R. Dubinsky, "Classification of essential tremor," Clin. Neuropharmacol. **15**, 81–87 (1992).
[13] A. Boose, S. Spieker, Ch. Jentgens, and J. Dichgans, "Long-term monitoring of agonist-antagonist interaction in pathological tremors," New Trends Clin. Neuropharmacol. **VIII**, 69 (1994).
[14] T. A. Larsen and D. B. Calne, "Review: Essential tremor," Clin. Neuropharmacol. **6**, 185–206 (1983).
[15] R. J. Elble, "Physiologic and essential tremor," Neurology **36**, 225–231 (1986).

Upright, correlated random walks: A statistical-biomechanics approach to the human postural control system

J. J. Collins and C. J. De Luca
NeuroMuscular Research Center and Department of Biomedical Engineering, Boston University,
44 Cummington St., Boston, Massachusetts 02215

(Received 24 May 1994; accepted for publication 2 August 1994)

The task of maintaining erect stance involves a complex sensorimotor control system, the output of which can be highly irregular. Even when a healthy individual attempts to stand still, the center of gravity of his or her body and the center of pressure (COP) under his or her feet continually move about in an erratic fashion. In this study, we approach the problem of characterizing postural sway from the perspective of random-walk theory. Specifically, we analyze COP trajectories as one-dimensional and two-dimensional random walks. These analyses reveal that over short-term intervals of time during undisturbed stance the COP behaves as a positively correlated random walk, whereas over long-term intervals of time it resembles a negatively correlated random walk. We interpret this novel finding as an indication that during quiet standing the postural control system utilizes open-loop and closed-loop control schemes over short-term and long-term intervals, respectively. From this perspective, our approach, known as stabilogram-diffusion analysis, has the advantage that it leads to the extraction of COP parameters which can be directly related to the steady-state behavior and functional interaction of the neuromuscular mechanisms underlying the maintenance of erect stance. © *1995 American Institute of Physics.*

I. INTRODUCTION

Upright stance is regulated by a complex control system that involves a number of different sensory systems, i.e., the visual, vestibular, and somatosensory systems. The net output of this control system can be highly irregular. For example, during quiet standing, the center of pressure (COP) under an individual's feet continually moves about in an erratic fashion. A plot of the time-varying coordinates of the COP is known as a stabilogram (Fig. 1). For several decades, researchers have studied the human postural control system by using force platforms to measure quiet-standing COP trajectories (Fig. 1). To date, however, the motor control insights gained from static posturography have been meager. This is due largely to the fact that, in most cases,[1-4] the analyses of the posturographic data have been limited to summary statistics, e.g., sway path length, average radial area, etc., which, in general, cannot be interpreted in a physiologically meaningful way. This situation is confounded by the fact that the COP is a measure of whole-body dynamics, and thereby represents the summed effect of a number of different neuromusculoskeletal components acting at a number of different joints. As a consequence of these factors, the utility of static posturography in the laboratory and clinic has been severely limited. Thus, there is a clear need to develop a reliable approach for extracting physiologically meaningful information from stabilograms.

We approach the problem of characterizing COP trajectories from a different perspective, namely, that of random-walk theory. In particular, we hypothesize that the output of the human postural control system under quiet-standing conditions can be modeled as a system of bounded, correlated random walks. Our approach, which is called *stabilogram-diffusion analysis*, is based on the assumption that the postural control system involves both deterministic and stochas-

tic components. One of our aims for this work is to develop a modeling framework that can be used to formulate and test hypotheses concerning the relative contributions of different sensorimotor subsystems and strategies to "quasistatic" postural control. Accordingly, in the present paper, we show that stabilogram-diffusion analysis leads to a series of COP parameters that can be directly related to the resultant steady-state behavior and functional interaction of the neuromuscular mechanisms underlying the maintenance of undisturbed stance. In this paper we review some of the main findings of our earlier studies.[5,6] A more complete description of stabilogram-diffusion analysis and our interpretation of its associated parameters can be found in Collins and De Luca.[5]

II. METHODS

A. Experimental methods

Ten healthy subjects—five males and five females—of similar age (19–24 yr, mean: 22±2 yr), height 1.60–1.80 m, mean: 1.69±0.08 m), and body weight (54.5–77.1 kg, mean: 64.3±8.4 kg) were included in the study. The subjects had no evidence or known history of a gait, postural, or skeletal disorder. Informed consent was obtained for each subject prior to participation, after the nature and possible consequences of the studies were explained. Postural sway was evaluated by using a Kistler 9287 multicomponent force platform and signal conditioner to collect COP trajectories under a subject's feet. Each subject was instructed to stand in an upright posture in a standardized stance on the platform. In the standardized stance, the subject's feet were abducted 10° and their heels were separated mediolaterally by a distance of 6 cm. During the testing, the subjects stood barefoot with their arms comfortably at their sides and their eyes open and fixed on a point in front of them. A series of five 90 s

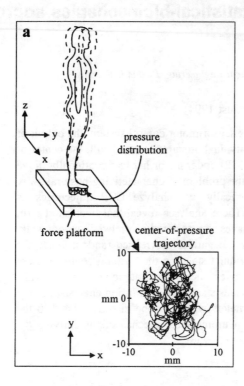

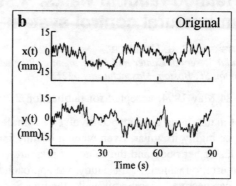

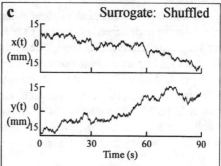

FIG. 1. (a) A schematic diagram of the experimental setup for examining quiet-standing postural stability. Shown also is a typical 90 s stabilogram for a healthy young individual. (b) The x-coordinate and y-coordinate time series corresponding to the stabilogram in (a). (c) Shuffled surrogate random-walk data sets that were generated from the original COP time series in (b).

trials was conducted for each subject. Rest periods of 2 min were provided between each trial. The COP signals were anti-aliased using a second-order lowpass filter (with a cutoff frequency of 34.1 Hz), and subsequently sampled at a rate of 100 Hz. The time series were then downsampled to a rate of 50 Hz, and the mean was subtracted from each time series to give an average COP position of (0,0).

B. Data analysis: Random-walk approach

The COP trajectories were studied as one-dimensional and two-dimensional random walks. In a classical random walk or, more generally, ordinary Brownian motion, past increments in displacement are uncorrelated with future increments, i.e., the system has no memory. In such cases, the mean square displacement of a random walker is linearly related to the time interval Δt by the general expression[7]

$$\langle \Delta j^2 \rangle = 2D_j\,\Delta t, \tag{1}$$

where $\langle \Delta j^2 \rangle$ is mean square displacement, D_j is the diffusion coefficient, and $j = x, y, r$. (In the present paper, x, y, and r denote mediolateral, anteroposterior, and planar displacements and measures, respectively.) In words, the diffusion coefficient is an average measure of the stochastic activity of a random walker, i.e., it is directly related to its jump frequency and/or amplitude.

In a correlated random walk or, more generally, fractional Brownian motion,[8] past increments in displacement

are correlated with future increments, i.e., the system has memory. In such cases, the relation given by Eq. (1) is generalized to the following scaling law:

$$\langle \Delta j^2 \rangle \sim \Delta t^{2H_j}, \tag{2}$$

where H_j is the scaling exponent, which can be any real number in the range $0 < H_j < 1$. Scaling exponents quantify the correlation between the step increments making up the trajectory of a random walker. This is best illustrated by considering the correlation function C for fractional Brownian motion, which is given by the expression[9]

$$C = 2(2^{2H_j - 1} - 1).$$

Note that for $H_j = 0.5$, the increments in displacement are statistically independent, i.e., $C = 0$. This is the result expected for classical Brownian motion. For $H_j > 0.5$, past and future increments are positively correlated, i.e., $C > 0$. In this case, a random walker moving in a particular direction for some t_0 will tend to continue in the same direction for $t > t_0$. In general, an increasing (decreasing) trend in the past implies an increasing (decreasing) trend in the future. This type of behavior is known as *persistence*.[9,10] For $H_j < 0.5$, on the other hand, the stochastic process is negatively correlated, i.e., $C < 0$. In this case, increasing (decreasing) trends in the past imply on the average decreasing (increasing) trends in the future. This type of behavior is referred to as *anti-persistence*.[9,10]

In order to calculate diffusion coefficients and scaling exponents from COP trajectories, we first generated plots of

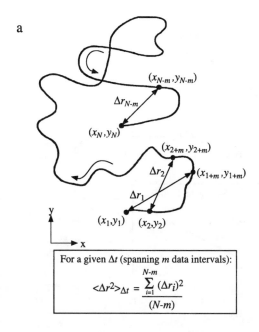

a

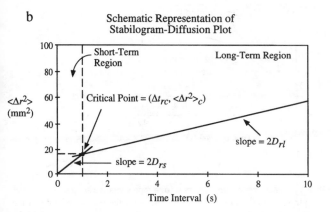

For a given Δt (spanning m data intervals):

$$\langle \Delta r^2 \rangle_{\Delta t} = \frac{\sum\limits_{i=1}^{N-m} (\Delta r_i)^2}{(N-m)}$$

b

Schematic Representation of Stabilogram-Diffusion Plot

FIG. 2. (a) Diagram showing the method for calculating mean square planar displacement $\langle \Delta r^2 \rangle$ as a function of time interval Δt for a COP trajectory made up of N data points $(x_1, y_1; x_2, y_2; \ldots; x_N, y_N)$. In this case, Δt does not represent the sampling interval; instead, Δt represents a moving time window spanning m data intervals. (b) A schematic representation of a typical resultant planar stabilogram-diffusion plot ($\langle \Delta r^2 \rangle$ vs Δt) generated from COP time series according to the method shown in (a). The diffusion coefficients D_{rs} and D_{rl} are computed from the slopes of the lines fitted to the short-term and long-term regions, respectively. The critical point, $(\Delta t_{rc}, \langle \Delta r^2 \rangle_c)$, is defined by the intersection of the lines fitted to the two regions of the plot. The scaling exponents H_{rs} and H_{rl} are calculated from the slopes of the log–log plots of the short-term and long-term regions, respectively (adapted from Collins and De Luca[5]).

mean square COP displacement versus Δt. (Such plots will be referred to as stabilogram-diffusion plots.) The displacement analysis was carried out by calculating the square of the displacements between all pairs of points separated in time by a specified time interval Δt [Fig. 2(a)]. The square displacements were then averaged over the number of Δt making up each COP time series. This process was repeated for increasing values of Δt.

Experimental studies concerned with diffusion-like processes typically analyze either long time series of data measurements or a large number of smaller time series of such

measurements.[11,12] In a posturographic investigation, it would be impractical, however, to have subjects stand on a force platform for extended periods of time. Physiological factors such as fatigue would tend to obscure the results. In the present study, it was therefore decided to collect a reasonable number of 90 s trials for each subject and analyze averaged sets of the results derived from these tests. Specifically, stabilogram-diffusion plots were computed for each subject trial, and then five such curves were averaged to obtain a resultant stabilogram-diffusion plot for a particular subject.

Diffusion coefficients [Eq. (1)] were calculated from the slopes of the resultant linear–linear plots of mean square COP displacement versus Δt. Similarly, scaling exponents [Eq. (2)] were computed from the resultant log–log plots of such curves. In all cases, the slopes were determined by utilizing the method of least squares to fit straight lines through defined portions of the aforementioned plots. All parameters were determined by a single investigator.

III. RESULTS

Resultant linear–linear and log–log plots of mean square planar COP displacement versus Δt for a representative subject are shown in Figs. 3(a) and 3(b), respectively. It should be noted that the stabilogram-diffusion curves changed slope after a critical point (or period) at some small Δt. This general feature was found in the resultant plots for all ten subjects who participated in this study. In order to parametrize such plots, two regions were identified—a short-term region and a long-term region [Fig. 2(b)]. These regions were separated by a transition period over which the slope of the stabilogram-diffusion plot changed considerably. (A third, distinct region over which mean square COP displacement saturates to some constant value is also expected after a sufficiently large time interval, given the fact that COP displacements are bounded by the base of support defined by an individual's feet, i.e., for bounded motion, $\langle \Delta j^2 \rangle$ saturates to a constant value after a sufficiently large Δt.[13] Unfortunately, the time series considered in this study were not long enough to characterize this region reliably.) Diffusion coefficients and scaling exponents were computed for each region [Fig. 2(b)].[14] Subscripts s and l will be used throughout the manuscript to denote the short-term and long-term regions, respectively. (The lines fitted for computation of D_{js}, D_{jl}, H_{js}, and H_{jl} had r^2 values that ranged from 0.91 to 1.00, 0.70–1.00, 0.97–1.00, and 0.74 to 1.00, respectively; the r^2 values for most data sets were all typically greater than 0.97.) An estimate for each critical point (or period) was determined as the intersection point of the regression lines fitted to the two regions of the linear–linear plots of $\langle \Delta j^2 \rangle$ vs Δt [Fig. 2(b)].[15]

The group means and standard deviations of the diffusion coefficients, scaling exponents and critical point coordinates for the ten subjects are given in bar-plot form in Fig. 4. Several general points should be noted. First, the short-term diffusion coefficients were considerably greater than the respective long-term diffusion coefficients [Fig. 4(a)]. In addition, the anteroposterior diffusion coefficients were larger than the respective mediolateral diffusion coefficients [Fig. 4(a)]. (This latter result was not unexpected, given that

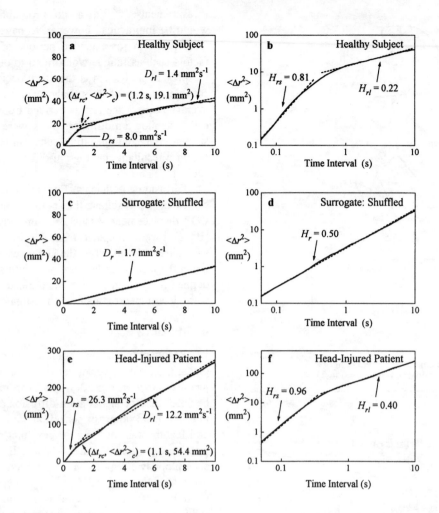

FIG. 3. Resultant (a) linear–linear and (b) log–log plots of mean square planar COP displacement versus time interval for a representative subject. Also shown in (a) and (b) are the fitted regression lines (dashed lines) for the short-term and long-term regions and the computed values for the respective stabilogram-diffusion parameters. (c) As in (a), but for shuffled surrogate random-walk data sets that were generated from the original COP time series. (d) As in (b), but for the surrogates in (c). (e) As in (a), but for a patient with a mild head injury. (f) As in (b), but for the patient in (e).

upright bipedal stance is considerably more stable in the frontal plane than in the sagittal plane.) Second, the short-term scaling exponents were considerably greater than 0.5 [Fig. 4(b)]. Thus, over short-term intervals of time during quiet standing, the COP behaves as a positively correlated random walk, i.e., the system exhibits persistence. On the other hand, the long-term scaling exponents were considerably less than 0.5 [Fig. 4(b)]. Thus, over long-term intervals of time, the COP behaves as a negatively correlated random walk, i.e., the system exhibits anti-persistence. Finally, the critical period occurred over relatively small time intervals, i.e., $\Delta t_{j_c} \approx 1.0$ s [Fig. 4(c)], and mean square displacements, i.e., $\langle \Delta j^2 \rangle_c$ was typically less than 20 mm^2 [Fig. 4(d)].

In order to determine whether the aforementioned correlations in the COP time series were artifacts of the data-set size and/or the amplitude distribution of the increments in displacement, we randomly shuffled the temporal order of the increments[16] making up the COP time series and then recombined the increments to form surrogate random-walk sequences [e.g., see Fig. 1(c)]. For each subject, an ensemble of ten different shuffled surrogate sets were generated from

each of the five original COP time series and subsequently analyzed. (The regression lines fitted for computation of the respective surrogate scaling exponents had r^2 values that ranged from 0.97 to 1.00.) We calculated the significance of the differences between the computed H_j values for the original COP time series and the surrogates according to the method described by Theiler et al.[17] (We also used techniques described therein to estimate error bars on the significance.) With this approach, the significance is defined by the difference between the value of H_j for the original COP time series and the mean value of H_j for the surrogates, divided by the standard deviation of the H_j values for the surrogates. We found that the double-logarithmic plots of mean square displacement versus Δt for the shuffled surrogates displayed only a single scaling region [e.g., see Fig. 3(d)], as would be expected for an uncorrelated random walk. The H_j values for the surrogates (range: 0.47–0.54, mean: 0.50±0.02) were also similar to those expected for a classical random walk [Figs. 5(a), 5(c), and 5(e)], and they were significantly different from those computed for the original COP time series [Figs. 5(b), 5(d), and 5(f)]. Thus, we were able to reject the

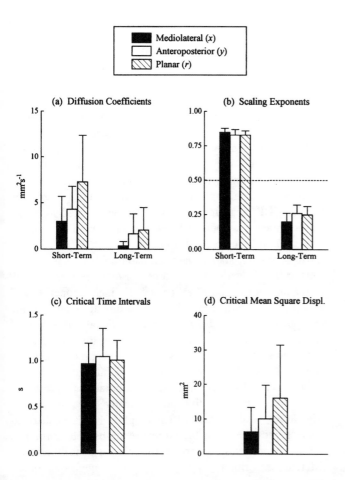

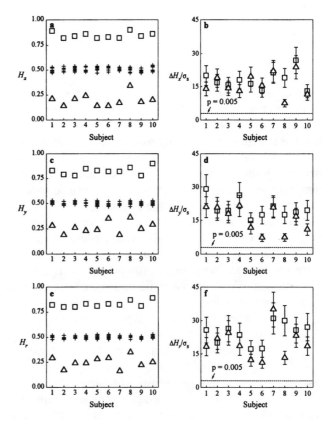

FIG. 4. Group means and standard deviations for the ten subjects: (a) diffusion coefficients, (b) scaling exponents, (c) critical time intervals, and (d) critical mean square displacements. In (b), a dashed line is drawn at the value expected for classical Brownian motion, i.e., $H_{ji}=0.50$.

FIG. 5. Random-walk analyses of COP time series and shuffled surrogate data sets. (a) Calculated values of H_x for the short-term ($\square$) and long-term ($\triangle$) scaling regions of the original COP time series and for the shuffled surrogates ($+$) for each of the ten subjects. (b) The significance of the differences between the computed H_x values for the original COP time series and the surrogates in (a). The significance values and error bars were calculated according to the techniques described by Theiler et al.[17] Here σ_s is the standard deviation of the H_x values for the surrogates, and ΔH_x is the difference between the value of H_x for the original COP time series and the mean value of H_x for the surrogates. A dashed line is plotted at the significance level that corresponds to a p value of 0.005. (c) As in (a), but for the anteroposterior scaling exponents (H_y). (d) As in (b), but for the computed values of H_y in (c). (e) As in (a), but for the planar scaling exponents (H_r). (f) As in (b), but for the computed values of H_r in (e).

null hypothesis that postural sway is an uncorrelated random walk. Importantly, these results suggest that the correlations in the COP time series were due to underlying dynamic processes and that they were not artifacts of the analysis.

Stabilogram-diffusion analysis may eventually be used to identify and/or diagnose individuals with balance disorders. As a preliminary indication of the possible clinical utility of this technique, we have included in Figs. 3(e) and 3(f) resultant planar stabilogram-diffusion plots for a patient (age: 36 yr) with a mild head injury. It is clear that some of the computed results for this patient were significantly different from those for the healthy subjects of the present study. For instance, the patient's short-term and long-term planar diffusion coefficients were more than three standard deviations greater than the respective group means given in Fig. 4(a). It can also be seen from Fig. 3(e) that the long-term region for the patient was characterized by small-amplitude, low-frequency oscillations. This finding suggests that some (or all) of the COP trajectories for this patient contained similar such oscillations. [It should be noted, however, that we have observed similar oscillations in the stabilogram-diffusion plots for a small number of healthy subjects, e.g., see Fig. 3(d) in Collins and De Luca.[5]] Further work with well-defined patient populations is obviously needed.

IV. DISCUSSION

In this work, we demonstrated that quiet-standing postural sway can be modeled as a system of bounded, correlated random walks. Specifically, we showed that over short-term intervals of time during undisturbed stance the COP behaves as a positively correlated random walk, whereas over long-term intervals of time it resembles a negatively correlated random walk. From a physiological standpoint, we interpret the presence of short-range positive correlations in the COP data as an indication that the postural control system utilizes open-loop control mechanisms over short-term intervals of time ($\Delta t < 1$ s) and small displacements. That is, the system allows the COP to "drift" for some time and/or displacement. This novel finding, which suggests that the system allows a certain amount of "sloppiness" in balance control, challenges the generally accepted notion that erect stance is always regulated by the action of feedback mechanisms.[18,19] It is important to note, however, that our analyses do not exclude the role of feedback mechanisms, such as the visual, vestibular, and proprioceptive systems, in the regulation of upright stance. In fact, the presence of longer-range negative correlations in the COP data suggests that closed-loop control mechanisms are utilized over long-term intervals of time ($\Delta t > 1$ s) and large displacements. That is, after some time and/or displacement, the postural control system shifts the COP back toward a relative equilibrium position. Within this conceptual model, the central nervous system still continually receives afferent information from peripheral sensory organs; however, such information is not used to modify the efferent signals transmitted to postural muscles unless, for example, some threshold value is exceeded. The integration of open-loop control schemes with closed-loop feedback mechanisms for balance regulation may have evolved to account for feedback-loop delays and inherent noise in the system (e.g., due to inherent muscle force fluctuations[20]), and to simplify the task of integrating vast amounts of sensory information when the body is not in jeopardy of instability.

Within the context of the above postural control hypothesis, the short-term and long-term diffusion coefficients approximate the effective stochasticity of the open-loop and closed-loop postural control mechanisms, respectively. The finding that the short-term diffusion coefficients were substantially greater than the long-term diffusion coefficients thus suggests that the open-loop control schemes (the output of which may take the form of descending commands to different postural muscles) exhibit an effectively higher level of stochasticity than the closed-loop feedback mechanisms. The short-term stochastic effects are likely due to the noise-like fluctuations that are produced across various joints of the body by the aforementioned open-loop activation signals. (Such fluctuations are a consequence of the fact that skeletal muscles are incapable of producing constant forces.[20]) The long-term stochastic effects may be related to the fact that the human body in upright stance can assume a number of different positions that are "statically stable." During quiet standing, an individual may switch between these different equilibrium positions in a stochastic manner.

Likewise, in light of the above hypothesis, the critical point coordinates approximate the temporal and spatial coordinates of the transition region over which the postural control system switches from open-loop control to closed-loop control. As noted in our earlier paper,[5] the position of the critical point may be set by a number of physiological/biomechanical factors and/or mechanisms, including (1) a proprioceptive "dead zone," i.e., a region over which slight variations in body-segment position and orientation are left unchanged; (2) a "dead zone" that arises from the interaction of postural responses with the body's inertia; or (3) fixed, preprogrammed central commands that are utilized in quiet stance. This issue requires further study.

Fractal measures, such as fractal dimensions, have been applied to several physiological systems and processes,[21,22] including the human postural control system.[23-25] However, in most cases, these measures have not been linked to the underlying physiology in a meaningful way; instead, their use has been limited primarily to describing and classifying time-series patterns and the shapes of biological objects. The

novelty of the present approach is that fractal-type parameters, i.e., scaling exponents, are interpreted from a motor control standpoint, i.e., they are linked in a mechanistic fashion to the dynamic characteristics of the postural control system. It would be erroneous to assume, however, that postural sway, given its fractal nature, is an instance of deterministic chaos. In a recent study,[6] we used surrogate-data techniques and algorithms from dynamical systems theory to show that COP trajectories are indistinguishable from correlated noise. We did not find any evidence that postural sway reflects a dynamical system with a low-dimensional attractor. We therefore concluded that balance regulation, as viewed through COP measurements, is better represented as a stochastic process, as opposed to a chaotic one. This work is consistent with our present findings.

In summary, stabilogram-diffusion analysis has the advantage that it leads to the extraction of three sets of COP parameters—diffusion coefficients, scaling exponents, and critical point coordinates—that can be directly related to the resultant steady-state behavior and functional interaction of the neuromuscular mechanisms underlying the maintenance of upright stance. It should also be noted that the majority of the stabilogram-diffusion parameters exhibit "good" to "excellent" reliability, as measured by intraclass correlation coefficients.[5] Thus, individuals typically have their own "signature" stabilogram-diffusion plots. This statistical-biomechanics approach therefore can be used to formulate and test hypotheses concerning the relative contributions of different sensorimotor subsystems and strategies to quiet-standing balance control.

ACKNOWLEDGMENTS

We thank Ann Pavlik and Mike Rosenstein for their assistance with software development and figure preparation. We also thank Dr. Casey Kerrigan of Spaulding Rehabilitation Hospital for her assistance with the recruitment and testing of the head-injured patient. This work was supported by the National Science Foundation (Grant No. BCS-9308659) and the Rehab R&D Service of the Department of Veterans Affairs.

[1] H. C. Diener, J. Dichgans, M. Bacher, and B. Gompf, "Quantification of postural sway in normals and patients with cerebellar diseases," Electroencephalogr. Clin. Neurophysiol. **57**, 134–142 (1984).

[2] R. L. Kirby, N. A. Price, and D. A. MacLeod, "The influence of foot position on standing balance," J. Biomech. **20**, 423–427 (1987).

[3] M. E. Norré, G. Forrez, and A. Beckers, "Posturography measuring instability in vestibular dysfunction in the elderly," Age Ageing **16**, 89–93 (1987).

[4] S. S. Hasan, M. J. Lichtenstein, and R. G. Shiavi, "Effect of loss of balance on biomechanics platform measures of sway: Influence of stance and a method for adjustment," J. Biomech. **23**, 783–789 (1990).

[5] J. J. Collins and C. J. De Luca, "Open-loop and closed-loop control of posture: A random-walk analysis of center-of-pressure trajectories," Exp. Brain Res. **95**, 308–318 (1993).

[6] J. J Collins and C. J. De Luca, "Random walking during quiet standing," Phys. Rev. Lett. **73**, 764–767 (1994).

[7] A. Einstein, "Über die von der molekularkinetischen Theorie der Wärme geforderte Bewegung von in ruhenden Flüssigkeiten suspendierten Teilchen," Ann. Phys. **322**, 549–560 (1905).

[8] B. B. Mandelbrot and J. W. van Ness, "Fractional Brownian motions, fractional noises and applications," SIAM Rev. **10**, 422–437 (1968).

[9] J. Feder, *Fractals* (Plenum, New York, 1988).

[10] D. Saupe, "Algorithms for random fractals," in *The Science of Fractal Images*, edited by H.-O. Peitgen and D. Saupe (Springer-Verlag, New York, 1988), pp. 71–136.

[11] M. F. Shlesinger and B. J. West (Editors), *Random Walks and Their Applications in the Physical and Biological Sciences* (American Institute of Physics, New York, 1984).

[12] E. W. Montroll and J. L. Lebowitz (Editors), *Fluctuation Phenomena* (North-Holland, Amsterdam, 1987).

[13] J. Theiler, "Some comments on the correlation dimension of $1/f^\alpha$ noise," Phys. Lett. A **155**, 480–493 (1991).

[14] The respective "endpoints" (near the transition period) used to fit regression lines to the short-term and long-term regions were determined by eye.

[15] The maximum time interval considered in the random-walk analysis was 10 s. This value was chosen because it was sufficient to characterize the transition period and the long-term region of the postural control system (as determined from a pilot study involving larger data sets, e.g., 240 s COP time series), and the inclusion of longer time intervals in the present analyses may have introduced spurious or unreliable results, given that we only considered 90 s COP time series.

[16] J. A. Scheinkman and B. LeBaron, "Nonlinear dynamics and stock returns," J. Business **62**, 311–337 (1989).

[17] J. Theiler, S. Eubank, A. Longtin, B. Galdrikian, and J. D. Farmer, "Testing for nonlinearity in time series: The method of surrogate data," Physica D **58**, 77–94 (1992).

[18] A. Ishida and S. Miyazaki, "Maximum likelihood identification of a posture control system," IEEE Trans. Biomed. Eng. **BE-34**, 1–5 (1987).

[19] R. Johansson, M. Magnusson, and A. Akesson, "Identification of human postural dynamics," IEEE Trans. Biomed. Eng. **BE-35**, 858–869 (1988).

[20] C. J. De Luca, R. S. LeFever, M. P. McCue, and A. P. Xenakis, "Control scheme governing concurrently active human motor units during voluntary contractions," J. Physiol. (London) **329**, 129–142 (1982).

[21] C. C. King, "Fractal and chaotic dynamics in nervous systems," Prog. Neurobiol. **36**, 279–308 (1991).

[22] T. Elbert, W. J. Ray, Z. J. Kowalik, J. E. Skinner, K. E. Graf, and N. Birbaumer, "Chaos and physiology: Deterministic chaos in excitable cell assemblies," Physiol. Rev. **74**, 1–47 (1994).

[23] T. Musha, "1/f fluctuations in biological systems," *Proceedings of the 6th International Conference on Noise in Physical Systems,* NSB Special Publication, 1981, Vol. 614, pp 143–146.

[24] J. B. Myklebust and B. M. Myklebust, "Fractals in kinesiology," Proc. 19th Annu. Mtg. Soc. Neurosci. **15**, 604 (1989).

[25] J. B. Myklebust, T. E. Prieto, B. M. Myklebust, and D. G. Lange, "Dimensionality of postural steadiness," Proc. 20th Annu. Mtg. Soc. Neurosci. **16**, 1315 (1990).

Self-organizing dynamics of the human brain: Critical instabilities and Sil'nikov chaos

J. A. Scott Kelso and Armin Fuchs

Program in Complex Systems and Brain Sciences, Center for Complex Systems, Florida Atlantic University, Boca Raton, Florida 33431

(Received 5 July 1994; accepted for publication 7 December)

Using a sensorimotor coordination task in conjunction with an array of SQUIDs (Superconducting QUantum Interference Devices) we demonstrate critical instabilities in human brain activity patterns. Analysis of the dominant spatial pattern of the brain and its time-varying amplitude displays a task-dependent geometry characteristic of Šil'nikov-like chaos, which changes qualitatively at the transition. © *1995 American Institute of Physics.*

I. INTRODUCTION

With respect to the issue of modeling the brain as a chaotic dynamical system it may be useful to make explicit the following points: (1) The human brain is a complex, dissipative system built from billions of subsystems: the neurons. (2) Under certain conditions, complex systems may exhibit low-dimensional behavior with only a small number of relevant degrees of freedom (say < 10 to put a number on it). Such is especially the case when the system is near instability points where it may switch from one state to another (nonequilibrium phase transitions). (3) Theoretically, nonlinear dynamical systems with more than two dimensions have the ability to enter a non-periodic state—a chaotic attractor—and show a phenomenon called deterministic chaos. (4) In dissipative systems there is always a certain amount of stochastic fluctuations present (the dissipation-fluctuation theorem). The influence of stochastic forces on the system's behavior is enhanced near transition points where it takes longer to relax from perturbations to the attractor. (5) In a rigorous sense the term "attractor" is defined only under *stationary* conditions and as time goes to infinity. For practical purposes, this definition may be weakened and an attractor defined assuming no changes in the parameters and in the external inputs to the system for a time much longer than the relaxation time. (6) Chaotic systems are sensitive to initial conditions. There are directions in the phase space where trajectories that are very close to each other diverge exponentially.

A consequence of the foregoing is that slight changes or fluctuations in a parameter may lead the system from a stable limit cycle to a chaotic attractor. However, the transient behavior for both is very similar and depends on the location and stability of the fixed points in the phase space. Here we provide some evidence suggesting that this geometry and the changes in this geometry are a key part of understanding the global dynamics of the brain.

Our central thesis is that the brain is fundamentally a pattern forming, self-organized system governed by nonlinear dynamical laws. Many people in the cognitive and brain sciences think the brain is like a computer manipulating symbols. Others, more concerned for the so-called "wetware" of the brain, liken it to an artificial neural network, a rugged landscape whose minima correspond to fixed point attractors.

Instead, inspired profoundly by Haken's synergetics,[1] we shall argue that the brain is a complex dynamical system in which, under certain conditions, spatiotemporal patterns emerge spontaneously and sustain themselves in a relatively autonomous fashion. In particular, rather than *settle* into attractors we shall show that the brain has a tendency to *dwell*— for variable amounts of time—in coherent metastable states. It is poised on the brink of instability where it can switch flexibly and quickly.

Synergetics provides essential theoretical concepts and methods for understanding the creation of pattern and form in open, nonequilibrium systems. Close to instabilities, complex systems containing many degrees of freedom (*material complexity*) exhibit low-dimensional behavior that may be described by collective variables (or *order parameters*) that characterize the emerging patterns—a cooperative effect. The resulting order parameter dynamics, though low-dimensional, are nevertheless *nonlinear* and hence capable of exhibiting enormous *behavioral complexity*. In other words, the underlying equations of motion may exhibit complicated solutions, including stochastic features and/or deterministic chaos.

An aspect that is often omitted from analyses of neural and behavioral function concerns how to find relevant collective variables in such complex systems. One philosophy, stemming perhaps from certain mathematical theorems is that *any* time series taken from the system, e.g. a single EEG recording of spontaneous brain activity, is enough to make meaningful inferences about the dynamics of the entire system. In the ideal case of mathematical models and precise physical experiments this may be true. However, calculations of the dimension of biological time series have not yielded much insight and are plagued with methodological problems.[2] Here we emphasize the significance of dynamic instabilities as a means of demarcating and identifying relevant collective states in the brain and the control parameters that promote switching among them. Not only is it possible to test predictions about the system's behavior around dynamic instabilities, but such instabilities also provide the system with a source of *flexibility*, i.e. as a way to enter and exit coherent, metastable states.

This paper is organized as follows. In Sec. II we describe an experimental paradigm that affords analysis of the spatiotemporal dynamics of the brain in relation to behavior.

While a subject performs a sensorimotor coordination task, the magnetic field generated by intracellular dendritic currents in the brain is measured using an array of SQUIDs (Superconducting QUantum Interference Devices). It turns out that during the task the magnetic field is extremely coherent in space and time and that certain aspects of both brain activity and overt behavior can be described by the same quantities. Remarkably, under these task conditions the brain exhibits predicted features associated with dynamic instabilities (critical slowing down, critical fluctuations) typical of other pattern forming complex systems in nature. Some of these results are reported in detail elsewhere.[3] Here we will focus on the spatial patterns (modes), and how they evolve in time. In particular, using phase space reconstruction techniques we will show how the modes may exhibit dynamics of the Šil'nikov type.[4] In Sec. III we provide a brief treatment of homoclinic trajectories in 3-D flows, a characteristic feature of the Šil'nikov scenario. In a final section, we draw out the implications of our results and analysis for understanding the brain-behavior relationship in terms of pattern formation and nonlinear dynamics.

II. SPATIOTEMPORAL PATTERNS OF THE BRAIN

How do we determine if the brain is a self-organized dynamical system? We need, at least, three things: an appropriate set of theoretical concepts and corresponding methodological strategies; a technology that affords analysis of the large scale, global dynamics of the brain in both space and time; and a clean experiment that prunes away complications but retains essential aspects.

A. The experiment

Below we give a brief description of the experimental setup. We refer the reader to Ref. 3 for more details. Periodic tones were presented to a subject at a frequency of 1 Hz, increasing every 10 cycles in steps of 0.25 Hz up to 3.0 Hz. The subject's task was to press a button between two consecutive tones i.e. to *syncopate* with the stimulus. Previous research[5] has established that when the rate of the stimuli exceeds a certain value subjects are no longer able to syncopate with the stimulus and switch spontaneously into a *synchronization* pattern. During the present experiment brain activity was also measured using an array of 37 SQUID sensors located over the left parieto-temporal cortex as indicated in Fig. 1(a). These detectors pick up neurally generated magnetic fields that are about 10^9 times weaker than the magnetic field of the earth. Figure 1(b) shows the averaged data from two sensors before and after the transition from syncopation to synchronization. Open squares mark the point in time where the stimulus occurred, solid squares correspond to the button press. Before the transition the stimulus and the response are anti-phase. After the transition, the subject's responses are nearly in-phase with the stimulus. The brain's magnetic field shows a strong periodicity during this perception-action task, especially in the pre-transition region. After the transition the amplitude drops and the signal looks noisier.

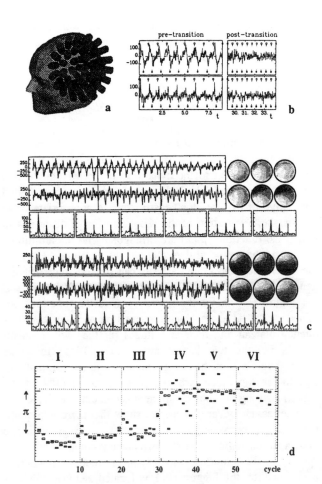

FIG. 1. (a) Reconstruction of the subject's head and location of SQUID sensors. (b) Time-series from single sensors before and after the transition. (c) *Upper part*: (right) Spatial dependence of the top mode on the first six frequency plateaus, each of which contains 10 cycles. Notice the change in the shape on plateaus five and six. (left) Amplitudes and spectra for the first six frequency plateaus (1 Hz to 2.25 Hz). *Lower part*: the same for the second mode. (d) Relative phases of the sensorimotor behavior (open squares) and the amplitude of the top mode of brain activity (solid squares) with respect to the stimulus. Notice the qualitative change at the beginning of plateau IV.

B. Analysis of the brain signals

The patterns of brain activity picked up by the SQUID array are very coherent in space. Thus, we treat the signals from the 37 sensors as a spatial pattern that evolves in time. The spatiotemporal signal $H(\mathbf{x},t)$ is decomposed into spatial, time-independent functions $\phi_i(\mathbf{x})$ and their corresponding amplitudes $\xi_i(t)$

$$H(\mathbf{x},t) = \sum_{i=1}^{N} \xi_i(t)\phi_i(\mathbf{x}). \qquad (1)$$

If the functions $\phi_i(\mathbf{x})$ are chosen properly, a truncation of this expansion at a small N (say $N < 5...10$) gives a good approximation of the original dataset. There are several ways to choose these spatial functions. One possibility, for instance, is to use a set of orthogonal functions like a spatial Fourier expansion. We used a basis calculated from a

Karhunen–Loève (KL) decomposition (see Ref. 3 for details) that is optimal in the sense that it minimizes a mean square error defined as

$$E_K = \int_T dt \int_\Omega d\mathbf{x} \left\{ H(\mathbf{x},t) - \sum_{k=1}^{K} \xi_k(t)\, \phi_k(\mathbf{x}) \right\}^2 \quad (2)$$

for every truncation level K.

We mention that this basis is not necessarily the best choice with respect to the dynamics of the system. In two recent papers Friedrich, Uhl, and Haken,[6,7] have provided alternative procedures for constructing an appropriate basis set. In one, a variation of the KL-expansion is discussed in which the functions $\phi_i(\mathbf{x})$ are orthogonal and the amplitude $\xi_{i-1}(t)$ is the temporal derivative of the amplitude $\xi_i(t)$. In the other, they show how a basis can be constructed if the general form of the order parameter dynamics is known.

Figure 1(c) shows the spatial form of the functions obtained by the KL expansion performed on each constant frequency plateau and their amplitudes for the two dominant modes, i.e. the two largest eigenvalues. These functions cover about 75% of the energy contained in the original signal. In the top mode (which represents about 60% of the signal) a strong periodic component is evident over the entire time series. However, the spectra show that there is a qualitative change between pre- and post-transition regions. In the pre-transition regime, the main frequency component corresponds to the stimulus (and response) frequency, whereas post-transition the biggest peak is located at twice this frequency. The spatial dependence of the top mode changes as well. Pre-transition there is one maximum located left of the center of the array. After the transition, the maximum of the pattern has shifted to the lower left-hand side and a local minimum emerges at the upper left. The temporal behavior of the second mode [Fig. 1(c) bottom] is much less periodic, and systematic differences between the regions before and after the transition are not so obvious.

As already mentioned, the (anti-phase) syncopation pattern is not stable above a certain frequency, and a spontaneous switch to an (in-phase) synchronization pattern is observed. Remarkably, we found a similar switching in the phase relation between the stimulus and the brain activity represented by the time series of the dominant mode. Open squares in Fig. 1(d) correspond to the phase relation of the sensorimotor behavior, solid squares represent the relative phase between the stimulus and the brain activity (time dependent mode amplitudes). The vertical dotted lines mark the points at which the control parameter (frequency) was increased. Horizontal dotted lines are separated by π rad. A clear qualitative change is observed at the beginning of plateau IV. More important, the phase of the brain signal and the sensorimotor behavior are almost identical in the pre-transition region. Post-transition, the brain signal becomes more diffuse even as the sensorimotor behavior becomes more regular. Another notable effect may be seen at the plateau boundaries before the transition. Near these points at which the frequency parameter is changed, the phase relation is perturbed and a "relaxation" occurs over a few cycles before the new stable value is reached. As the transition re-

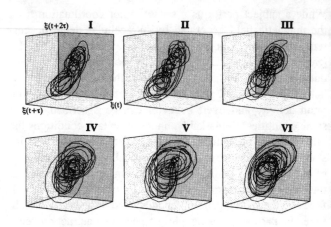

FIG. 2. Trajectories of the top mode in phase space (delay coordinates) for the six frequency plateaus from upper left to lower right.

gion is approached, this relaxation process takes longer, as a comparison between plateaus II and III reveals. This phenomenon of *critical slowing down* is a well-known signature of dynamic instabilities in non-equilibrium systems when a control parameter is changed.[1]

For the purpose of further analysis we plot the time series of the top mode's amplitude $\xi_1(t)$ in a three-dimensional phase space using delay coordinates. Figure 2 shows these displays on the first six frequency plateaus proceeding from upper left to lower right. Notice the trajectories never repeat or settle down, even though a clearly defined geometry is apparent. Moreover, this phase space image results in a very interesting structure with apparent changes in the geometry pre- and post-transition.

III. DYNAMIC MODELING

What type of dynamical system can be used to model the experimentally observed behavior? Recent work has successfully modeled the spatiotemporal behavior of the brain using nonlinearly coupled oscillators to represent the top two spatial modes, parametrically excited by an external driver (the periodically occurring tones).[8] Here we concentrate on the phase space trajectory of the top mode which, since it is one of several, may be chaotic in nature. We know from studies of a variety of nonequilibrium systems that chaotic behavior generated by mode interactions is a cooperative effect produced by the entire system. Isolated parts or single subsystems do not generally exhibit chaotic behavior on their own.

A chief characteristic of chaotic behavior generated by mode interactions in a spatially extended system is the existence of homoclinic and heteroclinic loops in the phase space of the collective modes. These loops or orbits exist for particular values of a control parameter and are composed of trajectories connecting saddle points. In particular, we consider a system that was investigated by Šil'nikov in 1965[4] which is one possible scenario for creating chaotic attractors. He analyzed a system in three dimensions for which the linear part in the vicinity of the saddle focus at the origin has the form

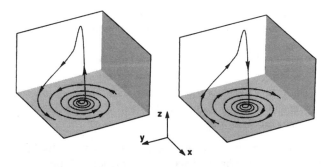

FIG. 3. Trajectories of a Šil'nikov-like system near the saddle focus at the origin (see text).

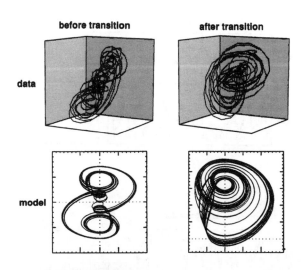

FIG. 4. *Top.* Phase space plots of top spatial mode using time delay coordinates before (plateau II) and after (plateau V) the transition. *Bottom* (Left). Model simulation of Šil'nikov system [Eq. (6)] with $\mu=0.65$, $\epsilon=0.55$, $b=0.65$, $a=0.008$. (Right). Model simulation of Šil'nikov system [Eq. (6)] with $a=0.2217$, same parameters as on the left.

$$\mathbf{L}=\begin{pmatrix} \lambda_r & -\omega & 0 \\ \omega & \lambda_r & 0 \\ 0 & 0 & \lambda_z \end{pmatrix}. \qquad (3)$$

In a region around the fixed point where this linear approximation is valid, the trajectories can be written in the form

$$r(t)\sim e^{\lambda_r t}, \quad z(t)\sim e^{\lambda_z t} \text{ where } r(t)=\sqrt{x(t)^2+y(t)^2}. \qquad (4)$$

Šil'nikov showed that if the fixed point has a homoclinic orbit and the condition

$$|\lambda_r|<|\lambda_z| \quad \text{(Šil'nikov condition)} \qquad (5)$$

is fulfilled, there exists an infinite number of unstable orbits in the system, allowing the system to enter a chaotic state.

A necessary (but not sufficient) prerequisite for the occurrence of chaos is an unstable direction in phase space. For the system $\mathbf{L}$ the Šil'nikov condition can be fulfilled in two different ways:

- $\lambda_z>0$, $\lambda_r<0$: The z-axis is an unstable one-dimensional manifold. The trajectory leaves the fixed point along this line and returns in a spiral to the xy-plane which is a stable two-dimensional manifold (Fig. 3, left).

- $\lambda_r>0$, $\lambda_z<0$: The xy-plane is a two-dimensional unstable manifold. The trajectory moves in a spiral away from the fixed point, and returns along the z-axis which is the stable direction in this case (Fig. 3, right).

Figure 3 displays these different geometries of the attractor. Sensitivity to initial conditions is most pronounced when the trajectory is in the vicinity of the origin. Recently Friedrich and Uhl[6] showed that the Šil'nikov condition is fulfilled for EEG signals recorded during a seizure of petitmal epilepsy. They found both types of the attractor in different data sets.

There is a wide class of dynamical systems that show chaos of the Šil'nikov type. The one we wish to focus upon here as a candidate for modeling of our SQUID data is due to Coullet, Tresser, and Arnéodo[9] and reads

$$\dot{x}=y,$$

$$\dot{y}=z, \qquad (6)$$

$$\dot{z}=\mu x-y-\epsilon z-ax^2-bx^3.$$

It is well known that for certain values of the parameters, a system described by Eq. (6) exhibits chaotic behavior. In fact, there are at least two different types of attractors depending on the values of the parameters a and b. If $a=0$, Eq. (6) is invariant under a substitution of x, y and z by their negative values. Solutions that contain this symmetry are shown in Fig. 4 (lower left). If $a \neq 0$ this symmetry is broken and the attractor is asymmetric [Fig. 4 (lower right)]. Visual inspection shows a remarkable similarity between these curves and the phase space portraits from our SQUID data on plateaus II and V shown in Fig. 4 (top). Not only are the phase space portraits very similar, there is an overall qualitative match between theory and experiment. Figure 5 compares time series and power spectra of the model and the SQUID data on plateaus II and V. In order to reduce noise in the data we applied the procedure introduced by Kostelich and Yorke.[10] In Fig. 5 the time series of the model look less noisy than the data but all the main features are still present. It is quite obvious that the dynamical system [Eq. (6)] generates the essential behavior of the brain's top mode. Indeed, the model underscores the fascinating connection between the geometry and the dynamics of the brain. Of course, further investigations are necessary to establish a quantitative correspondence between data and model and to clarify the underlying neural mechanisms.

IV. DISCUSSION

We focus this final discussion in terms of the main conceptual advantages that arise from our results and analysis. The brain possesses tremendous heterogeneity of structure, and its dynamics, in general are nonstationary. To obtain proof that chaos—as it is known in mathematics and physics— exists in the brain may be a futile quest. Nevertheless, under well-defined experimental conditions we have demonstrated that the brain exhibits low-dimensional dynamical behavior. From an incoherent spontaneous or rest

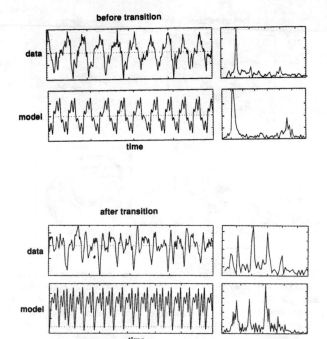

FIG. 5. *Top*. Time series and Fourier spectra (right) of top mode's behavior before the transition (plateau II) and corresponding model simulation. *Bottom*. Time series, Fourier spectra and model simulation after the transition is over (plateau V). Same parameters as in Fig. 4.

state the brain manifests coherent spatiotemporal patterns immediately a meaningful task is introduced. This result attests to both the *adaptability* and *information compression* capability conferred on the brain by its inherently pattern forming and nonlinear character.

It can hardly be overemphasized that the patterns formed by the brain that we have analyzed here exist only in relation to the environment or task context (cf. Fig. 1). If the brain is intrinsically chaotic, possessing, by definition, an infinite number of unstable periodic orbits, it has the capacity to match an equally unpredictable environment. Being chaotic at rest renders the brain access to any of these unstable orbits in order to satisfy functional requirements. Thus, when a task or environmental demand presents itself to the organism, the brain may utilize the chaotic motion to select and then stabilize an appropriate orbit or sequence of orbits.[11]

A further aspect of low-dimensional dynamical behavior in both brain and behavior pertains to critical instabilities. Like many of the complex, nonequilibrium systems studied by synergetics, we show that at critical values of a control parameter, the brain undergoes spontaneous changes in spatiotemporal patterns, measured e.g. in terms of relative phases, spectral properties of spatial modes etc. Remarkably, these quantities exhibit critical slowing down and fluctuation enhancement—predicted features of pattern forming instabilities in self-organizing (synergetic) systems.

Two comments are in order about these results:

(1) they highlight the importance of stochastic fluctuations in probing the stability of coherent patterns in the brain

and enabling the discovery of new patterns when the environmental, task, or internal conditions demand it; and

(2) nonequilibrium phase transitions provide the brain with a switching mechanism, essential for rapidly entering and exiting various coherent states. This ability—conferred on the brain by its phase transition character—is a hallmark of *flexibility*.

An even more flexible and fluid view of the brain emerges from phase space reconstruction of the spatial modes in which a class of behavior known as Šil'nikov chaos is revealed. Rather than requiring an active process to destabilize and switch the brain from one stable state to another, the presence of Šil'nikov chaos suggests that the brain possesses an inherently *intermittent* character. We had arrived at a similar inference some years ago based on empirical findings and theoretical considerations.[12] But more compelling here is that the actual trajectory of the main spatial pattern of the brain displays the geometry—a saddle focus connecting stable and unstable manifolds via homoclinic orbits—characteristic of Šil'nikov chaos. In this scenario the brain is never actually in a stable fixed point at all, but continuously evolves in the vicinity of a saddle focus. Thus, while patterns of brain activity are spatially coherent their temporal evolution is complex and, as we stressed here, task-dependent.

It is tempting to speculate that the brain operates globally using a relatively small (but not too small) set of basic modes whose contribution varies with experience and the functions brains (and people) have to perform. The clinical implications of this picture, e.g. in disorders such as schizophrenia, manic-depression and other brain diseases are tantalizing. In some cases the pathological brain may be restricted in its modal content and/or its dynamics. In others, too many modes may be excited and/or the dynamics never settle.

ACKNOWLEDGMENTS

Research support by NIMH (Neuroscience Research Branch) Grant No. MH42900, BRS Grant No. RR07258 and Contract No. N00014-88-J119 from the U.S. Office of Naval Research. Thanks to Tom Holroyd for his help with the figures.

[1] H. Haken, *Synergetics. An Introduction*, 3rd ed. (Springer-Verlag, Berlin, 1983); H. Haken, *Advanced Synergetics*, 2nd ed. (Springer-Verlag, Berlin, 1987); H. Haken, in *Synergetics of the Brain*, edited by E. Basar, H. Flohr, H. Haken, and A. J. Mandell (Springer-Verlag, Berlin, 1983).

[2] M. Ding, C. Grebogi, E. Ott, T. Sauer, and J. A. Yorke, Phys. Rev. Lett. **70**, 3872 (1993).

[3] A. Fuchs, J. A. S. Kelso, and H. Haken, Int. J. Bifurcation Chaos **2**, 917 (1992); J. A. S. Kelso, S. L. Bressler, S. Buchanan, G. C. DeGuzman, M. Ding, A. Fuchs, and T. Holroyd, Phys. Lett. A **169**, 134 (1992); J. A. S. Kelso, S. L. Bressler, S. Buchanan, G. C. DeGuzman, M. Ding, A. Fuchs, and T. Holroyd, in *Measuring Chaos in the Human Brain*, edited by D. Duke and W. Pritchard (World Scientific, Singapore, 1991).

[4] L. P. Šil'nikov, Sov. Math. Dokl. **6**, 163 (1965).

[5] J. A. S. Kelso, J. D. DelColle, and G. Schöner, in *Attention and Performance XIII*, edited by M. Jeannerod (Erlbaum, Hillsdale, NJ, 1990).

[6] R. Friedrich and C. Uhl, in *Evolution of Dynamical Structures in Complex Systems*, edited by R. Friedrich and A. Wunderlin (Springer-Verlag, Berlin, 1992).

[7] R. Friedrich, C. Uhl, and H. Haken, Z. Phys. B (in press).

[8] V. Jirsa, R. Friedrich, H. Haken, and J. A. S. Kelso, Biol. Cybern. **71**, 27 (1994).

[9] P. Coullet, C. Tresser, and A. Arnéodo, Phys. Lett. A **72**, 268 (1979).

[10] E. Kostelich and J. A. Yorke, Physica D **41**, 183 (1990).

[11] M. Ding and J. A. S. Kelso, in *Measuring Chaos in the Human Brain,* edited by D. Duke and W. Pritchard (World Scientific, Singapore, 1991).

[12] J. A. S. Kelso and G. C. DeGuzman, in *Tutorials in Motor Neuroscience,* edited by J. Requin and G. E. Stelmach (Kluwer, Dordrecht, 1991).

Characterizing the dynamics of auditory perception

Mingzhou Ding
Program in Complex Systems and Brain Sciences, Center for Complex Systems and Department of Mathematics, Florida Atlantic University, Boca Raton, Florida 33431

Betty Tuller and J. A. Scott Kelso
Program in Complex Systems and Brain Sciences, Center for Complex Systems, Florida Atlantic University, Boca Raton, Florida 33431

After listening to a sound that is presented repeatedly, subjects report hearing different transforms of the original sound. The frequency of reported transforms is a sensitive index of some speech disorders as well as cognitive flexibility in aging. In this paper, we propose and investigate quantitative measures that characterize the dynamics of this phenomenon, known as the verbal transformation effect. In particular, we show that the distribution of the dwell time, the time spent perceiving a string of a given phonemic form before switching to another form, obeys a power law for normal subjects with an exponent valued between 1 and 2. This result suggests that within this paradigm there is no characteristic time scale for the perceptual process. Additionally, we analyze the correlation properties of the transforms. We suggest that the complexity measures and techniques introduced here might be useful diagnostic tools for a number of speech and cognitive disorders. © *1995 American Institute of Physics.*

I. INTRODUCTION

In 1958, Warren and Gregory[1] made an interesting observation: When a person listens to a syllable (or a word or sentence) that is repeated over and over, with a relatively short separation between neighboring repetitions, the person's perception of the syllable is initially veridical. After a variable time period, however, the subject begins to perceive the syllable in a variety of alternate forms. These illusory changes, referred to as verbal (or phonemic) transforms,[2] have since received considerable attention. In general, the literature has concentrated on discovering statistical regularities relating stimuli or listeners to the reported transforms.[3–11] A main finding is that the transforms are sensitive to properties of the stimulus (semantic, phonological, and acoustic), as well as to those of the listener (age, gender, and phonetic training).

Admittedly, the conditions that enhance verbal transforms rarely occur during normal conversation and at first blush, the transforms might be attributed to fatigue of underlying neural processes. But other predicted features of neural fatigue do not occur; for example, listeners do not necessarily return to perceiving the presented stimulus veridically after a time perceiving an illusory alternative, and the reported transforms are much richer than suggested by fatigue of opponent phonetic processes.[12]

The verbal transformation effect is also reminiscent of the perceptual alternations that occur with visual reversible figures, but several important differences must be underscored. First, the auditory stimuli are not at all ambiguous except under repetitive conditions. Second, when perceptual switching occurs, the number of alternative phonemic structures reported is typically much greater than the two, or at most three, alternative percepts allowed by a visual display.

This second characteristic is of great interest because it is highly dependent on the listener's age. For college-age listeners, the number of switches between perceived forms continuously increases, or initially increases then levels off,

over the course of a 3 to 5 min trial. In contrast to the college-age listeners, older listeners show both a more restricted set of phonemic transforms and a slowed rate of switching among them.[2,13] Thus, the temporal measures examined in the present work may well provide a measure of the decrease in cognitive flexibility that occurs with normal aging and with the onset of Alzheimer's disease or other dementias of the non-Alzheimer's type.

The phenomenon of verbal transforms also shows promise in diagnosing the auditory/perceptual problems that occur in language disabled children and those with certain speech disorders. For example, many children with articulation disorders are also deficient in perception of time-dependent acoustic signals. Specifically, children who misarticulate /s/ also perceive fewer transforms of s-initial syllables (e.g., "sus") than do matched children with normal speech production.[14] These results, taken together with reports that verbal transforms are sensitive to second language and foreign language proficiency,[15] suggest that the verbal transformation effect provides a non-invasive behavioral measure of the perception-production link.

In this paper we seek quantitative measures that characterize the dynamics of verbal transforms. We depart from the traditional approach to the study of this phenomenon mainly by ignoring the identity of the perceived forms and treating the time-dependent perceptual changes as a dynamical process. We take this approach because of the large amount of variability in reported transforms to the same repeated syllable: Often there is no single transform heard by all listeners. Thus, we propose that the temporal evolution of transforms may be a better measure of perceptual flexibility than the transforms themselves. Although the techniques used are reminiscent of many previous studies, to make the dynamical analysis possible, we have modified the methodology in two important ways. First, we slow the rate of stimulus presentation so that the subject can record what is perceived on each presentation. This is crucial to the work described here since it allows an accurate measure of the time course of perceptual change. The technique also provides information concerning the phonemic relationship between each transform and the presented stimulus as well as the phonemic relationship between successive percepts. A detailed description of these relationships will be presented elsewhere.[16] Second, in order to evaluate whether temporal regularities characterize the evolving pattern of illusory changes and obtain better statistical resolution, we must examine very many such changes. For this reason, we extend the total number of repetitions in an experimental run substantially beyond that used in previous studies.

II. EXPERIMENTAL METHOD

Subjects. Ten Florida Atlantic University students volunteered as subjects. All of the students were native speakers of English with no known hearing deficit. The age range of the group was 22–32 years.

Stimuli. The syllables $[k\epsilon]$ and $[g\epsilon]$ were spoken by an adult male in a sound-insulated chamber, then digitized at 10 000 Hz. Each syllable was edited to a duration of 200 ms by truncating the vowel (by five pitch pulses or fewer) and ramping the amplitude of the final 50 ms for naturalness. Two stimulus sequences were constructed, each with a single syllable reproduced 1000 times with a 500 ms silent interval between successive tokens. Sequences were recorded onto audio tape for presentation to subjects.

Procedure. Subjects were told that they would hear 12-minute segments of auditory material, that certain sounds might be repeated over and over, but that other sounds might also be heard. The subject's task was to listen to each sound and, during the short silence between sounds, to write down what they heard. Subjects were tested individually in a quiet room. Six subjects listened to each stimulus sequence once in a single session. A 5 min rest break occurred between sequences, during which the subject annotated their response sheet, describing more fully any shorthand responses. Stimulus presentation was through headphones at a comfortable listening level (approximately 65 dB SPL). Based on preliminary results, we recruited four additional subjects who each participated in ten listening sessions, spaced throughout a two-week period. Sequence order was varied across subjects and sessions.

All subjects reported hearing changes in the syllables presented. The total number of variants in a single trial ranged from a low of 2 to a high of 26 across subjects and stimuli.

III. RESULTS AND DISCUSSION

In the present paper, we ignore the phonemic identity of the perceived forms and instead focus on the temporal characteristics of perceptual change. The event that we are particularly interested in is the length of time (denoted by the variable L) that any given percept is maintained before the perceived phonemic string switches to some other form. This quantity (hereafter referred to as the "dwell time") is of general interest because it reflects the putative interaction between two competitive perceptual processes. That is, on

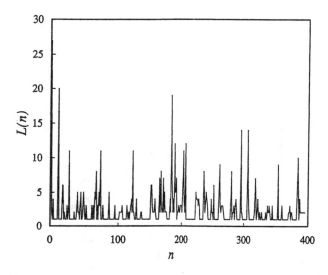

FIG. 1. $L(n)$ versus n for a typical experimental run. The stimulus is $[k\epsilon]$.

the one hand, perceptual systems exhibit a resistance to change when the stimulus itself is unchanging. On the other, perceptual systems become increasingly sensitized to aspects of the environment in which the stimulus is embedded so that the originally established percept is more likely to be replaced by another as time progresses. We believe that it is the interplay between these factors that underlies the phenomena we describe below and that it is the relative weight of the factors that changes with age.

The question we ask is whether listeners tend to maintain each percept for a characteristic length of time (with some variability) before switching to another phonemic form. Figure 1 plots the dwell time of the nth phonemic string $L(n)$ for a single typical experimental run of repeating $[k\epsilon]$ as a function of the ordering index n. Note the tremendous variation in the values of L. To be specific, the subject first reported a string of 27 consecutive $[k\epsilon]$ syllables [dwell time $L(1)=27$], followed by 2 $[k\text{æ}]$ syllables $[L(2)=2]$, followed by 1 instance of $[k\epsilon]$ $[L(3)=1]$, followed by 4 instances of $[k\text{æt}]$ $[L(4)=4]$, and so on. Treating $L(n)$ as a random variable, we examine the distribution of dwell times by plotting in Fig. 2(a) the histograms of $\ln N(L)$ versus $\ln L$. Here $N(L)$ is the total number of occurrences of phonemic strings that persisted for time L. To increase the statistical resolution we have collapsed our data across 10 sessions of single 1000-token trials for all of the 10 subjects. Data from trials of repeated $[k\epsilon]$ (square) are shown separately from those of repeated $[g\epsilon]$ (diamond). We arbitrarily connect the data points from the same stimulus sequence to guide the eye. Evidently the function of $N(L)$ versus L can be roughly fit by a power law,

$$N(L) \sim L^{-\alpha}, \qquad (1)$$

where α is the scaling exponent whose value is about 1.6. Plots for individual sessions show similar power law behavior, although with more variability in the straight line fits, thus justifying the use of collapsed data in Fig. 2(a). The

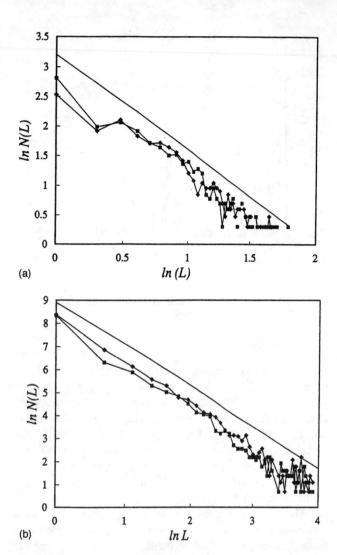

(a)

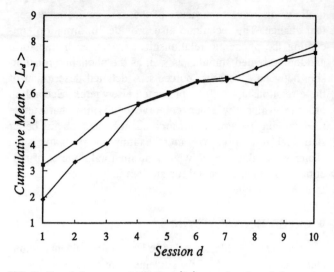

FIG. 3. Cumulative mean dwell time $\langle L_d \rangle$ as a function of the session number d. See text for more details. ■ $=[k\epsilon]$; ♦ $=[g\epsilon]$.

(b)

FIG. 2. (a) ln $N(L)$ versus ln L for ten subjects, each given one presentation of each stimulus sequence. The slope of the straight line is 1.6. (b) ln $N(L)$ versus ln L for four subjects, each given ten presentations of each stimulus sequence. The slope of the straight line is 1.8. In both graphs, ■ $=[k\epsilon]$ and ♦ $=[g\epsilon]$.

quantity $P(L)=N(L)/N$, with N the total number of perceived strings, approximates the probability that a given percept persists for the length of L. Thus,

$$P(L)\sim L^{-\alpha}. \tag{2}$$

Equation (2) appears to be a general attribute of the present experimental paradigm and bears several interesting consequences. If the strings of identical percepts have a finite average dwell time, $\langle L \rangle$, then its value could be considered a reference scale by which to measure time. In particular, switches among percepts could be said to occur with an average rate of $1/\langle L \rangle$. But, when $\alpha < 2$ in Eq. (2), the first moment $\langle L \rangle$ is in fact infinite due to the divergent sum

$$\sum_1^\infty LP(L)\sim\sum_1^\infty L^{1-\alpha}=\infty. \tag{3}$$

For the data displayed in Fig. 2(a), the slope α for both the $[k\epsilon]$ and $[g\epsilon]$ distributions is less than 2. This means that a

characteristic time scale cannot be established for the shifting perceptions. In the literature, such processes have been referred to as fractal times.[17]

One might consider that the nonexistence of a finite average $\langle L \rangle$ is caused by the experimental methodology not allowing the perceptual system sufficient time to establish a consistent time scale. In order to evaluate this, we present further results from four subjects who each participated in ten listening sessions. As shown in Fig. 2(b), the larger dataset collected over a prolonged time period leads to a smoother distribution of ln $N(L)$ versus ln L, which again shows a power law relationship with $\alpha < 2$. This suggests that there is indeed a power law governing the switching events in the phonemic transformations with no characteristic time scales.

In practice, Eq. (3) implies that the computed average dwell time increases when more data are collected. To verify this experimentally we separate the data in Fig. 2(b) according to the session (day) in which they were gathered. We then calculate the mean length of time that percepts persist $\langle L_1 \rangle$ for the data of the first experimental session, the mean $\langle L_2 \rangle$ for the combined data of session 1 and session 2, the mean $\langle L_3 \rangle$ for the combined data of sessions 1, 2 and 3, and so on. The result is shown in Fig. 3. As one can see, the cumulative means form generally increasing functions as the dataset increases in size for both $[k\epsilon]$ and $[g\epsilon]$ (the squares and diamonds, respectively), indicating the nonexistence of a finite average $\langle L \rangle$. It is important to note that this behavior is intrinsic to the distribution of L, and without a proper understanding of this, one may erroneously ascribe a mean to the collected data and draw unwarranted conclusions.

In the above analysis only the distribution of L is considered. Our next objective is to study the correlation of L over time. By directly inspecting the data one observes an apparent trend that a long $L(n)$ tends to be followed by a short $L(n+1)$, and likewise a short $L(n)$ tends to be followed by a long $L(n+1)$. To demonstrate this we introduce a new variable which is the nth step increment (or decrement) $I(n)=L(n+1)-L(n)$. In Fig. 4 we plot $I(n+1)$ ver-

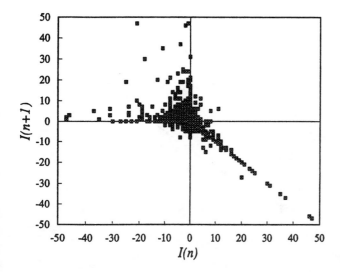

FIG. 4. $I(n+1)$ versus $I(n)$ for a typical subject. The stimulus is $[k\epsilon]$.

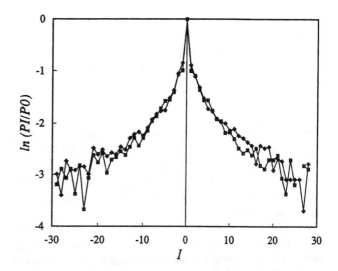

FIG. 5. The normalized distribution of $I(n)$. PI is the number of occurrences of the value I and $P0$ is the number of occurrences of 0 in the increments and decrements data. $\blacksquare = [k\epsilon]$; $\blacklozenge = [g\epsilon]$.

sus $I(n)$ collapsed over all the runs with the stimulus $[k\epsilon]$ for a typical subject. The displayed points have a stronger concentration in the second and fourth quadrants, indicating that a positive $I(n)$ is more likely to be followed by a negative $I(n)$, and vice versa. Data sequences exhibiting this character have been called anticorrelated. Recently, there have been reports in the literature showing that in certain physiological systems such as the heart,[18] not only are the relevant variables anticorrelated, but the correlation seems to have an extremely long range. To study this issue for our system we employ a systematic method introduced by Peng et al.[18] based on the increments $I(n)$. Specifically, a mean fluctuation function $F(n)$ is computed which is defined as

$$F(n) \equiv \overline{|L(n'+n) - L(n')|}$$
$$= \overline{|I(n') + I(n'+1) + \cdots + I(n'+n-1)|}. \quad (4)$$

The overbar indicates an ensemble average, which in the present context is the average over all dwell times n' in a given session, and then averaged across sessions. Operationally, this is equivalent to setting a fixed distance n (initially 1), moving the beginning point sequentially from $n'=1$ to $n'=2$ to $n'=3$, and so on, then calculating the quantity $F(n)$ for n ranging from 1 to 50. The average across the ten sessions is then calculated for each subject. (Another approach is to concatenate the results from all sessions to create a single time series for each subject. The drawback is that it introduces artificial effects at the conjunction points between different sessions.) As explained in Ref. 19, the behavior of $F(n)$ for large n is indicative of the nature of the correlation property in the time series. In particular, if

$$F(n) \sim n^{\beta}, \quad (5)$$

for large n, then $0 \leq \beta < 1/2$ means that the time series is long-range anticorrelated, $\beta = 1/2$ indicates that the time series is uncorrelated or the correlation decays very fast, and $\beta > 1/2$ corresponds to a long-range, positively correlated time series. If the time series is anticorrelated one can suspect that the system is controlled by some stabilizing process. In the case of positive correlation the opposite happens

in that a positive $I(n)$ is more likely to be followed by another positive $I(n+1)$, and a negative $I(n)$ is more likely to be followed by a negative $I(n+1)$, suggesting an underlying destabilizing process.

The distributions of $I(n)$ for both stimulus sequences in our experiment are highly similar and are shown in Fig. 5. Thus far we have not determined what type of distribution fits the data best, but this will not affect the correlation result below. Figure 6 shows the log–log plot of $F(n)$ versus n calculated using Eq. (4). Evidently the curve can be roughly fit by a straight line with a slope close to zero. This seems to indicate long-range anticorrelation. But, upon further reflection of the method, we find that this type of plot may have more than one explanation. Specifically, consider a stationary time series $x(t)$ with $\overline{x(t)} = 0$. The mean fluctuation function is defined as

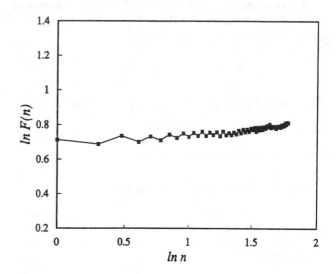

FIG. 6. $\ln F(n)$ versus $\ln n$ averaged over all listening sessions and both stimulus sequences for four subjects.

$$F(T) \equiv \sqrt{\overline{[x(t+T)-x(t)]^2}},$$

where the overbar indicates ensemble average. [To facilitate analysis we adopt here the equivalent definition of $F(T)$ using the variance.] After simple algebra we get

$$F(T) = \sqrt{2\sigma^2 - 2C(T)},$$

where $\sigma^2 = \overline{x(t)^2}$ is a constant and $C(T) = \overline{x(t+T)x(t)}$ is the autocorrelation function. If $x(t)$ is uncorrelated, $C(T) = 0$ for $T > 0$, then $F(T)$ can be viewed as an algebraic function of T with an exponent $\beta = 0$. While this type of time series will yield a plot similar to that of Fig. 6 it is clearly not long-range anticorrelated.

A more direct way to quantify the correlation between the $L(n)$'s is to compute the autocorrelation function itself. But this function tends to be more variable when compared to the following method. The technique we employ is similar to that of Peng *et al.* but treats $L(n)$ as the relevant variable instead of $I(n)$. This technique can be considered as a variant of the Hurst rescaled range analysis commonly used in studying the fractal character of time records.[19,20] Again the results can be accounted for without assuming long-range correlation.

Define a mean range function $G(n)$ as

$$G(n) \equiv \sqrt{\overline{[L(n')+L(n'+1)+\cdots+L(n'+n-1)]^2}}. \quad (6)$$

The overbar indicates the average over all strings n' in a given session, and then across sessions. Essentially, what is being done here is to treat the $L(n)$'s as the step taken in a random walk and examine the variance of the walker's position after the nth step. This is an indirect way to study the correlation among $L(n)$'s, but since the definition involves more averaging, the results tend to be less noisy. Figure 7 shows $\ln G(n)$ versus $\ln n$ calculated for the perception data. It can be seen that, while for relatively large n the log–log curve shows a scaling region with a slope close to 1, for relatively small n there is a markedly smaller slope. We present theoretical arguments explaining this empirical observation.

Suppose that we have a total of N perceived strings of identical phonemic forms. From Eq. (2), the number of strings $N(L)$ with dwell time L is

$$\frac{N(L)}{N} \sim L^{-\alpha}.$$

The longest dwell time L_m in this dataset is thus

$$L_m \sim N^{1/\alpha}.$$

Using this L_m we calculate $\overline{L}$ to be

$$\overline{L} \sim \sum_{L=1}^{L_m} L L^{-\alpha} \sim \frac{1}{2-\alpha} L_m^{2-\alpha} \sim N^{(2-\alpha)/\alpha},$$

and $\overline{L^2}$ to be

$$\overline{L^2} \sim N^{(3-\alpha)/\alpha}.$$

Since our aim here is to obtain order of magnitude estimates, the sums above are replaced by integrals. Other approxima-

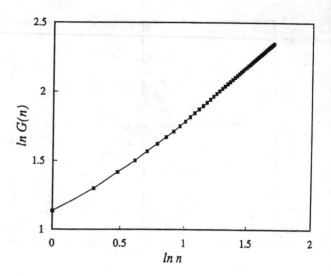

FIG. 7. $\ln G(n)$ versus $\ln n$ averaged over all listening sessions and both stimulus sequences for four subjects.

tions are valid for large N and for $1 < \alpha < 2$. Assuming that $L(n)$'s are uncorrelated [similar analysis can be carried out for short-range correlated $L(n)$'s], the mean fluctuation function $G(n)$ defined in Eq. (6) can be written as

$$G(n) = \sqrt{n\overline{L^2} + n(n-1)\overline{L}^2}$$
$$\sim \sqrt{nN^{(3-\alpha)/\alpha} + n(n-1)N^{(4-2\alpha)/\alpha}}. \quad (7)$$

Comparing $\overline{L^2}$ and $\overline{L}^2$ one has

$$\overline{L^2}/\overline{L}^2 \sim N^{(\alpha-1)/\alpha}.$$

Namely, when N is large, $\overline{L^2}$ dominates $\overline{L}^2$. Reflected in Eq. (7), this means that when n is small the first term dominates, consistent with the observation in Fig. 7 that the slope is smaller in the small n region. The second term, however, grows faster and can overtake the first when n becomes large. Thus, as n increases, the $\ln G(n)$ versus $\ln n$ plot will have an increasing slope, approaching one. Again this conforms with the data shown in Fig. 7.

IV. SUMMARY

In this paper we show that when several different percepts arise from the same physical stimulus, the distribution of the time spent within each phonemic form, the dwell time, obeys a power law whose exponent lies between 1 and 2. This finding, together with other evidence, suggests that within the present paradigm, perception does not possess a characteristic time scale. Such temporal power laws with noninteger exponents occur in an array of natural systems of practical interest (see Ref. 17 and references therein) but are not typically explored in studies of perceptual systems (but see Ref. 21).

In our attempt to ascertain the correlation properties among the successive dwell times we found that the outcome of a commonly used method can have more than one explanation. We analyze the cause of this and show that for our system the correlation present on the short time scale is unlikely to be long-ranged.

Finally, we mention that although the results of this paper are interesting in their own right from a psychological point of view, a more important consequence may be that they form the basis for investigations of special populations. In particular, the analysis technique may have wide implications for assessing the loss of cognitive flexibility with aging, Alzheimer's disease, and non-Alzheimer's dementias, and for assessing the strength of the perception-production interaction in normal and disordered language acquisition. Theoretically, the present results constrain the type of models that can be built in attempts to explain normal auditory perceptual processes and their breakdown. This latter point is particularly relevant and timely given the increasing trend toward using physically motivated theories to understand higher brain functions.[22,23]

ACKNOWLEDGMENTS

We thank Larry Liebovitch for discussions. This work was supported by the NIH, NIMH, and ONR.

[1] R. M. Warren and R. Gregory, Am. J. Psychol. **71**, 612 (1958).

[2] R. M. Warren, Brit. J. Psychol. **52**, 249 (1961).

[3] J. M. Clegg, Brit. J. Psychol. **62**, 303 (1971).

[4] N. J. Esposito, Percept. Mot. Skills **61**, 1019 (1985).

[5] L. M. Goldstein and J. R. Lackner, Cognition **2**, 279 (1974).

[6] R. N. Ohde and D. J. Sharf, J. Acoust. Soc. Am. **66**, 30 (1979).

[7] R. N. Ohde and D. J. Sharf, J. Acoust. Soc. Am. **68**, 1266 (1980).

[8] N. J. Lass and R. M. Gasperini, Brit. J. Psychol. **64**, 183 (1973).

[9] R. M. Warren, Am. J. Psychol. **74**, 506 (1961).

[10] R. M. Warren and R. P. Warren, J. Verbal Learn. Verbal Behavior **5**, 142 (1966).

[11] R. L. Diehl, K. R. Kluender, and E. M. Parker, J. Exp. Psychol.: Human Percept. Perf. **11**, 209 (1985).

[12] R. M. Warren and M. D. Meyers, J. Phonetics **15**, 169 (1987).

[13] J. Débigaré, R. Desaulniers, H. Mercier, and M.-C. Ouellette, Rev. Can. Psychol. **40**, 29 (1986).

[14] J. R. Edmonson, J. M. Hutchinson, and M. A. Nerbonne, J. Aud. Res. **21**, 85 (1981).

[15] K. Henn-Reinke, Doctoral dissertation, University of Wisconsin—Milwaukee, 1986.

[16] B. Tuller, M. Ding, and J. A. S. Kelso, in preparation.

[17] M. F. Shlesinger, Ann. Rev. Phys. Chem. **39**, 269 (1988).

[18] C.-K. Peng, J. Mietus, J. M. Hausdorff, S. Havlin, H. E. Stanley, and A. L. Goldberger, Phys. Rev. Lett. **70**, 1343 (1993).

[19] J. Feder, *Fractals* (Plenum, New York, 1988).

[20] J. B. Bassingthwaighte, L. S. Liebovitch, and B. J. West, *Fractal Physiology* (Oxford University Press, New York, 1994).

[21] J. A. S. Kelso, P. Case, T. Holroyd, E. Horvath, J. Rączaszek, B. Tuller, and M. Ding, "Multistability and metastability in perceptual and brain dynamics," in *Multistability in Cognition*, edited by M. Stadler and P. Kruse (Springer-Verlag, Berlin, in press).

[22] J. A. S. Kelso, *Dynamic Patterns: The Self-Organization of Brain and Behavior* (MIT Press, Cambridge, MA, in press).

[23] T. M. McKenna, T. A. McMullen, and M. F. Shlesinger, Neuroscience **60**, 587 (1994).

Nonlinear dynamics in pulsatile secretion of parathyroid hormone in normal human subjects

Klaus Prank,[a] Heio Harms, Georg Brabant, and Rolf-Dieter Hesch[b]

Abteilung Klinische Endokrinologie, Medizinische Hochschule Hannover, Konstanty-Gutschow-Str. 8, D-30625 Hannover, Germany

Matthias Dämmig and Fedor Mitschke

Institut für Quantenoptik, Universität Hannover, Welfengarten 1, D-30167 Hannover, Germany

(Received 10 May 1994; accepted for publication 8 August 1994)

In many biological systems, information is transferred by hormonal ligands, and it is assumed that these hormonal signals encode developmental and regulatory programs in mammalian organisms. In contrast to the dogma of endocrine homeostasis, it could be shown that the biological information in hormonal networks is not only present as a constant hormone concentration in the circulation pool. Recently, it has become apparent that hormone pulses contribute to this hormonal pool, which modulates the responsiveness of receptors within the cell membrane by regulation of the receptor synthesis, movement within the membrane layer, coupling to signal transduction proteins and internalization. Phase space analysis of dynamic parathyroid hormone (PTH) secretion allowed the definition of a (in comparison to normal subjects) relatively quiet "low dynamic" secretory pattern in osteoporosis, and a "high dynamic" state in hyperparathyroidism. We now investigate whether this pulsatile secretion of PTH in healthy men exhibits characteristics of nonlinear determinism. Our findings suggest that this is conceivable, although on the basis of presently available data and techniques, no proof can be established. Nevertheless, pulsatile secretion of PTH might be a first example of nonlinear deterministic dynamics in an apparently irregular hormonal rhythm in human physiology. © *1995 American Institute of Physics.*

I. INTRODUCTION

Deterministic chaos has been proposed as the underlying principle of organization in many systems, including biological ones.[1,2] The possibility of chaotic behavior has been discussed for the dynamics of the electrical activity of the human heart[3,4] and the brain.[5] In simple organisms, the detection of nonlinear behavior in information transfer is associated with differentiation and proliferation.[6] Modulation of the amplitude and/or the frequency of the hormone pulses in higher organisms can modify intracellular signaling pathways,[7] gene expression,[8] cell proliferation,[9] and cellular function.[10]. Changes in the mean serum concentration are generated by this amplitude and/or frequency modulation.[11,12] Since episodic hormone secretion and negative feedback control are recognized as general phenomena,[13,14] we investigated whether nonlinear determinism can be identified in information transfer of the endocrine regulation.

Recently, we were able to demonstrate[15] that the low dynamic pattern of parathyroid hormone (PTH) secretion in osteoporosis is associated with a loss of both trabecular bone connectivity and bone mass. This result is in accordance with animal experiments: Tam *et al.*[16] showed that if the circulating hormonal pool of PTH is artificially kept constant in rats, there is a disruption of bone apposition and resorption, resulting in a loss of the normal trabecular bone structure. On the other hand, discontinuous injection of PTH increased trabecular bone network and enhanced bone mass. The same

results could be found when the experiments were repeated in the greyhound.[17] It was also demonstrated recently[18] that a loss of bone mass in rats due to ovarian hormone deficiency could be reversed through discontinuous injection of PTH.

In contrast to the situation with osteoporosis, patients with hyperparathyroidism, a condition under which an increase of trabecular bone network can be observed,[19] show a characteristic high dynamic secretion of PTH.[15] The secretion of PTH in normal human subjects is characterized by frequent burst-like pulses with high amplitudes, as demonstrated independently by several groups.[20–22] Our purpose was to determine whether the secretory pattern of PTH could be described by a nonlinear deterministic process. Such characterization might help in modeling the secretory dynamics of PTH and explain the disruption of the normal secretory pattern in osteoporotic and hyperparathyroid patients.

II. SUBJECTS AND METHODS

A. Subjects

Here we report studies on three healthy young male volunteers (aged 20–30 yr). Our studies were approved by the local Committee on Medical Ethics, and all subjects gave their informed written consent. All study subjects had an unremarkable personal and family medical history and were nonsmokers. Physical examination, white blood count, differential, protein, creatinine clearance, albumin, total calcium, sodium, potassium, phosphate, magnesium, chloride,

---

[a]Present address: Seestrasse 1, D-78464 Konstanz, Germany.
[b]Author to whom correspondence should be addressed.

creatinine, triglycerides, cholestoral, glucose, nitrogen, alkaline phosphatase activity, and electrocardiogram were normal in all subjects.

B. Sampling protocol

Blood sampling and further processing of samples was carried out by three trained persons. PTH concentration was measured from 1800–1800 h in *subjects 1 and 3,* and from 1800–1500 h in *subject 2.* Blood samples (1 ml) were drawn every 2 min via a central venous catheter within 3 s. The specimens were then centrifuged at 4 °C and frozen at −20 °C within 45 min. Twenty-four hours before sampling no alcohol intake, medication, or caffeine was permitted. The central venous catheter was placed one hour before the initiation of blood sampling. Throughout the study, the subjects rested in bed.

C. Determination of hormone concentration

The PTH concentrations were measured in duplicate using a two-site chemiluminometric (sandwich) immunoassay (Magic Lite Intact PTH, Ciba-Corning Diagnostics Corporation, Medfield, MA; intra-assay coefficient of variation 3.0%). This assay comprises acridiniumester-labeled sheep antihuman amino-terminal PTH (1-34) antibodies and mouse monoclonal antihuman PTH (44-68) regional antibodies covalently coupled to paramagnetic particles and synthetic human PTH (1-84) standards.

D. Data analysis

With a very small amount of data as we have here, one has no choice but to proceed with the assumption that the underlying process is stationary in the statistical sense. In the Sec. III we will have to come back to this assumption.

Quasiperiodicity was ruled out by examination of the Fourier spectrum of the time series (calculated with a standard NAG library routine) of PTH concentration. A distinction between nonlinear deterministic and random data cannot be done by merely calculating dimensions, because several pitfalls can easily create a mirage.[23] In particular, finite point size effects[24] or linear correlations[25,26] may result in spurious convergence of the dimension estimate, even for purely stochastic data. Therefore, we made use of the "surrogate technique" advocated by Theiler.[27] This technique involves the creation of dummy, or surrogate, data sets that represent randomized versions of the original, to benchmark the original against. To generate such surrogates, Theiler suggests two procedures that emphasize on different statistical aspects of the data.

The original is Fourier transformed to obtain magnitude and phase spectra. The phases are then replaced with independent, identically distributed random numbers taken from a $[0,2\pi]$ interval. After transforming back to the time domain, one obtains a randomized data set that has, however, precisely the same power spectrum as the original. This kind of surrogate data is suitable to determine whether the signal can be described by a stationary Gaussian linear stochastic model.

The second procedure, slightly more complicated, permutes the original data points (hence the amplitude distribution of the original is preserved in the surrogates) in such a way that the power spectrum remains very similar. This kind of surrogate data is to be preferred whenever the original data are far from Gaussian distributed.

In either case, several surrogate data sets are prepared for each original to allow for a quantitative evaluation of the comparison. A measure for the amount of deterministic structure that has been destroyed by the randomization is given by the significance S, defined as

$$S = \frac{\langle X_{\text{surr}} \rangle - X_{\text{orig}}}{\sigma},$$ (1)

where X is an estimate of either the correlation dimension D_2, the correlation entropy K_2, or some other suitable statistical measure of the data. Here $\langle\ \rangle$ denotes the average over all surrogates, and sigma is the standard deviation of the scatter of the surrogates.

Any use of low pass filters to improve the signal-to-noise ratio can create systematic errors in the dimension calculation. Therefore, all calculations were performed on nonfiltered data, with one exception (see Sec. III). In that case, we used an acausal filter that avoids filter-induced errors.[28]

The trajectory of the PTH secretory dynamics in phase space was reconstructed by time delayed variables[29,30] from the PTH time series. All data sets were evaluated for the correlation dimension D_2 and correlation entropy K_2 by the algorithm of Grassberger and Procaccia.[31] The relevance of D_2 is that for a random process, one expects not to find any finite value for D_2, whereas in a deterministic system the first integer larger than D_2 provides a lower bound of the number of degrees of freedom in the underlying dynamical system. In particular, noninteger values of D_2 are considered as evidence for the existence of an underlying attractor, which is then a fractal invariant set in phase space.

It is important, however, to understand the limitations of a correlation dimension estimation using the algorithm of Grassberger and Procaccia. There exists a minimum amount of data points for any required degree of accuracy.[32,24]

The algorithm of Grassberger and Procaccia also yields an estimate of the correlation entropy K_2^{33}. This quantity is zero for periodic or quasiperiodic signals, and infinite for delta-correlated noise. It also is an estimator for the information entropy K_1, which equals the sum of the positive Lyapunov exponents. Therefore K_2 will be useful for a consistency check of the Lyapunov exponents.

Lyapunov exponents are the average exponential rates of divergence or convergence of nearby orbits in phase space. There are as many Lyapunov exponents λ_i, as there are degrees of freedom in the dynamical system.

From the PTH data, we calculated the most positive exponent λ_+ with an algorithm proposed by Wolf *et al.*[34] Note that if the algorithm returns a positive value for λ_+, this does not prove chaos by itself, since positive results can readily occur for random signals.[35] After temporal inversion, the same algorithm was used for calculating the most negative exponent λ_-. For any stable dissipative deterministic sys-

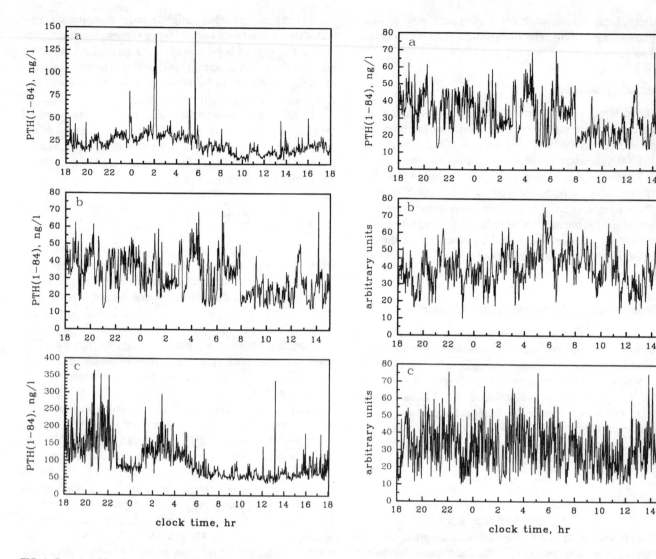

FIG. 1. Representative time series of PTH (1-84) concentrations in plasma of three healthy young male subjects. (a) *subject 1*; (b) *subject 2*; and (c) *subject 3*.

FIG. 2. (a) Time series of PTH (1-84) concentrations in plasma of *subject 2*; (b) time series of one surrogate data set corresponding to the original time series shown in (a) (generated by *procedure 1*); and (c) time series of one surrogate data set corresponding to the original time series shown in (a) (generated by *procedure 2*).

tem, $\Sigma_{\lambda_i<0}|\lambda_i|>\Sigma_{\lambda_i>0}\,\lambda_i$ must hold. Therefore, in cases of low-dimensional chaos, one would typically expect $|\lambda_-|>\lambda_+$.

III. RESULTS

Figure 1 shows the time series of the PTH concentration in plasma, taken from three healthy subjects. Examples of corresponding surrogates generated by *procedures 1 and 2* are shown for *subject 2* in Fig. 2. Visual inspection reveals that either type of surrogates has its specific merits.

Procedure 1 (same power spectrum) yields a better overall similarity in appearance, but the tendency to strong sharp spikes is somewhat reduced. On the other hand, *procedure 2* reproduces the spikiness well, but tends to enhance the high-frequency content. The power spectrum (Fig. 3) of the same data consists of a broadband continuum with no prominent features. The same result was found upon analysis of the data from the other subjects. As long as we maintain the assumption of stationarity, this rules out quasiperiodicity, and therefore the choices how to classify our data are narrowed down

to either chaotic or random signals. We emphasize at this point that the spectra contain considerable power density up to the highest frequencies (Nyquist limit), indicating that a sample interval of two minutes is certainly not too short.

While current technology does not allow shorter sampling intervals, it is conceivable that future continuous data acquisition might reveal further information.

In Fig. 4(a), the estimate of the correlation dimension D_2 is plotted as a function of the embedding dimension for the same data from *subject 2*. For comparison, the results for ten surrogate data sets with identical power spectrum (*procedure 1*) are represented through their confidence range, defined as the mean value plus/minus one standard deviation. Figure 4(b) shows the same, except that *procedure 2* (identical value histogram) was used. The curve for the original data converges in the neighborhood of $D_2=5$, whereas for the surrogates of either case, there is a steady increase with embedding dimension up to values where point number effects render the results meaningless. It is quite apparent that there

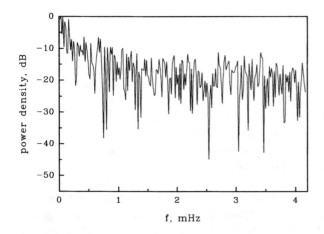

FIG. 3. Fourier power spectrum of the time series of PTH concentration (*subject 2*).

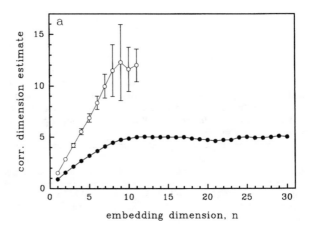

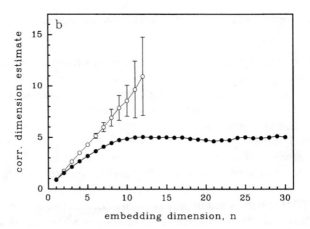

FIG. 4. Diagram of correlation dimension estimates (slope of correlation integral) versus the embedding dimension n. Filled circles: Original data (*subject 2*). Open circles: mean value $\pm$ one standard deviation for ten corresponding surrogate data sets. (a) Surrogate data sets generated with *procedure 1* (see Sec. II D). The scaling region for all data was chosen to range from 0.13 to 0.17 in units of global maximum distance. The original exhibits a clear convergence near $D_2=5$, while the surrogates climb up to a saturation value set by the limited point number, until, above embedding dimension $n \approx 20$, the algorithm fails to return well-defined slopes for the surrogates; (b) surrogate data sets generated with *procedure 2* (see Sec. II D). The scaling region was the same as for (a). The original converges as in (a), while the surrogates climb up until above $n \approx 12$, the algorithm fails to return well-defined slopes for the surrogates.

is a difference of the order of two standard deviations between surrogates, and original for both procedures. While the first procedure might be fooled due to non-Gaussian distribution of the original, this source of error is ruled out with the second procedure. This comes at the price that the second procedure does not leave the power spectrum totally unchanged, but tends to enhance high-frequency spectral components. While this is hard to judge from a broadband spectrum, there is, in fact, a somewhat faster decay in autocorrelation, in comparison to the original data.

To convince ourselves that this effect is not the cause for the observed significant differences between original and surrogates, we also artificially enhanced high-frequency components of the original, such that its autocorrelation matched that of the surrogates, and found that the convergence of the dimension estimate to a value of about 5 was not affected.

Our results therefore strongly support an interpretation that there is nonlinear determinism in the signal. Table I lists the results for similar calculations involving data from all subjects, and also for calculations of the entropy K_2 and the Lyapunov exponents λ_+ and λ_-. Note that the surrogate technique is not applicable to Lyapunov calculations.[35]

For *subject 3*, the raw data yield poor convergence for the dimension estimate. The D_2 value given in Table I was obtained from filtered data (see above). All other entries are based on unfiltered data. Following Smith,[32] we find that for 721 data points, a 30% wide "scaling region," and correlation dimensions up to $D_2=5$, as we encounter here, the best estimate for D_2 has a 20% error margin. This renders distinction of post-decimal digits pointless. Similarly, the error bars on the Lyapunov exponents are considerable. This caveat notwithstanding, it is reassuring to find that consistently $|\lambda_-|>\lambda_+$. Also, comparisons of λ_+ with K_2 show that the computational results are mutually consistent.

IV. DISCUSSION

The self-organization of cellular structures, organs, and organisms needs encoding of biological information in deterministic systems. The hormonal system is the major biologi-

cal system, which by modulation of membrane/nuclear receptors and ion channels communicates developmental and regulatory programs in mammalian organisms. Nonlinear information transfer in experimental biological systems and simple organisms influences differentiation and proliferation by its regulation of gene expression.

It was unknown, however, whether nonlinear determinism might be responsible for the rich structural and functional organization of higher mammalian organisms. Our results suggest such a possibility.

Our analysis leads to the following conclusion: For the observed oscillatory dynamic fluctuations of intact PTH in the circulating blood of our three healthy subjects, simple stochastic models were shown not to explain the observed convergence of the dimension estimate. Thus, an interpreta-

TABLE I. Results of data analysis. D_2: correlation dimension; K_2: correlation entropy; λ_+: the most positive Lyapunov exponent; λ_-: the most negative Lyapunov exponent; orig: the original measured data; surr: average of ten surrogate data sets generated according to *procedure 2*; A qualitatively different convergence behavior was found for original and surrogate data: for most cases, there was no convergence for the surrogates (symbol: *). S: significance as defined in Eq. (1), calculated with the same computational parameters (attractor reconstruction parameters and length scale chosen for the determination of the slope of the correlation integral) as for the corresponding original data. *n/a*: not applicable since Lyapunov exponents are not suitable for the surrogate technique.

Subject	D_2	S	K_2 bit/2 min	S	λ_+ bit/2 min	λ_- bit/2 min
1 orig	2...2.5	5	0.09...0.12	2.4	0.12	−0.20
surr	*		*		n/a	n/a
2 orig	5	2.5	0.14...0.17	2.2	0.16	−0.32
surr	*		*		n/a	n/a
3 orig	4...5	2	0.14...0.19	2.4	0.09	−0.11
surr	*		0.50		n/a	n/a

tion of the dynamics as being due to an underlying deterministically chaotic process is conceivable as an explanation.

We must caution that with the presently available means, nonstationary stochastic processes cannot be ruled out. It stands to reason, though, that strong nonstationarity would likely have wiped out fractal phase space structure. The fact that we do detect convergence to a finite correlation dimension, if only over a small scaling region, suggests that stationarity might be reasonable as a first assumption.

While the situation awaits further clarification, one may discuss whether an interpretation of chaos would make good physiological sense. Indeed, chaotic systems presumably allow an optimal adaptation to their fluctuating environmental parameters.

See, e.g. Ref. 36, where it has been shown that chaotic optimization is potentially superior to other optimization schemes. It is therefore conceivable that organisms organized by chaos might have had a competitive edge over different designs in the process of evolution.

It is thus tempting to speculate that chaotic dynamics of PTH secretion provide the optimal stimulation pattern for the functional coupling of osteoclasts and osteoblasts in the physiological bone remodeling process, which determines the three-dimensional trabecular architecture of bone.

Our findings would then suggest a new interpretation of osteoporosis and hyperparathyroidism as dynamical diseases,[37] associated with the loss of an adaptive hormonal rhythm.

It has been argued recently that chaotic signals can be controlled by applying judiciously chosen, minute perturbations precisely because chaos is highly sensitive to initial conditions.[38] Following this point of view, an evolutionary advantage of controlled chaos has been discussed by Doebeli.[39]

This approach has been employed successfully, among other experiments, to stabilize cardiac arrhythmias induced in the rabbit ventricle: By administering weak electric stimuli to the heart at certain times, the arrhythmia could be converted to periodic beating.[40]

Following this line of thought, any proof of chaos in some process of a living organism might gain clinical relevance in the future, because it opens an avenue toward a strategy of its control.

Let us finally point out that it has been proposed to consider health in biological systems as an "information-rich" broadband state,[41] as opposed to pathological situations, which would be characterized by a loss of information (narrow-band state).[42] We have advanced the hypothesis of a "dynamic code."[43,44] This term is meant to signify the functional coding of biological information in time, which would be complementary to the structural coding of information by the "genetic code." While this hypothesis must be regarded as speculative for the moment, we do feel that it can help to explain the physiological linkage of functional programs of the developing and the mature organism to genetic programs.

ACKNOWLEDGMENTS

This work was supported in part by a travel grant from the *Deutsche Forschungsgemeinschaft*.

[1] L. Glass and M. C. Mackey, *From Clocks to Chaos: The Rhythms of Life* (Princeton University Press, Princeton, NJ, 1988).

[2] H. Degn, A. V. Holden, and L. F. Olsen, *Chaos in Biological Systems* (Plenum, New York, 1987).

[3] L. Glass, A. L. Goldberger, M. Courtemanche, and A. Shrier, "Nonlinear dynamics, chaos, and complex cardiac arrhythmias," Philos. Trans. R. Soc. London Ser. 1 A **413**, 9–26 (1987).

[4] A. Babloyantz and A. Destexhe, "Is the normal heart a periodic oscillator?" Biol. Cybernet. **58**, 203–211 (1988).

[5] A. Babloyantz and A. Destexhe, "Low-dimensional chaos in an instance of epilepsy," Proc. Natl. Acad. Sci. USA **83**, 3513–3517 (1986).

[6] A. Goldbeter and Y. X. Li, "Frequency coding in intercellular communication," in *Cell to Cell Signaling: From Experiments to Theoretical Models*, edited by A. Goldbeter (Academic, London, 1989), pp. 415–432.

[7] C. Schöfl, A. Sanchez-Bueno, G. Brabant, P. H. Cobbold, and K. S. R. Cuthbertson, "Frequency and amplitude enhancement of calcium transients by cyclic AMP in hepatocytes," Biochem. J. **273**, 799–802 (1991).

[8] D. J. Waxman, N. A. Pampori, P. A. Ram, A. K. Agrawal, and B. H. Shapiro, "Interpulse interval in circulating growth hormone patterns regulates sexually dimorphic expression of hepatic cytochrome P450," Proc. Natl. Acad. Sci. USA **88**, 6868–6872 (1991).

[9] J. Isgaard, L. Carlsson, O. G. Isaksson, and J. O. Jansson, "Pulsatile intravenous growth hormone (GH) infusion to hypophysectomized rats increases insulin-like growth factor I messenger ribonucleic acid in skeletal tissues more effectively than continuous GH infusion," Endocrinology **123**, 2605–2610 (1988).

[10] E. Knobil, "The neuroendocrine control of the menstrual cycle," Rec. Prog. Horm. Res. **36**, 53–88 (1980).

[11] G. Brabant, K. Prank, U. Ranft, T. Schuermeyer, T. O. F. Wagner, H. Hauser, B. Kummer, H. Feistner, R. D. Hesch, and A. von zur Mühlen, "Physiological regulation of circadian and pulsatile thyrotropin secretion in normal man and woman," J. Clin. Endocrinol. Metab. **70**, 403–409 (1990).

[12] J. D. Veldhuis, A. Iranmanesh, G. Lizarralde, and M. L. Johnson, "Amplitude modulation of a burstlike mode of cortisol secretion subserves the circadian glucocorticoid rhythm," Am. J. Physiol. **257**, E6–E14 (1989).

[13] W. F. Crowley and J. G. Hofler, *The Episodic Secretion of Hormones* (Wiley, New York, 1987).

[14] G. Brabant, K. Prank, and C. Schöfl, "Pulsatile patterns in hormone secretion," Trends Endocrinol. Metab. **3**, 183–190 (1992).

[15] H. M. Harms, K. Prank, U. Brosa, E. Schlinke, O. Neubauer, G. Brabant, and R. D. Hesch, "Classification of dynamical diseases by new mathematical tools: Application of multi-dimensional phase space analyses to the pulsatile secretion of parathyroid hormone," Eur. J. Clin. Invest. **22**, 371–377 (1992).

[16] C. S. Tam, J. N. Heersche, T. M. Murray, and J. A. Parsons, "Parathyroid hormone stimulates the bone apposition rate independently of its resorptive action: Differential effects of intermittent and continuous administration," Endocrinology **110**, 506–512 (1982).

[17] R. Podbesek, C. Edouard, P. J. Meunier, J. A. Parsons, J. Reeve, R. W. Stevenson, and J. M. Zanelli, "Effects of two regimes with synthetic human parathyroid hormone fragment on bone formation and the tissue balance of trabecular bone in greyhounds," Endocrinology **112**, 1000–1006 (1983).

[18] C. C. Liu, D. N. Kalu, E. Salerno, R. Echon, B. W. Hollis, and M. Ray, "Preexisting bone loss associated with ovariectomy in rats is reversed by parathyroid hormone," J. Bone Min. Res. **6**, 1071–1080 (1991).

[19] M. Parisien, S. J. Silverberg, E. Shane, L. de la Cruz, R. Lindsay, J. P. Bilezikian, and D. W. Dempster, "The histomorphometry of bone in primary hyperparathyroidism: Preservation of cancellous bone structure," J. Clin. Endocrinol. Metab. **70**, 930–938 (1990).

[20] H. Harms, U. Kaptaina, W. R. Külpmann, G. Brabant, and R. D. Hesch, "Pulse amplitude and frequency modulation of parathyroid hormone in plasma," J. Clin. Endocrinol. Metab. **69**, 843–851 (1989).

[21] N. Kitamura, C. Shigeno, K. Shiomi, K. Lee, S. Ohta, T. Sone, S. Katsushima, E. Tadamura, T. Kousaka, I. Yamamoto, S. Dokoh, and J. Konishi, "Episodic fluctuation in serum intact parathyroid hormone concentration in men," J. Clin. Endocrinol. Metab. **70**, 252–263 (1990).

[22] M. H. Samuels, J. Veldhuis, C. Cawley, R. J. Urban, M. Luther, B. Bauer, and G. Mundy, "Pulsatile secretion of parathyroid hormone in normal young subjects: assessment by deconvolution analysis," J. Clin. Endocrinol. Metab. **76**, 399–403 (1993).

[23] J. Theiler, "Estimating fractal dimension," J. Opt. Soc. Am. A **7**, 1055–1073 (1990).

[24] J. P. Eckmann and D. Ruelle, "Fundamental limitations for estimating dimensions and Lyapunov exponents in dynamical systems," Physica D **56**, 185–187 (1992).

[25] A. R. Osborne and A. Provenzale, "Finite correlation dimension for stochastic systems with power-law spectra," Physica D **35**, 357–381 (1989).

[26] J. Theiler, "Some comments on the correlation dimension of $1/f^{\alpha}$ noise," Phys. Lett. **155**, 480–493 (1991).

[27] J. Theiler, B. Galdrikian, A. Longtin, S. Eubank, and J. D. Farmer, "Using surrogate data to detect nonlinearity in time series," in *Nonlinear Modeling and Forecasting*, edited by M. Casdagli and S. Eubank (Addison-Wesley, Redwood City, CA, 1992), pp. 163–188.

[28] F. Mitschke, "Acausal filters for chaotic signals," Phys. Rev. A **41**, 1169–1171 (1990).

[29] N. H. Packard, J. P. Crutchfield, J. D. Farmer, and R. S. Shaw, "Geometry from a time series," Phys. Rev. Lett. **45**, 712–716 (1980).

[30] F. Takens, "Detecting strange attractors in turbulence," in *Dynamical Systems and Turbulence*, edited by D. A. Rand and L. S. Young, Lecture Notes in Mathematics (Springer-Verlag, Berlin, 1981), Vol. 898, pp. 366–381.

[31] P. Grassberger and I. Procaccia, "Characterization of strange attractors," Phys. Rev. Lett. **50**, 346–349 (1983).

[32] L. A. Smith, "Intrinsic limits on dimension calculations," Phys. Lett. A **133**, 283–288 (1988).

[33] P. Grassberger and I. Procaccia, "Estimation of the Kolmogorov entropy from a chaotic signal," Phys. Rev. A **28**, 2591–2593 (1983).

[34] A. Wolf, J. B. Swift, H. L. Swinney, and J. A. Vastano, "Determining Lyapunov exponents from a time series," Physica D **16**, 285–317 (1985).

[35] F. Mitschke and M. Dämmig, "Chaos versus noise in experimental data," Int. J. Bifurcation Chaos **3**, 693–702 (1993).

[36] G. Mantica and A. Sloan, "Chaotic optimization and the construction of fractals: Solution of the inverse problem," Complex Syst. **3**, 37–62 (1989).

[37] M. C. Mackey and J. G. Milton, "Dynamical diseases," Ann. NY Acad. Sci. **504**, 16–32 (1987).

[38] T. Shinbrot, E. Ott, C. Grebogi, and J. A. Yorke, "Using small perturbations to control chaos, " Nature **363**, 411–417 (1993).

[39] M. Doebeli, "The evolutionary advantage of controlled chaos," Proc. R. Soc. London Ser. B **254**, 281–285 (1993).

[40] A. Garfinkel, M. L. Spano, W. L. Ditto, and J. N. Weiss, "Controlling cardiac chaos," Science **257**, 1230–1235 (1992).

[41] A. L. Goldberger, V. Bhargava, B. J. West, and A. J. Mandell, "Some observations on the question: Is ventricular fibrillation 'chaos'?," Physica D **19**, 282–289 (1986).

[42] A. L. Goldberger, L. J. Findley, M. R. Blackburn, and A. J. Mandell, "Nonlinear dynamics in heart failure: Implications of long-wavelength cardiopulmonary oscillations," Am. Heart. J. **107**, 612–615 (1984).

[43] R. D. Hesch, "Classification of cell receptors," in *Current Topics in Pathology. Cell Receptors*, edited by G. Seifert (Springer-Verlag, Berlin, 1991), pp. 13–51.

[44] K. Prank, H. Harms, C. Kayser, G. Brabant, and R. D. Hesch, "The dynamic code: Information transfer in hormonal systems," in *Complexity, Chaos and Biological Evolution*, edited by E. Mosekilde and L. Mosekilde (Plenum, New York, 1992), pp. 95–118.

Quantification of scaling exponents and crossover phenomena in nonstationary heartbeat time series

C.-K. Peng
Cardiovascular Division, Harvard Medical School, Beth Israel Hospital, Boston, Massachusetts 02215 and Center for Polymer Studies and Department of Physics, Boston University, Boston, Massachusetts 02215

Shlomo Havlin
Department of Physics, Bar Ilan University, Ramat Gan, Israel

H. Eugene Stanley
Center for Polymer Studies and Department of Physics, Boston, Massachusetts 02215

Ary L. Goldberger
Cardiovascular Division, Harvard Medical School, Beth Israel Hospital, Boston, Massachusetts 02215

(Received 28 June 1994; accepted for publication 7 December 1994)

The healthy heartbeat is traditionally thought to be regulated according to the classical principle of homeostasis whereby physiologic systems operate to reduce variability and achieve an equilibrium-like state [Physiol. Rev. **9**, 399–431 (1929)]. However, recent studies [Phys. Rev. Lett. **70**, 1343–1346 (1993); *Fractals in Biology and Medicine* (Birkhauser-Verlag, Basel, 1994), pp. 55–65] reveal that under normal conditions, beat-to-beat fluctuations in heart rate display the kind of long-range correlations typically exhibited by dynamical systems far from equilibrium [Phys. Rev. Lett. **59**, 381–384 (1987)]. In contrast, heart rate time series from patients with severe congestive heart failure show a breakdown of this long-range correlation behavior. We describe a new method—detrended fluctuation analysis (DFA)—for quantifying this correlation property in non-stationary physiological time series. Application of this technique shows evidence for a crossover phenomenon associated with a change in short and long-range scaling exponents. This method may be of use in distinguishing healthy from pathologic data sets based on differences in these scaling properties. © *1995 American Institute of Physics.*

I. INTRODUCTION

Clinicians often describe the normal activity of the heart as "regular sinus rhythm." But in fact cardiac interbeat intervals normally fluctuate in a complex, apparently erratic manner[1,2] [Fig. 1(a)]. This highly irregular behavior has recently motivated researchers[3,4] to apply time series analyses that derive from statistical physics, especially methods for the study of critical phenomena where fluctuations at all length (time) scales occur. These studies show that under healthy conditions, interbeat interval time series exhibit long-range power-law correlations reminiscent of physical systems near a critical point.[5,6] Furthermore, certain disease states may be accompanied by alterations in this scale-invariant (fractal) correlation property. Here we explore the potential utility of such scaling alterations in the detection of pathological states.

Our analysis in this paper is based on the digitized electrocardiograms of beat-to-beat heart rate fluctuations recorded with an ambulatory (Holter) monitor. The time series obtained by plotting the sequential intervals between beat i and beat $i+1$, denoted by $B(i)$, typically reveals a complex type of variability [Fig. 1(a)]. The mechanism underlying such fluctuations appears to be related primarily to countervailing neuroautonomic inputs. Parasympathetic stimulation decreases the firing rate of pacemaker cells in the heart's sinus node. Sympathetic stimulation has the opposite effect. The nonlinear interaction (competition) between the two branches of the autonomic nervous system is the postulated

mechanism for the type of erratic heart rate variability recorded in healthy subjects.[1,7]

An immediate problem facing researchers applying time series analysis to interbeat interval data is that the heartbeat time series is often highly non-stationary. One question is whether this heterogeneous structure arises trivially from changes in environmental conditions having little to do with the intrinsic dynamics of the system itself. Alternatively, these fluctuations may arise from a complex nonlinear dynamical system rather than being an epiphenomenon of environmental stimuli.

From a practical point of view, if the fluctuations driven by uncorrelated stimuli can be decomposed from intrinsic fluctuations generated by the dynamical system, then these two classes of fluctuations may be shown to have very different correlation properties. If that is the case, then a plausible consideration is that only the fluctuations arising from the dynamics of the complex, multiple-component system should show long-range correlations. Other responses should give rise to a different type of fluctuation (although highly non-stationary) having characteristic time scales (i.e. frequencies related to the stimuli). This type of "noise," although physiologically important, can be treated as a "trend" and distinguished from the more subtle fluctuations that may reveal intrinsic correlation properties of the dynamics. To this end, we introduced a modified root mean square analysis of a random walk—termed *detrended fluctuation analysis* (DFA)[8,9]—to the analysis of physiological data. The advan-

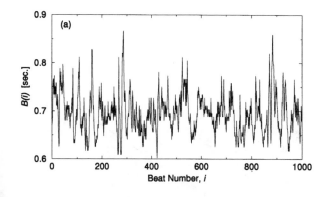

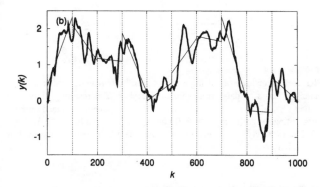

FIG. 1. (a) The interbeat interval time series $B(i)$ of 1000 beats. (b) The integrated time series: $y(k) = \sum_{i=1}^{k} [B(i) - B_{ave}]$, where $B(i)$ is the interbeat interval shown in (a). The vertical dotted lines indicate box of size $n = 100$, the solid straight line segments represent the "trend" estimated in each box by a least-squares fit.

tages of DFA over conventional methods (e.g. spectral analysis and Hurst analysis) are that it permits the detection of long-range correlations embedded in a seemingly non-stationary time series, and also avoids the spurious detection of apparent long-range correlations that are an artifact of non-stationarity. This method has been validated on control time series that consist of long-range correlations with the superposition of a non-stationary external trend.[8] The DFA method has also been successfully applied to detect long-range correlations in highly heterogeneous DNA sequences,[8,10,11] and other complex physiological signals.[12]

II. DETRENDED FLUCTUATION ANALYSIS COMPUTATION

To illustrate the DFA algorithm, we use the interbeat time series shown in Fig. 1(a) as an example. Briefly, the interbeat interval time series (of total length N) is first integrated, $y(k) = \sum_{i=1}^{k} [B(i) - B_{ave}]$, where $B(i)$ is the ith interbeat interval and B_{ave} is the average interbeat interval. Next the integrated time series is divided into boxes of equal length, n. In each box of length n, a least-squares line is fit to the data (representing the *trend* in that box) [Fig. 1(b)]. The y coordinate of the straight line segments is denoted by $y_n(k)$. Next we detrend the integrated time series, $y(k)$, by subtracting the local trend, $y_n(k)$, in each box. The root-mean-square fluctuation of this integrated and detrended time series is calculated by

$$F(n) = \sqrt{\frac{1}{N} \sum_{k=1}^{N} [y(k) - y_n(k)]^2}. \qquad (1)$$

This computation is repeated over all time scales (box sizes) to provide a relationship between $F(n)$, the average fluctuation as a function of box size, and the box size n (i.e. the number of beats in a box which is the size of the window of observation). Typically, $F(n)$ will increase with box size n. A linear relationship on a double log graph indicates the presence of scaling. Under such conditions, the fluctuations can be characterized by a scaling exponent α, the slope of the line relating $\log F(n)$ to $\log n$. Consider first a process where the value at one interbeat interval is completely uncorrelated from any previous values, e.g. white noise. This can be achieved by using a time series for which the order of the points has been shuffled (so-called "surrogate" data set). For this type of uncorrelated data, the integrated value, $y(k)$, corresponds to a random walk, and therefore $\alpha = 0.5$.[13] If there are only short-term correlations, the initial slope may be different from 0.5, but α will approach 0.5 for large window sizes. An α greater than 0.5 and less than or equal to 1.0 indicates persistent long-range power-law correlations such that a large (compared to the average) interbeat interval is more likely to be followed by large interval and vice versa. In contrast, $0 < \alpha < 0.5$ indicates a different type of power-law correlation such that large and small values of the time series are more likely to alternate.[14] A special case of $\alpha = 1$ corresponds to $1/f$ noise.[5,15] For $\alpha \geq 1$, correlations exist but cease to be of a power-law form; $\alpha = 1.5$ indicates *Brown* noise, the integration of white noise. The α exponent can also be viewed as an indicator that describes the "roughness" of the original time series: the larger the value of α, the smoother the time series. In this context, $1/f$ noise can be interpreted as a "compromise" between the complete unpredictability of white noise (very rough "landscape") and the very smooth "landscape" of Brownian noise.[16,17]

Figure 2 compares the DFA analysis of representative 24 hour interbeat interval time series of a healthy subject (O) and a patient with congestive heart failure (△). Notice that for large time scales (asymptotic behavior), the healthy subject interbeat interval time series shows almost perfect power-law scaling over two decades ($20 \leq n \leq 10000$) with $\alpha = 1$ (i.e., $1/f$ noise) while for the pathologic data set $\alpha \approx 1.3$ (closer to Brownian noise). This result is consistent with our previous finding that there is a significant difference in the long-range scaling behavior between healthy and diseased states.[3,4]

III. NORMAL VS PATHOLOGIC TIME SERIES

To test for statistical significance using the DFA method, we re-analyzed cardiac interbeat data from two different groups of subjects reported in our previous work:[3] 12 healthy adults without clinical evidence of heart disease (age range: 29–64 years, mean 44) and 15 adults with severe heart failure (age range: 22–71 years; mean 56).[18] Data from each subject comprise approximately 24 hours of ECG recording. Data from patients with heart failure due to severe left ven-

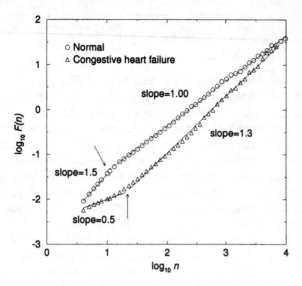

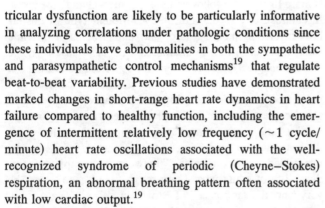

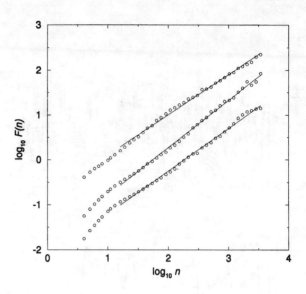

FIG. 2. Plot of log $F(n)$ vs log n (see description of DFA computation in text) for two very long interbeat interval time series (~ 24 hours). The circles are from a healthy subject while the triangles are from a subject with congestive heart failure. Arrows indicate "crossover" points in scaling.

FIG. 3. Plot of log $F(n)$ vs log n of 3 data subsets (each contains approximately 8 hours of data) from the same subject. The resulting plots were shifted vertically for purpose of display. The α exponents obtained over the same fitting range (from 16 to 3400 beats) are very similar: 0.90, 1.05 and 0.95, respectively. Note that not all three data sets exhibit crossover in scaling behavior.

tricular dysfunction are likely to be particularly informative in analyzing correlations under pathologic conditions since these individuals have abnormalities in both the sympathetic and parasympathetic control mechanisms[19] that regulate beat-to-beat variability. Previous studies have demonstrated marked changes in short-range heart rate dynamics in heart failure compared to healthy function, including the emergence of intermittent relatively low frequency (~ 1 cycle/minute) heart rate oscillations associated with the well-recognized syndrome of periodic (Cheyne–Stokes) respiration, an abnormal breathing pattern often associated with low cardiac output.[19]

We observe the following scaling exponent (for time scale $10^2 \sim 10^4$ beats) for the group of healthy cardiac interbeat interval time series (mean value $\pm$S.D.): $\alpha = 1.00 \pm 0.11$.[20] This result is consistent with previous reports of $1/f$ fluctuations in healthy heart rate (by spectral analysis).[21,22] The pathologic group shows a significant ($p < 0.01$ by Student's t-test) deviation of the long-range correlation exponent from normal. For the group of heart failure subjects, we find that $\alpha = 1.24 \pm 0.22$. Of interest, some of the heart failure subjects show an α exponent very close to 1.5 (Brownian noise), indicating random walk-like fluctuations, also consistent with our previous findings in this group. The group-averaged exponent α is less than 1.5 for the heart failure patients, suggesting that pathologic dynamics may only transiently operate in the random walk regime or may only approach this extreme state as a limiting case. We obtained similar results when we divided the time series into three consecutive subsets (of ~ 8 hours each) and repeated the above analysis. Therefore our findings are not simply attributable to different levels of daily activities (see Fig. 3).

IV. CROSSOVER PHENOMENA

Although this asymptotic scaling exponent may serve as a useful index for selected diagnostic purposes, a drawback is that very long data sets are required (at least 24 hours) for statistically robust results. For practical purposes, clinical investigators are usually interested in the possibility of using substantially shorter time series. In this regard, we note that for short time scales, there is an apparent *crossover* exhibited for the scaling behavior of both data sets (arrows in Fig. 2). For the healthy subject, the α exponent estimated from very small n (<10 beats) is larger than that calculated from large n (>10 beats). This is probably due to the fact that on very short time scales (a few beats to ten beats), the physiologic interbeat interval fluctuation is dominated by the relatively smooth heartbeat oscillation associated with respiration, thus giving rise to a large α value. For longer scales, the interbeat fluctuation, reflecting the intrinsic dynamics of a complex system, approaches that of $1/f$ behavior as previously noted. *In contrast, the pathologic data set shows a very different crossover pattern* (Fig. 2). For very short time scales, the fluctuation is quite random (close to white noise, $\alpha \approx 0.5$). As the time scale becomes larger, the fluctuation becomes smoother (asymptotically approaching Brownian noise, $\alpha \approx 1.5$). These findings are consistent with our previous report of altered correlation properties under pathologic conditions.[3,4] At present it is unclear why we observe such alteration. Nevertheless, a good quantitative description can probably advance our understanding.

V. STOCHASTIC MODEL FOR PATHOLOGIC DATA

The physiologic mechanism for the long-range correlations represented by the $1/f$ spectrum of normal interbeat intervals remains to be established. Both stochastic and deterministic models have been proposed to account for such scale-invariant behavior in physical systems. We introduce a simple three-parameter stochastic model (without relating to actual neuroautonomic control mechanisms) that can quantitatively describe the crossover scaling behavior *under extreme pathologic conditions.* The simple stochastic model is based on two assumptions:

(i) For short time scales (less than $10-20$ beats) the cardiac interbeat intervals with congestive heart failure can be described as white noise. Consider that the sinus node tends to maintain a constant ("homeostatic") firing rate. However, the actual beat-to-beat time intervals will deviate from a perfectly regular oscillation due to random fluctuations described by a distribution with a zero mean value and a well-defined variance (Δ^2). The typical period (the characteristic time) that the sinus node keeps its firing rate constant is denoted by τ.

(ii) The system responds to other driving forces (environmental influences or intrinsic factors) by increasing or decreasing the firing rate. The typical change of the firing rate is characterized by a parameter δ. Once the sinus node adjusts its firing rate, it will tend to maintain it for a period of τ beats as described in (i).

Figure 4 shows the comparison of the actual interbeat data for one of the heart failure subjects to that generated by the model. The effect of assumption (i) is to generate white noise for time-scale less than τ, i.e., if we let $\tau \to \infty$ then the DFA plot of this model will be a straight line with slope 0.5 for all ranges of n. On the other hand, the effect of (ii) is to create the kind of noise associated with Brownian motion ("brown noise"), i.e., if we set τ very small (~ 1 beat) then the DFA plot will be a straight line with slope 1.5. In order to simulate the observed *crossover* between these two regimes, we need to set τ in the model to be of the same order as the crossover time observed in Fig. 4(c). Beside the parameter τ, we only need to select the other two parameters, Δ^2 and δ, to fit the observed data.

The simple model described above is useful because it shows how two apparently different pathologic scaling mechanisms are in fact connected by the emergence of a characteristic time, corresponding to the observed "crossover" behavior of the real data. However, this model is limited in its scope because it (i) does not account for the $1/f$ ($\alpha = 1$) scaling behavior of the healthy heart rate dynamics, and (ii) it does not relate the parameters to specific neuroautonomic control mechanisms. We note that this model implies that under extreme pathologic conditions, the system attempts to maintain a constant interbeat interval for short time scales while responding to other factors over longer time scales by a smooth variation of the interbeat interval. This behavior is dramatically different from the observed dynamics of interbeat interval under normal (healthy) condition which shows a more complex pattern of sinus rhythm fluctuations than can be accounted for with traditional homeostasis models.[23]

VI. CLINICAL APPLICATION: PRELIMINARY RESULTS

The above observation of a differential crossover pattern for healthy versus pathologic data motivated us to extract

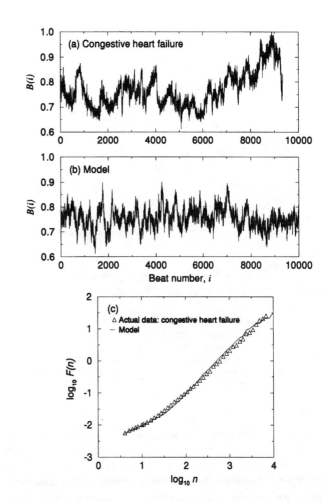

FIG. 4. (a) Interbeat interval time series from a patient with heart failure (the same subject described in Fig. 2). (b) Time series generated by model. Only part of the total time series is shown here. (c) The DFA of the interbeat interval function $B(i)$ for data in (a) and (b). The triangles represent actual data from the subject and the solid lines are generated by the model. The actual simulation of the model is carried out as follows: (i) Choose a firing rate, R_1, such that $B(1)$ equal to the average value, $\bar{B}$, of the real interbeat data set. (ii) The subsequent interbeat values will be $B(1)$ plus a random fluctuation (described by a distribution with zero mean and a finite variance, Δ^2). (iii) With a probability $1/\tau$, the firing rate R_1 will change to a new value $R_2 = R_1 + \xi$. The magnitude of this drift, ξ, is random and described by a distribution with zero mean and standard deviation δ. For this simulation, the value of the parameters are: $\tau = 20$ beats, $\Delta = 0.011$ s and $\delta = 0.008$ s. The parameter τ is chosen to fit the crossover time, where Δ and δ are chosen for fitting the data over short and long time scales, respectively. To account for the physiological constraint that the firing rate cannot become arbitrarily large or small, we also add a instantaneous restoring force that is proportional to the difference between the current firing rate and the mean (average) firing rate (measured from the actual data). This restoring force only affects very long time scales ($\sim 10^4$) fluctuations.

two parameters from each data set by fitting the scaling exponent α over two different time scales: one short, the other long. To be more precise, for each data set we calculated an exponent α_1 by making a least squares fit of $\log F(n)$ vs $\log n$ for $4 \leq n \leq 16$. Similarly, an exponent α_2 was obtained from $16 \leq n \leq 64$. Since these two exponents are not extracted from the asymptotic region, relatively short data sets are sufficient, thereby making this technique applicable to "real world" clinical data.

We applied this quantitative fluctuation analysis to the two different groups of subjects mentioned above to measure

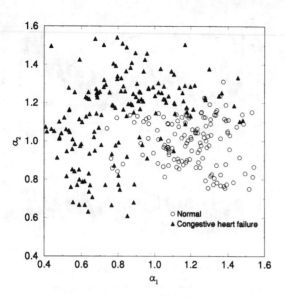

FIG. 5. Scatter plot of scaling exponents α_1 vs α_2 for the healthy subjects (O) and subjects with congestive heart failure ($\triangle$). The α's were calculated from interbeat interval data sets of length 8192 beats. Longer data set records were divided into multiple data sets (each with 8192 beats). Note good separation between healthy and heart disease subjects, with clustering of points in two distinct "clouds."

the two scaling exponents α_1 and α_2. The two exponents were calculated for each data set of length $N = 8192$ beats (~ 2 hours) and longer data set records were divided into multiple subsets (each with 8192 beats). For healthy subjects, we find the following exponents (mean value $\pm$ S.D.) for the cardiac interbeat interval time series: $\alpha_1 = 1.201 \pm 0.178$ and $\alpha_2 = 0.998 \pm 0.124$. For the group of congestive heart failure subjects, we find that $\alpha_1 = 0.803 \pm 0.259$ and $\alpha_2 = 1.125 \pm 0.216$, both significantly ($p < 0.0001$ for both α_1 and α_2) different from normal. Furthermore, we show in Fig. 5 that fairly good discrimination between these two groups can be achieved by using these two scaling exponents. We note that not all subjects in our preliminary study show an obvious crossover in their scaling behavior. Only 8 out of 12 healthy subjects exhibited this crossover, while 11 out of 15 pathologic subjects exhibited a "reverse" crossover. However, the two scaling exponents (α_1 and α_2) measured from relatively short data sets can still be potentially useful indicators to distinguish normal from pathologic time series.[24]

To test the effect of data length on these calculations, we repeated the same DFA measurements for longer data sets ($N = 16384$) and also for shorter data sets ($N = 4096$). As expected, the results for shorter data sets are less reliable (more overlap between two groups) due to anticipated statistical error related to finite sample size.[25] On the other hand, longer data sets result in little improvement for the distinction between groups. Therefore, the data length of 8192 seems to be a statistically reasonable choice.[26]

Furthermore, we note that data from normal interbeat interval time series are tightly clustered suggesting that there may exist a "universal" scaling behavior for physiologic interbeat time series. In contrast, the pathologic data show more variation, a finding which may be related to different

clinical conditions and varying severity of the pathologic states.

VII. CONCLUSION

In summary, we apply a new fluctuation analysis (modified from classical random walk analysis) to the nonstationary heartbeat time series from healthy subjects and those with severe heart disease (congestive heart failure). We show that this method is capable of identifying crossover behavior due to differences in scaling over short versus long time scales. This finding is of interest from a physiologic viewpoint since it motivates new modeling approaches to account for the control mechanisms regulating cardiac dynamics on different time scales. From a practical point of view, quantification of these scaling exponents may have potential applications for bedside and ambulatory monitoring.

ACKNOWLEDGMENTS

We wish to thank J. M. Hausdorff, J. E. Mietus and G. B. Moody for helpful discussions. Partial support was provided to CKP by a NIMH National Research Service Award, to HES by the National Science Foundation and to ALG by the G. Harold and Leila Y. Mathers Charitable Foundation, the National Institute on Drug Abuse, and the National Aeronautics and Space Administration.

[1] R. I. Kitney and O. Rompelman, *The Study of Heart-Rate Variability* (Oxford University Press, Oxford, 1980).
[2] A. L. Goldberger, D. R. Rigney, and B. J. West, Sci. Am. **262**, 42–49 (1990).
[3] C.-K. Peng, J. Mietus, J. M. Hausdorff, S. Havlin, H. E. Stanley, and A. L. Goldberger, Phys. Rev. Lett. **70**, 1343–1346 (1993).
[4] C.-K. Peng, S. V. Buldyrev, J. M. Hausdorff, S. Havlin, J. E. Mietus, M. Simons, H. E. Stanley, and A. L. Goldberger, in *Fractals in Biology and Medicine*, edited by T. F. Nonnenmacher, G. A. Losa, and E. R. Weibel (Birkhaüser-Verlag, Basel, 1994), pp. 55–65.
[5] P. Bak, C. Tang, and K. Wiesenfeld, Phys. Rev. Lett. **59**, 381–384 (1987).
[6] H. E. Stanley, *Introduction to Phase Transitions and Critical Phenomena* (Oxford University Press, London, 1971).
[7] M. N. Levy, Circ. Res. **29**, 437–445 (1971).
[8] C.-K. Peng, S. V. Buldyrev, S. Havlin, M. Simons, H. E. Stanley, and A. L. Goldberger, Phys. Rev. E **49**, 1691–1695 (1994).
[9] Computer software of DFA algorithm is available upon request; contact C.-K. Peng (e-mail: peng@chaos.bih.harvard.edu).
[10] S. V. Buldyrev, A. L. Goldberger, S. Havlin, C.-K. Peng, H. E. Stanley, and M. Simons, Biophys. J. **65**, 2675–2681 (1993).
[11] S. M. Ossadnik, S. V. Buldyrev, A. L. Goldberger, S. Havlin, R. N. Mantegna, C.-K. Peng, M. Simons, and H. E. Stanley, Biophys. J. **67**, 64–70 (1994).
[12] J. M. Hausdorff, C.-K. Peng, Z. Ladin, J. Y. Wei, and A. L. Goldberger, J. Appl. Physiol. **78**, 349–358 (1995).
[13] E. W. Montroll and M. F. Shlesinger, in *Nonequilibrium Phenomena II. From Stochastics to Hydrodynamics*, edited by J. L. Lebowitz and E. W. Montroll (North-Holland, Amsterdam, 1984), pp 1–121.
[14] S. Havlin, R. B. Selinger, M. Schwartz, H. E. Stanley, and A. Bunde, Phys. Rev. Lett. **61**, 1438–1441 (1988).
[15] W. H. Press, Comments Astrophys. **7**, 103–119 (1978).
[16] C.-K. Peng, S. Buldyrev, A. L. Goldberger, S. Havlin, F. Sciortino, M. Simons, and H. E. Stanley, Nature **356**, 168–170 (1992).
[17] S. V. Buldyrev, A. L. Goldberger, S. Havlin, C.-K. Peng, and H. E. Stanley, in *Fractals in Science*, edited by A. Bunde and S. Havlin (Springer-Verlag, Berlin, 1994), pp. 48–87.
[18] ECG recordings of Holter monitor tapes were processed both manually and in a fully automated manner using our computerized beat recognition

algorithm (Aristotle). Abnormal beats were deleted from each data set. The deletion has practically no effect on the DFA analysis since less than 1% of total beats were removed. Patients in the heart failure group were receiving conventional medical therapy prior to receiving an investigational cardiotonic drug; see D. S. Baim *et al.*, J. Am. Coll. Cardiol. **7**, 661–670 (1986).

[19] A. L. Goldberger, D. R. Rigney, J. Mietus, E. M. Antman, and S. Greenwald, Experientia **44**, 983–987 (1988).

[20] Typical regression fit shows excellent linearity of double log graph (indicated by correlation coefficient $r > 0.97$) for both groups. However, usually data from healthy subjects show even better linearity on log–log plots than data from subjects with heart disease. Our estimate of α is consistent with the previous analysis in Ref. 3. Note, however, that in Ref. 3 the analysis was performed on the interbeat *increment* data to avoid the problem of non-stationarity. Therefore, the scaling exponent computed in Ref. 3 is smaller than the α exponent computed by DFA by a value of 1 (due to the integration process in DFA).

[21] A. L. Goldberger and B. J. West, Yale J. Biol. Med. **60**, 421–435 (1987).

[22] M. Kobayashi and T. Musha, IEEE Trans. Biomed. Eng. **BE-29**, 456–457 (1982).

[23] W. B. Cannon, Physiol. Rev. **9**, 399–431 (1929).

[24] A further refinement (not presented here) may be obtained by not arbitrarily setting the crossover scale to be 16 beats for all data sets. Instead, each individual data set could have its own ranges for fitting α_1 and α_2 that depend on the specific crossover point in the given data set.

[25] C.-K. Peng, S. V. Buldyrev, A. L. Goldberger, S. Havlin, M. Simons, and H. E. Stanley, Phys. Rev. E **47**, 3730–3733 (1993).

[26] We also tested these calculations by varying the fitting range for α_2. We find that the results are very similar when we measure α_2 from 16 beats to 128 beats. However, when we move the upper fitting range for α_2 from 128 beats to 256 beats or more, the pathologic data sets show larger variation of α_2 leading to less obvious separation from normal subjects. This is partly due to the fact that, for finite length data sets, the calculation error of $F(n)$ increases with n.[25] Therefore, scaling exponents obtained over larger values of n will have greater uncertainty.

Quantitative analysis of heart rate variability

J. Kurths
*Arbeitsgruppe Nichtlineare Dynamik der Max-Planck-Gesellschaft an der Universität Potsdam, Pf. 601553,
D-14415 Potsdam, Germany*

A. Voss
MDC, Franz-Volhard-Klinik, Wiltbergstrasse 50, D-13125 Buch, Germany

P. Saparin
Saratov State University, Astrakhanskaja U1. 40, Russia

A. Witt
*Arbeitsgruppe Nichtlineare Dynamik der Max-Planck-Gesellschaft an der Universität Potsdam,
Pf. 601553, D-14415 Potsdam, Germany*

H. J. Kleiner and N. Wessel
MDC, Franz-Volhard-Klinik, Wiltbergstrasse 50, D-13125 Buch, Germany

(Received 19 May 1994; accepted for publication 8 August 1994)

In the modern industrialized countries every year several hundred thousands of people die due to sudden cardiac death. The individual risk for this sudden cardiac death cannot be defined precisely by common available, noninvasive diagnostic tools like Holter monitoring, highly amplified ECG and traditional linear analysis of heart rate variability (HRV). Therefore, we apply some rather unconventional methods of nonlinear dynamics to analyze the HRV. Especially, some complexity measures that are based on symbolic dynamics as well as a new measure, the renormalized entropy, detect some abnormalities in the HRV of several patients who have been classified in the low risk group by traditional methods. A combination of these complexity measures with the parameters in the frequency domain seems to be a promising way to get a more precise definition of the individual risk. These findings have to be validated by a representative number of patients. © 1995 American Institute of Physics.

I. INTRODUCTION

Ventricular arrhythmia, especially ventricular tachycardia (VT) and ventricular fibrillations are in many cases the cause of sudden cardiac death of patients after myocardial infarction. The improved identification of patients highly threatened by these severe rhythm disturbances is an important and very actual clinical problem.

Short as well as long-range fluctuations in the heart rate are related to the autonomic nervous system control of heart activity and vasomotion. Recent studies have shown that a low heart rate variability (HRV) is a clear indication of an increased risk for severe ventricular arrhythmia and sudden cardiac death. These phenomena seem to be associated with a structural change of the beat to beat interval dynamics.

Kleiger[1] showed that a reduced HRV carries an adverse prognosis in patients who have survived an acute myocardial infarction. Malik[2] examined HRV in those patients to find the optimum time and duration of recording of the ambulatory ECG for the prediction of the risk of a sudden cardiac death, or serious arrhythmic events. It has been reported that patients after an acute myocardial infarction have a reduced parasympathetic function which causes an increased sympathetic tonus.

Therefore, several well-known techniques have been applied to detect such high risk patients from ECG (cf. Fig. 1). First, some rather simple time domain measures of heart rate variability have been proven useful for clinical purposes. Second, the spectral analysis of the RR time series that expresses HRV in the frequency domain exhibits different oscillating sources of the variability of heart beat generation.

The different regions in the power spectrum are related to special physiological phenomena. We have considered the following: The frequency band < 0.0033 Hz (ultra low frequency power ULF) and the frequency band 0.0033 ... 0.05 Hz (very low frequency power VLF) represents humoral, vasomotion and thermo regulations and reflects also the activity of the renin–angiotensin–aldosteron system. The frequency band 0.05 ... 0.15 Hz (low frequency power LF) reflects modulation of sympathetic or parasympathetic tone by baroflex activity (blood pressure regulation) and the frequency band 0.15 ... 0.45 Hz (high frequency power HF) represents the modulation of vagal activity especially influenced by respiration. Bigger[3] showed that the day-to-day stability of the measure of heart period variability makes it possible to detect small changes due to progression, regression of diseases or treatment effects. Further on he pointed out that according to Kleiger's results the ULF of the spectrum especially has the strongest association with mortality in post-infarction patients. Another approach to detect such high risk is the analysis of very late potentials (VLP) obtained from ECG.[4,5]

However, the traditional techniques of data analysis in time and frequency domain are often not sufficient to characterize the complex dynamics of heart beat generation. Hence, different attempts have been reported to apply the concept of nonlinear dynamics to this problem.[6] After some optimism in the 1980s, it has become clear that the HRV cannot be generally characterized by low fractal dimensions. The purpose of this contribution is, therefore, to analyze the HRV by means of other methods of nonlinear dynamics

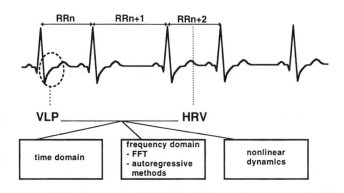

FIG. 1. Scheme of different techniques for the analysis of ECG.

which are based on the concept of symbolic dynamics and on a renormalized entropy.

The organization of this paper is as follows: The kind of the data and the traditional techniques to analyze them are described in Sec. II. In Sec. III we introduce different complexity measures. Their efficiency to detect high risk patients is discussed in Sec. IV which also includes a comparison with the results obtained from traditional techniques. Section V concludes the paper.

II. DATA AND PRE-PROCESSING

A. Data

The ECG recording has been done as follows: A 30 to 60 min 4 channel high resolution ECG (Frank leads and an additional diagonal lead) with a sampling frequency of 2000 Hz and 16 bit resolution (PC system with commercial available fast digitizing board) was obtained under rest conditions. The Simson method[7] was used to calculate the sum vector magnitude from the three highly amplified (digital high pass filter, Butterworth characteristics 40 Hz) leads X, Y, and Z.

After digitizing and extracting of RR intervals by automatic procedures all RR time series have been checked by a technician and if necessary edited. The software RR detection algorithm is based on the cross-correlation technique.

B. Patients

In this preliminary study, we have included a sample of 43 patients subdivided in 3 groups (cf. Fig. 2). The first group consists of 21 healthy persons. In the second group there are 9 patients after myocardial infarction (MI) with low electrical risk (arrhythmias of low degree). Group 3 represents those 13 cardiac patients after MI for whom severe ventricular arrhythmias (sustained ventricular tachycardia) have been documented.

C. Traditional analysis

These techniques can be divided into time and frequency domains (see Fig. 1).

In the time domain we have calculated the following standard parameters: the quotient of mean and standard deviation, the standard deviation of averages of NN intervals over 1 and over 5 minutes as well as the proportion of NN-interval-differences >50 and >100 ms and the root mean square of successive differences.

From the estimated power spectrum we have determined the power of the 4 above-mentioned frequency bands (ULF, VLF, LF, HF) and the ratios LF/whole power and LF/HF.

All these quantities that are based on linear statistics are rather simple to calculate, but they do not lead to a satisfying detection of high risk patients. The rapid development in the theory of nonlinear dynamical systems has caused some optimism for a more appropriate understanding of such complex rhythms, as expressed in the HRV.

III. COMPLEXITY MEASURES

In the 1980s the wide-spread hope arose that many complicated systems observed in nature can be described by a few nonlinear coupled modes. The properties of these systems are characterized by fractal dimensions, Lyapunov exponents, or Kolmogorov–Sinai entropy.[8] However, we now know that such a low dimensionality can be expected only for rather coherent phenomena, such as observed in laser systems. Physiological data, as studied here, seem to have a more complex structure, may be due to high-dimensional processes or due to the influence of random-like fluctuations. In this section, we present rather unconventional approaches to find some characteristics in these records.

A. Symbolic dynamics

Symbolic dynamics is based on a coarse-graining of the measurements, i.e., the data t_n are transformed into a pattern whose elements are only a few symbols (letters from some alphabet). This way, the study of the dynamics simplifies to the description of symbol sequences. In doing so one loses some amount of detailed information, but some of the invariant, robust properties of the dynamics may be kept (Hao[9]).

The first step is to find a suitable symbolic description. If we do not know a generating partition, there is no straightforward procedure for this problem, but it is context dependent (Kurths *et al.*[10]). Hence, we have to look for a coding procedure which is suitable for our purpose. From various tests we have found that for our purpose at least 4 different symbols are necessary. This leads us to use two different kinds to transform the HRV records into symbol sequences. The first transformation refers to three given levels,

$$s_n = \begin{cases} 0, & \text{if } t_n > (1+a)\mu, \\ 1, & \text{if } t_n > \mu \quad \text{and } t_n \leq (1+a)\mu, \\ 2, & \text{if } t_n > (1-a)\mu \quad \text{and } t_n \leq \mu, \\ 3, & \text{if } t_n \leq (1-a)\mu, \end{cases} \quad (1)$$

where μ denotes the mean RR-interval and a is a special parameter specified in Sec. IV. The second transformation considers the kind of difference between two adjacent measurement values; it especially reflects dynamical properties of the record:

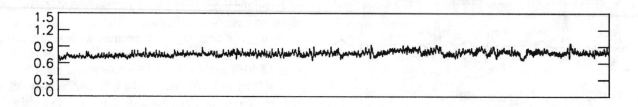

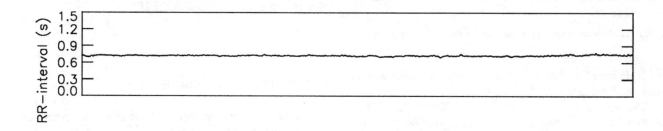

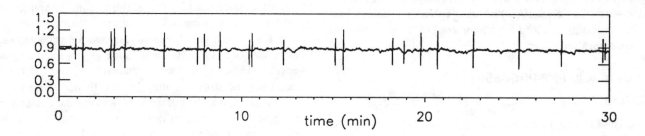

FIG. 2. Tachograms of a healthy (top) and two ill persons.

$$\tilde{s}_n = \begin{cases} 0, & \text{if } \Delta t_n > 1.5\sigma_\Delta, \\ 1, & \text{if } \Delta t_n > 0 \quad \text{and } \Delta t_n \leq 1.5\sigma_\Delta, \\ 2, & \text{if } \Delta t_n > -1.5\sigma_\Delta \quad \text{and } \Delta t_n \leq 0, \\ 3, & \text{if } \Delta t_n \leq -1.5\sigma_\Delta, \end{cases} \quad (2)$$

with $\Delta t_n = t_{n+1} - t_n$ and σ_Δ is the variance of Δt_n. In the following we check, which of these transformations is more appropriate for our purpose.

Next, some classical parameters, which quantify different aspects of the behavior of such a symbolic string s_n are presented.

The first approach is to calculate the frequencies of occurring symbols. To investigate a rather broad range of dynamics, one should analyze long words. However, our data sets only contain about 2000 RR-intervals and the number of all possible words of length l basing on the alphabet, as introduced in Eq. (1), is 4^l. We, therefore, count length-3 words as a good compromise between including some dynamics and the reliability in estimating the frequencies. With these frequencies one can distinguish rather uniform distributions from more complicated ones. This leads to the first measure of complexity which simply counts the number of forbidden words. For statistical reasons, we modify this idea

somewhat and test for the number of words with a low probability of occurrence (probability less than 0.001).

A classical measure of symbol sequences is the Shannon entropy. From the probabilities $p(s^k)$ of words of length k we get the Shannon entropy of kth order as follows:

$$H_k = -\sum_{s^k, p(s^k) > 0} p(s^k) \log_2 p(s^k). \quad (3)$$

This H_k measures the average number of bits needed to specify an arbitrary word of length k in the symbolic string.

The concept of Renyi[11] entropy was introduced as a generalization of Shannon's ansatz

$$H_k^{(q)} = (1-q)^{-1} \log_2 \left(\sum_{s^k} p(s^k)^q \right) \quad (4)$$

where q is a real number and $q \neq 1$. It includes different averaging of probabilities. $H_k^{(q)}$ converges to Shannon entropy H_k as $q \rightarrow 1$. Both, the Shannon entropy and the spectrum of Renyi entropies are measures of complexity which characterize systems as follows:[12–14]

(1) The complexity is zero for constant sequences.

(2) In case of periodicity with prime period $m, m < k$ one gets $H = \log_2 m$.

(3) For uniform distributions it takes its maximum value $H = k \log_2 \alpha$ where α is the number of symbols.

(4) $H_k^{(q)}$ decreases with growing q.

(5) If $q > 1$ those words of length k with large probability dominantly influence the Renyi entropy. This behavior is strengthened for larger q values. Vice versa, if $0 < q < 1$ then words with small probability mainly determine the value of $H_k^{(q)}$.

In order to get reliable estimates of these H_k or $H_k^{(q)}$, which are also based on counting the frequencies of substrings, we calculate here entropy of order 3 only. A possible inhomogeneous structure inherent the data is checked by determining the Renyi entropies for $q = 4$ and $q = 0.25$.

It is important to note that all special complexity measures mentioned above do not include long-range correlations.

B. Renormalized entropy

The main purpose of this paper is the comparison of the HRV of different persons to get some judgement of their risk for sudden cardiac death. As is well-known, the underlying system that generates the HRV is not closed, but an open one. From the viewpoint of general system theory, this means that different persons may have different mean energy. In such a case the immediate comparison of measures, such as Shannon entropy, may lead to some difficulties. Basing on a recent suggestion of Klimontovich,[15] we, therefore, introduce here another complexity measure, the renormalized entropy. This approach, loosely speaking, renormalizes the entropy obtained from a time series $x(t)$ of a certain person in such a manner that the mean effective energy coincides with that of a reference person $x_r(t)$.

Starting from these two time series, we can easily estimate the corresponding probability distributions $f(z)$ and $f_r(z)$. By using formal arguments from thermodynamics the effective energy is defined as:

$$h_{\text{eff}}(z) = -\log f_r(z). \tag{5}$$

The renormalization of f_r into $\tilde{f}_r$ is constructed such that the mean effective energies $\langle h_{\text{eff}} \rangle$ of f and $\tilde{f}_r$ are equal. To make this idea operational, we first represent the distribution in terms of the canonical Gibbs distribution

$$\tilde{f}_r(z) = \exp\left(\frac{\Phi(T_{\text{eff}}) - h_{\text{eff}}(z)}{T_{\text{eff}}} \right) \tag{6}$$

which can be rewritten as

$$\tilde{f}_r(z) = C(T_{\text{eff}}) \cdot \exp(-h_{\text{eff}}(z)/T_{\text{eff}}), \tag{7}$$

where T_{eff} and $\Phi(T_{\text{eff}})$ are the effective temperature, respectively, the free effective energy. Because h_{eff} can be calculated from Eq. (5), there are two unknowns in Eq. (7): $C(T_{\text{eff}})$ and T_{eff}. They are determined from the following two conditions.

(a) Normalization:

$$\int \tilde{f}_r(z) dz = 1;$$

(b) equality of mean effective energy:

$$\int h_{\text{eff}}(z) \tilde{f}_r(z) dz = \int h_{\text{eff}}(z) f(z) dz.$$

Hence, $\tilde{f}_r$ fulfills the properties wanted. Consequently, we can compare the Shannon entropies of f and $\tilde{f}_r$

$$H = -\int f(z) \log f(z) dz$$

and

$$\tilde{H}_r = -\int \tilde{f}_r(z) \log \tilde{f}_r(z) dx. \tag{8}$$

For that the renormalized entropy difference

$$\Delta \tilde{H} = H - \tilde{H}_r \tag{9}$$

is introduced. It is important to note that $\Delta \tilde{H}$ is a relative measure that depends on the reference person (system) chosen. Applying it to the logistic map, we have recently found that this renormalized entropy is the only complexity measure which clearly indicates all transitions between different regimes which are caused by this map (Saparin *et al.*[16]). Therefore, this new measure can also be a good tool to detect high risk patients.

IV. RESULTS AND DISCUSSION

We calculate all characteristics of the three main different approaches mentioned above from the HRV records described in Sec. II. The parameters in the time and in the frequency domain are determined as usually, i.e., 5 parameters in the time domain and 6 parameters in the frequency domain (as described in Sec. II C) (see Table I).

Next, we describe some details of the estimate of the complexity measures introduced in Sec. III. It comes out that the first transformation [Eq. (1)] into a symbol sequence is for our purpose more appropriate than the dynamical transformation [Eq. (2)]. The optimum value of a in Eq. (1) is about 0.1. For persons with cardiac risk, the distribution of length-3 words is concentrated on about 10 words (of 64 possible ones), whereas healthy persons are characterized by a more uniform distribution. An efficient criterion to distinguish both is then: persons have a risk if there are more than 44 words which seldom occur. As expected, the Shannon entropy is not so useful as the generalized Renyi entropies. Due to the higher variability of healthy persons, we expect that Renyi entropies for a rather small q is much higher for this group than for the high risk group. The special criterion

TABLE I. Number of subjects found as risk by different techniques (Secs. II B and III).

Group	No. of subjects	Time domain	Frequency domain	Renyi information	Frequency of words	$\Delta \bar{S}$
Healthy	21	0	1	0	0	0
Low risk	9	3	4	6	5	6
High risk	13	6	9	7	11	8

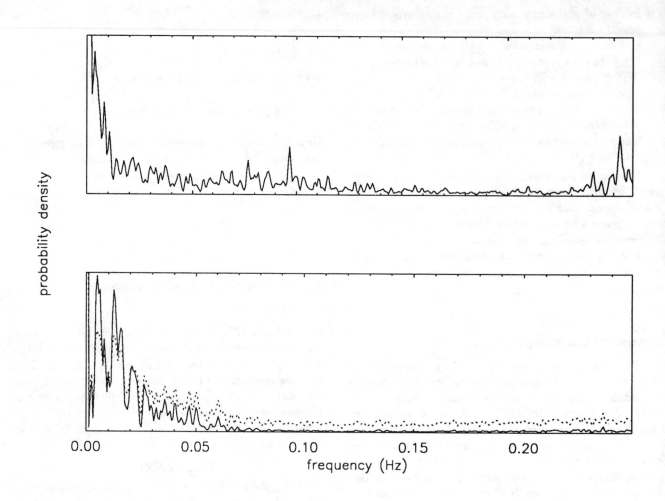

FIG. 3. Renormalization of distributions in the power spectrum: top—original distribution of the reference person; bottom—original (solid line) and renormalized (dashed) distribution of another person.

reads then: $H_3^{0.25} < 3.6$ is an indication for cardiac risk. We also apply this kind of complexity measure for strings obtained from transformation equation (2).

Our calculation of the renormalized entropy $\Delta \tilde{H}$ is based on the distribution of the trigonometric components, i.e., especially the power spectrum in the range 0–0.25 Hz. We have tested several healthy probands as reference persons and have chosen that with the largest renormalized entropy. The corresponding power spectrum is shown in Fig. 3 (upper panel). Note that this choice of a reference subject does not sensitively influence the results. Figure 3 (lower panel) demonstrates how the renormalization procedure influences a distribution. After choosing this reference person, the $\Delta \tilde{H}$ of all healthy persons under consideration is in the interval $(-0.75,0)$. Hence, an indication for cardiac risk is if $\Delta \tilde{H}$ is outside of this interval. We indeed find values in both directions; a very low $\Delta \tilde{H}$ expresses a strongly reduced variability.

It is important to note that no healthy proband is misinterpreted by means of these complexity measures. To determine, on the other hand, the individual cardiac risk, it is more suitable if we consider an integrated risk that includes all 4 criteria discussed above. This is in accordance with the

use of the special parameters in the time and frequency domain. Hence, we can compare three different risk estimates (Fig. 4 and Table I):

(a) As expected, the parameters in the time domain are less efficient than the other ones. By means of this risk, about 40% of the high risk patients are detected only. Therefore, this approach will not be further included.

(b) The analysis in the frequency domain leads to a rather good distinction of the three groups. This seems to be due to the physiological meaning of some bands in the power spectrum.

(c) The risk basing on the complexity measures gives the best detection rate of the high risk patients.

Because the persons detected in the frequency domain and by complexity measures are not completely overlapping, we combine both. This way, a very good detection rate of high risk patients is obtained.

The evaluation of persons for whom only a low risk has so far been reported is an open problem. Here, we get an important difference between both kinds of tools. To check which techniques better fit to find high risk patients from this group, a more sophisticated medical characterization than the electric risk (LOWN4) is necessary.

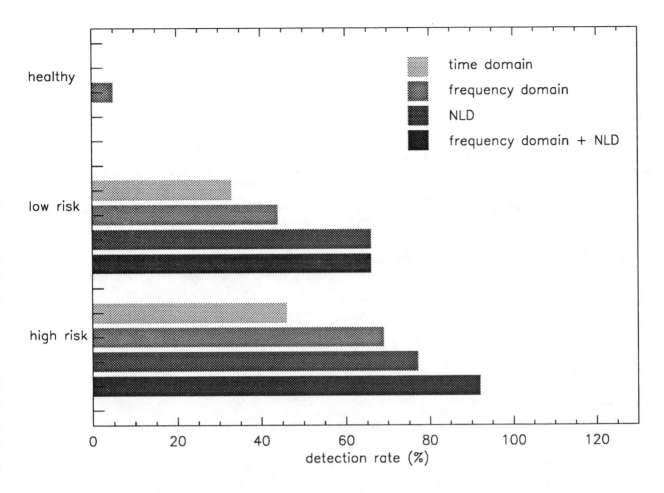

FIG. 4. Comparison of the detection rate for high cardiac risk by means of different techniques. The subjects are subdivided in 3 groups classified by usual methods. NLD refers to comlexity measures obtained from nonlinear dynamics.

V. SUMMARY

We have applied the concept of complexity measures to determine the risk for sudden cardiac death from the HRV, a very actual clinical problem. By means of classical methods, especially parameters in the time domain, the individual risk cannot be defined precisely enough.

We have found some indications that two kinds of complexity measures are very promising:

(a) Renyi entropies and the number of forbidden words, both of which are based on the notion of symbolic dynamics as well as (b) a renormalized entropy which we have recently analyzed in the framework of complexity measures.[16]

In combination with some parameters in the frequency domain, these quantities seem to define a rather precise definition of the individual risk. In contrast to this, the parameters in the time domain which are in broad use do not improve the detection rate.

It is important to note that one cannot find an optimum complexity measure. We guess that a combination of some such quantities which refer to different aspects, such as structural or dynamical properties, seems to be the most promising way. The complexity measure proposed by Pincus[17] as well as the criteria that are based on the description of long-range correlations (cf. Peng *et al.*[18]) should also be included to define the individual risk.

Finally, we would like to emphasize that our findings have to be validated by a larger and more representative number of patients, especially to check our optimized nonstandard techniques. We also think that the study of the heart rhythms are in its infancy and should by continued by modeling the underlying processes and further analyses of measurements.

ACKNOWLEDGMENTS

This research was supported in part by funding of the Ministerium für Wissenschaft, Forschung und Kultur des Landes Brandenburg. We are indebted to the unknown referees for their helpful remarks.

[1] R. E. Kleiger, J. P. Miller, J. T. Bigger, and A. J. Moss, "Decreased heart rate variability and its association with increased mortality after acute myocardial infaction," Am. J. Cardiol. **59**, 256–262 (1987).

[2] M. Malik, T. Farell, and A. J. Camm, " Circadian rhythm of heart rate variability after acute myocardial infarction and its influence on the prognostic value of heart rate variability," Am. J. Cardiol. **66**, 1049–1054 (1990).

[3] J. T. Bigger, J. L. Fleiss, L. M. Rolnitzky, and R. C. Steinmann, "Stability

over time of heart period variability in patients with previous myocardial infarction and ventricular arrhythmias," Am. J. Cardiol. **69**, 718–723 (1992).

[4] A. Voss, J. Kurths, H. Fiehring, and H. J. Kleiner, "Frequenzanalyse hochverstaerkter EKGs mit Hilfe der Maximum-Entropie-Spektralschaetzung," Z. Klin. Med. **43**, 1403–1406 (1988).

[5] A. Voss, J. Kurths, and H. Fiehring, "Frequency domain analysis of the highly amplified ECG on basis of maximum entropy spectral estimation," Med. Biol. Eng. Comput. **30**, 277–282 (1992).

[6] A. L. Goldberger, "Fractal mechanisms," IEEE EMBS **11**, 47–52 (1992); "Is the normal heartbeat chaotic or homeostasis," New Physiol. Sci. **6**, 87–91 (1991).

[7] M. B. Simson, "Use of signals in the terminal QRS complex to identify patients with ventricular tachycardia after myocardial infarction," Circulation **64**, 235–242 (1982).

[8] J. P. Eckmann and D. Ruelle, "Ergodic theory of chaos and strange attractors," Rev. Mod. Phys. **57**, 617 (1985).

[9] B.-L. Hao, "Symbolic dynamics and characterization of complexity," Physica D **51**, 161–176 (1991).

[10] J. Kurths, A. Witt, H. Atmanspacher, F. Feudel, H. Scheingraber, and R. Wackerbauer, "General remarks on complexity," in *Inside versus Outside*, edited by H. Atmanspacher and J. Dalenaort (Springer-Verlag, Berlin, 1994), pp. 219–234.

[11] A. Renyi, *Wahrscheinlichkeitsrechnung. Mit einem Anhang über Informationstheorie* (Deutscher Verlag der Wissenschaften, Berlin, 1977).

[12] R. Wackerbauer, A. Witt, H. Atmanspacher, J. Kurths, and H. Scheingraber, "Quantification of structural and dynamical complexity," Chaos, Solitons Fractals **4**, 133–173 (1994).

[13] A. Witt, J. Kurths, F. Krause, and K. Fischer, "On the reversals of the Earth's magnetic field," Geophys. Astrophys. Fluid Dyn. (in press).

[14] A. Hempelmann and J. Kurths, "Dynamics of the outburst series of SS Cygni," Astron. Astrophys. **232**, 356–360 (1990).

[15] Yu. L. Klimontovich, *Turbulent Motion and the Structure of Chaos* (Kluwer–Academic, Dordrecht, 1991).

[16] P. Saparin, A. Witt, J. Kurths, and V. Anishenko, "The renormalized entropy—An appropriate complexity measure," Chaos, Solitons Fractals (in press).

[17] S. Pincus, "Approximate entropy (ApEn) as a complexity measure," Chaos **5**, 110–117 (1995).

[18] C.-K. Peng, J. Mietus, J. M. Hausdorff, S. Havlin, H. E. Stanley, and A. L. Goldberger, "Long-range correlations and non-Gaussian behaviour of the heartbeat," Phys. Rev. Lett. **70**, 1343–1346 (1993).

Nonlinear time series analysis of electrocardiograms

A. Bezerianos,[a] T. Bountis,[b] G. Papaioannou,[b] and P. Polydoropoulos[a]
University of Patras, 261 10 Patras, Greece

(Received 8 June 1994; accepted for publication 21 September 1994)

In recent years there has been an increasing number of papers in the literature, applying the methods and techniques of Nonlinear Dynamics to the time series of electrical activity in normal electrocardiograms (ECGs) of various human subjects. Most of these studies are based primarily on correlation dimension estimates, and conclude that the dynamics of the ECG signal is deterministic and occurs on a chaotic attractor, whose dimension can distinguish between healthy and severely malfunctioning cases. In this paper, we first demonstrate that correlation dimension calculations must be used with care, as they do not always yield reliable estimates of the attractor's "dimension." We then carry out a number of additional tests (time differencing, smoothing, principal component analysis, surrogate data analysis, etc.) on the ECGs of three "normal" subjects and three "heavy smokers" at rest and after mild exercising, whose cardiac rhythms look very similar. Our main conclusion is that no major dynamical differences are evident in these signals. A preliminary estimate of three to four basic variables governing the dynamics (based on correlation dimension calculations) is updated to five to six, when temporal correlations between points are removed. Finally, in almost all cases, the transition between resting and mild exercising seems to imply a small increase in the complexity of cardiac dynamics. © *1995 American Institute of Physics.*

I. INTRODUCTION

As is well known, the usual electrocardiogram (ECG) records the electrical activity of a large mass of atrial and ventricular cells.[1] Since cardiac depolarization and repolarization normally occur in a synchronized fashion, the ECG is able to record these electrical activities in the form of certain well-defined waves, as shown in Fig. 1.

The P wave reflects the excitation of the atria stimulated by the so-called sinoatrial (SA) node action potential, the QRS complex describes the excitation of the ventricles of the His-Purkinje network, and the T wave is associated with the recovery of the initial electrical state of the ventricles.

The human ECG, even in the case of a resting subject, displays a considerable amount of fluctuations in time (the so-called heart rate variability), as well as in amplitude. It has been shown that conventional statistical measures of these variabilities have significant prognostic implications in cases of myocardial infractions, and are useful for detecting arrythmias.[2]

In recent years, considerable attention has been devoted to unifying various aspects of cardiac pathophysiology using nonlinear dynamics, particularly through applications of chaos theory and fractal geometry.[3,4] The main efforts, so far, have concentrated on the analysis of the QRS complex and heart rate variability, and not so much on the full ECG time series.[5]

In this paper, we have used the methods and techniques of nonlinear time series analysis to compute the correlation dimension[6-9] of an ECG time series of six male subjects, three of whom are "normal" (ages 20–30) and three heavy smokers (ages 20–40). At first, a straightforward calculation suggests that the dynamics of the full ECG signal (sampled

at 300 Hz), in all of these cases, has a deterministic component and lies on a chaotic attractor of dimension as low as three to four.

After a more careful investigation of these time series, however, we find that they contain a significant amount of "noise" (or, randomness) in the high-frequency part of the power spectrum; see Fig. 2. This is demonstrated by the behavior of the time "derivative" of the signal[10] (i.e., the series of successive time differences), containing the high-frequency fluctuations of the data. In all cases studied, this time differenced series was found to have a higher dimension than the original ECG. Still, this increase brings the dimension of the signal to a value near five to six, which remains fixed, even when the embedding dimension is raised to 10.

Moreover, eliminating dynamically neighboring points in correlation dimension calculations[11] shows that the apparent low-dimensionality of ECGs at small scales, is most likely due to *temporal* rather than *spatial* correlations between the points. Here, again, when dynamically neighboring points are removed from the calculation of the correlation dimension, its value grows by one to two units, suggesting that the principal components governing the dynamics may be as many as five to six. This is in agreement with results obtained using singular value decomposition[12] (or principal component analysis).

Several researchers have suggested that the specialized cardiac conduction network (i.e., the His-Purkinje system) has a fractal geometry, and consequently that the normal QRS complex is a broadband waveform with a power spectrum that obeys an inverse power law.[13] Furthermore, some studies have shown that the human heart rate, in the case of healthy subjects, displays a considerable amount of fluctuations. In fact, a decrease in heart rate variability has been observed in patients at high risk of sudden death due to a left ventricular malfunction.[14]

Goldberger *et al.*,[15] owing to the narrow band spectrum

---

[a]At the School of Medicine, Department of Medical Physics.
[b]At the Department of Mathematics, Section of Applied Analysis.

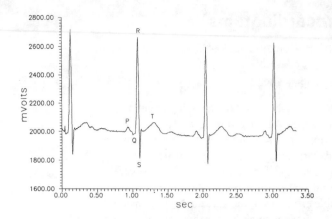

FIG. 1. Typical ECG pattern of a "normal" person

of ventricular fibrillation, concluded that it is not chaotic, since chaos is characterized by broadband frequency spectra. Later studies[16] have sought to explain these results, while there have been continuing attempts to settle the question of whether ventricular fibrillation is chaotic or not.[17,18]

On the other hand, in a recent paper[19] it is claimed that the transition from the sinus rhythm to fully developed ventricular fibrillation is accompanied by an increase in the complexity of the ECG dynamics. This is shown by calculating the correlation dimension of the time series and finding that its value steadily increases from nearly 2.1 to 3.7 to larger than 7.8, corresponding to sinus rhythm, ventricular extrasystoles and fibrillation, respectively.

How can one be sure about these values, however? The slopes of the correlation integrals must be examined at a judiciously chosen range, and even there they fluctuate significantly, making an accurate estimation of the dimension rather delicate. In fact, it is even questionable that one may even speak about the "dimension" of an "attractor," since the shape of the curves cannot even distinguish the results from what one would get in the case of Gaussian noise!

Perhaps the only meaningful interpretation one could attach to such correlation dimension estimates is that of an

indicator, or a statistic, which may be of some value when used to compare different subjects under different physiological conditions.

We will argue that the correlation dimension of an ECG signal does not *by itself* constitute a reliable measure of the complexity of a system's chaotic dynamics. For the sinus rhythm of a single person, for example, it typically varies between 2 and 4, and does not appear to depend on whether the subject is a heavy smoker, resting, or has been mildly exercising.

We have, therefore, supplemented dimension calculations with a number of tests in order to obtain a more complete picture of ECG dynamics. Such tests include time differentiation,[10] smoothing out of high frequencies and principal component analysis. What we find is that a straightforward computation yields an underestimate of the correlation dimension of the ECG signal, which appears to be five to six, i.e., closer to the range of the correlation dimension of the time-differenced series.

Finally, we observed, for almost all subjects, that this value typically increases by about 1, between resting and mild exercising. This seems to indicate that cardiac dynamics does become more "complex" (i.e., higher dimensional) under conditions of physical stress.

The plan of the paper is as follows: In Sec. II we briefly outline the principles and techniques of chaotic dynamics used in this work; in Sec. III we describe the cases we have studied and the main results, while our conclusions are discussed in Sec. IV.

II. THE APPROACH OF NONLINEAR TIME SERIES ANALYSIS

Let us assume that the ECG signal we wish to study can be described by a deterministic flow of n generally coupled, nonlinear ordinary differential equations (ODEs),

$$\dot{\mathbf{x}} = \mathbf{f}(\mathbf{x}), \quad \mathbf{x} = [x_1(t),...,x_n(t)], \tag{1}$$

where $\mathbf{f} = (f_1,...f_n)$ are unknown functions of the coordinates $x(t)$.

Now, let $V(t) = V[\mathbf{x}(t)]$ be a scalar observable depending on the state of the system $\mathbf{x}(t)$ and obtained by a well-defined measurement process. More specifically, in our case, this scalar is the electrostatic potential average of a 12-lead ECG recording of human subjects.

According to a celebrated theorem by Takens,[20] given the time series of a scalar observable,

$$[V(t_1),V(t_2),...,V(t_i),...], \quad \Delta t_i \equiv t_i - t_{i-1}, \tag{2}$$

recorded at successive intervals, $i = 1,2,...,N$ (here $\Delta t_i = \Delta t = 1$ step), one constructs a vector $\mathbf{X}(t)$, whose coordinates are time-delayed copies of $V(t)$, as follows:

$$\mathbf{X}(t_i) = [V(t_i),V(t_i+\tau),...,V(t_i+(m-1)\tau)], \tag{3}$$

where τ is the delay time (see below) and $m = 1,2,3,...$. The content of the theorem is that, under some general conditions, the orbit followed by $\mathbf{X}(t)$ in this m-dimensional embedding space (for $m \geq n$) differs from the actual solution $\mathbf{x}(t)$ of (1) only by a smooth change of coordinates.

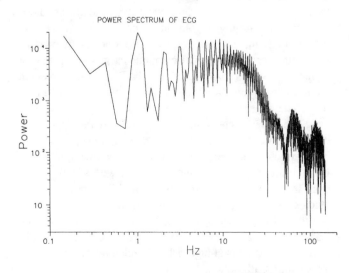

FIG. 2. Power spectrum of an ECG signal.

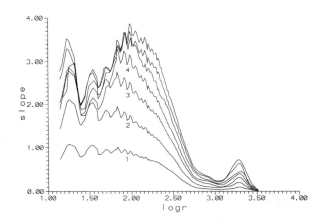

FIG. 3. The slope of $\log C(m,r)$ vs $\log r$; see (6) and (7) for embedding space dimensions $m = 1, 2, ..., 8$.

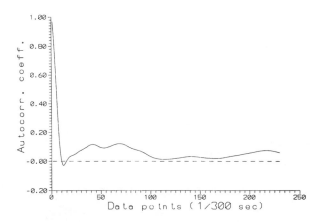

FIG. 4. The autocorrelation coefficient of a typical ECG signal. Note that the signal decorrelates at $\tau_d \approx 10$.

Clearly, if the dimension m of the embedding space is too small, the orbit $\mathbf{X}(t)$ constitutes a projection, which will tend to "fill" completely the available m-dimensional space. On the other hand, if m increases beyond a critical integer value d, some of the main geometric properties of the dynamics are expected to remain unchanged. ($d \leq n$ is called the embedding dimension of the "attractor" of the time series.)

One such geometric property is the correlation dimension ν, which can be measured by the Grassberger–Procaccia method[6] as follows: Consider N points $\mathbf{X}_j \equiv \mathbf{X}(t_j)$ in an m-dimensional space and define the correlation function around the ith point by

$$C_i(m,r) \equiv (1/N)(\text{number of points } \mathbf{X}_j$$

$$\text{with } |\mathbf{X}_j - \mathbf{X}_i| < r), \tag{4}$$

$|\cdots|$ being the Euclidean norm, $i, j = 1, 2, ..., N$, for some $r > 0$. Summing (4) over i and averaging over N we obtain the correlation integral

$$C(m,r) = \frac{1}{N} \sum_{i=1}^{N} C_i(m,r), \tag{5}$$

which is expected to scale as a power of the radius r,

$$C(m,r) \propto r^{\nu(m)}, \quad \text{as } r \to 0. \tag{6}$$

The slope of the curve of $\log C(m,r)$ vs $\log r$ (all logs are with base 10),

$$\nu(m) \equiv \lim_{r \to 0} d[\log C(m,r)]/d(\log r), \tag{7}$$

is called the correlation dimension of our data. Now, if this data indeed lies on an attractor and the dynamics is characterized by deterministic chaos, ν is expected to be a (close) lower bound of the *fractal dimension* D of the attractor, i.e., $\nu \leq D$.[7,8]

We have plotted $\log C(m,r)$ vs $\log r$ for our ECG signals, for several values of the embedding space dimension m and delay τ, and have observed a tendency of the results to approach a definite curve over a scaling region in the middle part of the figure. To estimate the slope of that curve, we numerically plot in Fig. 3 the derivative (7), in the typical

case of a normal subject, and find that it oscillates near $\nu = 3$.

Note that these curves are obtained by increasing the dimension of the embedding space to $m = 8$. We did, of course, test the dependence of these results on the number of data points and found that for $N \geq 16\ 000$ values our results did not differ significantly.

Regarding the number of data points N used in these calculations, we point out that, according to a formula proposed in Ref. 21, $N \geq N_{\min}$, with $N_{\min} = 10^{2+0.4D}$, where D is the fractal dimension of the attractor. In our case, taking $D = 5$, one obtains $N_{\min} = 10\ 000$, and thus our number of $N \geq 16\ 000$ points is quite satisfactory for this study.

As far as the value of the delay time τ is concerned, this was chosen larger than the so-called decorrelation time, τ_d, where the autocorrelation function of the signal has its first zero;[22] see Fig. 4. As τ_d was found in most cases to be $10 \leq \tau_d \leq 40$, choosing a delay $\tau = 50$, 100, or 150 did not significantly affect the results.

It is also clear that when τ is very small, say $\tau = 1$, the dynamics (in a two-dimensional embedding space) is strongly correlated along the diagonal; see Fig. 5(a). However, when τ is set larger than τ_d, say $\tau = 100$, the orbits are free to explore the full extent of the attractor, as shown in Fig. 5(b).

Now, although, with increasing embedding dimension m, the function (7) is seen to converge to a definite curve, it is often not easy to observe a well-defined "plateau" on this curve, even after varying τ. In such cases, one cannot be sure that there is indeed a low-dimensional attractor governing the dynamics, since similar results can be obtained from the signal with power-law noise.[10] Clearly a much more detailed study of the data is needed.

Let us analyze these results in more detail to find how they depend on a number of other parameters present in the system. For example, what happens if we eliminate from the calculation (4) points $\mathbf{X}_j$ that lie *dynamically* close to $\mathbf{X}_i$, i.e., occur at j time intervals before and after $\mathbf{X}_i$?

What we discover—when throwing out all points with $j = \pm 1, \pm 2, ..., \pm W$, in (4)—is that there is a clear increase in the correlation dimension, by about two units, see Fig. 6(a), for $W \geq 5$. This demonstrates that (at small $\log r$) a low

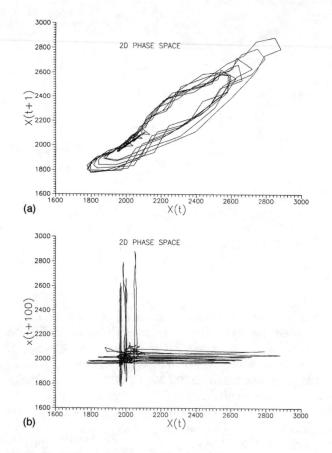

(a)

(b)

FIG. 5. The ECG attractor in a two-dimensional phase space. (a) Note how the points are correlated for time delay $\tau=1$, while (b) for $\tau > \tau_d$ (here $\tau=100$) they explore more completely the actual attractor.

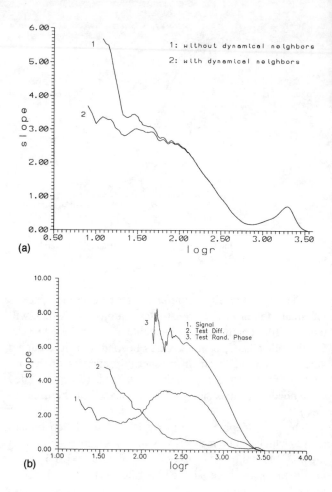

(a)

(b)

FIG. 6. The same as for Fig. 3, for $m=7$. (a) Curve 1 is obtained by including all dynamical neighbors, while curve 2 shows the increase in correlation dimension when some of these neighbors $j=\pm1,\pm2,...,\pm10$ have been removed. (b) Comparison between correlation dimension estimates of the input ECG signal (curve 1), time-differenced signal (curve 2), and phase-randomized data.

value of ν may be due to temporal rather than geometrical proximity between points on the attractor. On the other hand, the fact that the shape of the function (7) and the value of $\nu \approx 6$ remain unaffected for $m=8,9,10$ may indicate that the proper number of principal components governing the dynamics of the ECG signal is five to six rather than three to four.

In order to further study the chaotic versus random and low- versus high-dimensional character of our ECG signals, we will now apply a number of tests pointed out in the recent literature.[10]

The first one is the test of phase randomization, which examines whether the apparent low-dimensionality of a time series is due to a power-law behavior of its Fourier amplitudes, $|A(\omega)|^2 \sim \omega^\alpha$ whose phases are randomly distributed. To check whether this is the case here, we Fourier analyze our data,

$$V(t_i)=\sum_{k=1}^{N/2} A(\omega_k)\cos(\omega_k t_i + \varphi_k), \quad i=1,...,N, \quad (8)$$

with $\omega_k=2\pi k/(N \Delta t)(\Delta t=1)$, and proceed to randomize the phases φ_k in (8), thus constructing a surrogate series $[V(t_i),i=1,2,...,N]$. If the correlation dimension of this series, $\bar\nu$, is nearly equal to the one obtained by (6) and (7), we will then have detected randomness in the Fourier phases of our original series.

The correlation exponent $\bar\nu$, however, behaves quite differently than the ν of the original series: It shows no tendency to saturate and continues to increase, with increasing m, as shown in Fig. 6(b) (also see Table I). This result clearly implies that the Fourier phases of our series are not

TABLE I. Correlation dimension of input signal (ν), time-differenced series (ν_Δ) and phase randomized series ($\bar\nu$).

Case		ν	ν_Δ	$\bar\nu$
N1	Resting	3.04±0.626	3.79±0.078	6.56±0.905
	exercise	3.58±0.846	5.68±0.518	6.50±0.432
N2	Resting	2.63±0.640	4.23±0.549	6.75±0.525
	exercise	2.79±0.396	6.14±0.743	6.22±0.635
N3	Resting	2.61±0.470	4.33±0.225	6.19±1.152
	exercise	3.20±1.092	4.66±1.086	7.26±2.327
S1	Resting	2.08±0.704	4.21±0.404	6.58±0.305
	exercise	3.01±0.877	5.21±0.776	6.65±0.662
S2	Resting	2.21±0.503	4.71±0.435	6.58±0.505
	exercise	3.49±0.452	5.91±0.478	6.81±0.642
S3	Resting	2.74±0.292	5.31±0.348	6.01±0.834
	exercise	2.71±0.725	4.81±0.484	6.58±0.924

completely uncorrelated, and hence do not constitute a source of randomness for our signal.

Owing to the singular distribution of our data [see Fig. 5(b)], it is possible that phase randomization changes length scales in these calculations, which may explain why the corresponding curve in Fig. 6(b) reaches its maximum and terminates at higher log r values than the other two curves. It is clear, however, that it does yield a considerably longer correlation dimension estimates, characteristic of random data.

So what is going on? Is there noise in our signals, and if so, where does it reside? A clear answer to this question is provided by the test of time differentiation, i.e., by studying the time-differenced series $[\Delta V(t_i)]$, defined by

$$\Delta V(t_i) = V(t_i) - V(t_{i-1}), \quad i = 1, 2, ..., N, \quad (9)$$

whose dynamics turns out to differ significantly from that of the original series $[V(t_i)]$.

Note that, if the series $[V(t_i)]$ had been derived from a purely deterministic flow, described by a system of ODEs like (1), the dynamics of the signal itself and its derivative would be expected to have very similar geometrical and statistical properties. This is indeed what happens, e.g., with the time-differenced signal, $\Delta x(t) = x(t + \Delta t) - x(t)$, of the x component of the Lorentz model.[10]

In our case, however, things are different. We have computed the correlation dimension, ν_Δ, of (9), for a number of ECG signals taken from resting as well as exercising subjects, and found that it typically increases by about two units compared with the ν value of the original series [see Fig. 6(b) and Table I]. Moreover, there values do not significantly change if dynamical neighbors are also removed from the calculations.

This shows that there is indeed "noise" present in the high-frequency part of the data, which is probably due to the fact that the heart is not an isolated mechanism, operating independently of any other function of the human body. Rapid changes in the values of these differences may also be responsible for the high-frequency content of our spectra. It is interesting that in most cases studied, this measure of "randomness" in our series, ν_Δ increases by about one unit under mild exercising conditions (see Table I).

It is also possible to "temper" this high-frequency, nondeterministic component by applying to our series a smoothing procedure, according to which every point $V(t_i)$ is replaced by an average over 1 forward and 1 backward neighbor in time, and consider the series of "moving averages,"

$$V(t_i) \rightarrow S(t_i) = \tfrac{1}{4}[V(t_i - \Delta t) + 2V(t_i) + V(t_i + \Delta t)]. \quad (10)$$

This procedure indeed produces a smoother power spectrum and exhibits correlation dimension plots very similar to those of Fig. 3.

Thus we may choose to abandon the original ECG signal $[V(t_i)]$ and consider instead the averaged series $[S(t_i)]$, (10), which is, to a large extent, free from high-frequency random fluctuations. This is evidenced by the fact that if we now apply time differentiation to the "smoothed" data (2.10), the resulting series $[\Delta S(t) = S(t_i) - S(t_{i-1})]$ has a $\nu_\Delta \approx \nu$ of the

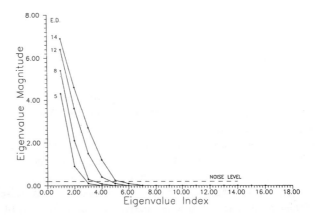

FIG. 7. Computation of eigenvalues of the $m \times m$ covariance matrix of SVD analysis, for $m = 5, 8, 12, 14$. Note how, as m increases, four to five eigenvalues are raised above the noise level, indicating that the dynamics is governed by four to five principal components.

original series $[S(t_i)]$ (removing dynamical neighbors has, of course, the same effect of raising the dimension as before).

Finally, we examine our ECG signals from the viewpoint of singular value decomposition (SVD) or principal component analysis.[12] According to this approach, one constructs first the trajectory matrix,

$$Z = (1/N^{1/2})[\mathbf{X}^T(1), \mathbf{X}^T(2), ..., \mathbf{X}^T(M)], \quad (11)$$

where

$$\mathbf{X}(i) = [V(t_i), V(t_i + \delta), ..., V(t_i + (M-1)\delta)]; \quad (12)$$

cf. (3), where $\delta = k \, \Delta t$ is a suitably chosen lag parameter and $(M-1)k + M = N$. Then, one considers the covariance matrix $Z^T Z$ with elements

$$(Z^T Z)_{i,j} = \frac{1}{N}\mathbf{X}(i)\mathbf{X}^T(j), \quad i, j = 1, 2, ..., m \leqslant M \quad (13)$$

(in an m-dimensional embedding space), and computes its eigenvalues and eigenvectors for several values of $m = 5, 8, 12, 14, ...$ etc.

What we find is that the number of significant eigenvalues (also corresponding to the number of principal components) above the noise level increases from four to five, see Fig. 7. The value of δ we have used in (12) is $\delta = 1$, following a criterion proposed in Ref. 12. According to this criterion, $m\delta\gamma_s \approx 1/f_*$, where m is the embedding dimension, γ_s is the sampling time, and f_* is the frequency at which the power of the signal is significantly reduced (in our case, $m = 7$, $\gamma_s = 1/300, f_* = 30$).

III. STUDY CASES AND RESULTS

The cases studied in this paper consist of three healthy young men of ages 20–30 and of three heavy smokers, 20–40 yr old. Their ECG signals were recorded at the clinical ECG laboratory of the University of Patras Hospital, under M.D. monitoring.

No evidence of cardiovascular disease was observed in any of the cases, as assessed by history, clinical examination, resting, and exercise tests concluded by 12-lead ECG recordings.

One ECG lead, with clearly visible P and T waves and QRS complexes of large-amplitude (corresponding to lead V) was recorded continuously for 10–15 min, in supine (resting) and upright (exercise) positions. The exercise test was carried out with a treadmill speed of 2.5 km/h and 10% inclination, while the recording period started after the heart rate and blood pressure of the subject had been stabilized.

The ECGs were amplified using a CASE 15 exercise system (Marquette, OH) with standard amplification and filters set between 0.04 and 80 Hz. The signals were digitized on line (12-bit Metrabyte DAS 16F, ADC board) at a rate of 300 Hz and stored on hard disk for further processing. Each resulting file of 900–1500 heart beats finally consist of ten sets of 22 000 points each. In this work, we analyze several of these sets independently and found that all yielded statistically very similar results.

The results for one of these sets are summarized in Table I. As is evident from the second column of Table I, the correlation dimension of all subjects, "normal" or heavy smokers, resting or exercising, lies between 2–4, when computed, using the Grassberger–Procaccia algorithm, without removing dynamically neighboring points.

However, as seen in column 3, this dimension increases, when studying the "derivative" (or time-differenced) signal, to a value between 4 and 6 and remains there, even for embedding space dimensions $m = 8, 9, 10$. Similar results are obtained when one removes a number of dynamical neighbors (before and after each point) in the correlation dimension calculations.

This is to be contrasted with the behavior of the correlation dimension of "surrogate" data, obtained by randomizing the phases of the Fourier components of the original series. Here the dimension is, in all cases, larger than 6, and the series clearly displays features of random noise. It appears, therefore, reasonable to say that the dynamics of our ECG signals lies on a five- to six-dimensional deterministic attractor. Finally, it is interesting to note that the correlation dimension ν_Δ increases by 1 in the transition from resting to mild exercising conditions. This suggests typically that under physical stress the human heart may find it more efficient to increase the complexity of its dynamics.

IV. DISCUSSION

Babloyantz and Destexhe[5] were among the first to study ECGs at rest, in normal sinus rhythms, using the techniques of chaotic dynamics. They found that the correlation dimension of an ECG varies between 3.6 and 5.2, and thus suggested that the dynamics occurs on a low-dimensional deterministic attractor. They did not, however, have the opportunity to test the sensitivity of their results on a number of parameters, commonly used nowadays, to probe more deeply into the dynamical properties of a given signal.

Ravelli and Andolini[19] also calculated the correlation dimension, of human cardiac activity ranging from sinus rhythm to ventricular fibrillation. They found that ν increases, as one proceeds from sinus rhythm to fully developed ventricular fibrillation, and concluded that this indicates an increase in the complexity of the dynamics of the corresponding ECG signal.

However, as is well known, the autonomous nervous system controls only sinus rhythms and not fibrillation. Thus, the claim that, in the transition from one to the other, chaotic properties become stronger is rather ill-founded, since it refers to phenomena caused by entirely different physiological processes.

There are, of course, also the earlier studies of Goldberger *et al.*[23] on the power spectrum of the QRS complex, suggesting that the power law obeyed by that spectrum is a consequence of the apparent fractal nature of the His-Purkinje system. This view, however, has been challenged by a recent study,[13] which shows that QRS spectra for beats not conducted by the His-Purkinje system follow a power law as well, if not better, than His-Purkinje conducted beats, and do so with similar power-law exponents.

All this makes it clear that, although there are few who doubt the existence of low-dimensional deterministic dynamics in human ECGs, there is a wide variety of methodologies, as well as interpretations of the results, in connection with different physiological or pathological conditions.

Our intention in this paper was to concentrate on a full ECG time series and examine the usefulness and reliability of a number of recently proposed tools for the analysis of chaotic behavior present in the data. This was done using a number of subjects, with different life histories and different rates of deregulation of their autonomic cardiac tone.

Our results demonstrate that there are no major differences in the dynamics of ECG signals taken from "normal" versus heavily smoking subjects, under resting or (mild) exercising conditions. There is strong evidence of a deterministic attractor, whose correlation dimension is seen to be nearly five or six, when the high-frequency part of the spectrum is taken into account, and effects due to temporal correlations between its points are removed. This is also consistent with singular value decomposition results, which show that an ECG signal is well described by the interaction of five to six principal components, and with the fact that our data does not show features of Gaussian or fractal Brownian noise.

In our view, dimension calculation such as we have presented here can only be used as a hint that a small number of variables is responsible for the main behavior of the cardiac dynamics. At best, they provide an indicator that may be used to distinguish between ECG signals obtained under very different circumstances.

A lot still remains to be done in the study of cardiac dynamics, especially in clinically more critical cases. For example, it is known that power spectrum analysis of heart rate variability (the statistics of R–R intervals) can quantify the cardiac autonomic tone.[24] Thus, changes in the frequency domain of R–R intervals may, in fact, be related to the onset of myocardiac infraction,[25] or even the so-called retrospected cardiac death.[4] Such studies, however, suffer from the unavailability of long enough time series (for nearly 5000 data points one requires a continuous ECG of one hour).

Currently, we are in the process of obtaining data sets, which are sufficiently long to permit a more detailed study of the dynamics of R–R intervals in cases with strong clinical interest, and results will be presented in future publications.

ACKNOWLEDGMENTS

Part of this work was supported by a grant from the G.S.R.T. (General Secretariat of Research and Technology) of the Greek Ministry of Industry, Energy, and Technology. We wish to thank one of the referees, whose valuable comments helped us look more critically in the interpretation of some of our results. We also thank A. Tsonis for many stimulating discussions.

[1] A. M. Kalz, *Physiology of the Heart* (Raven, New York, 1992).

[2] E. L. Michelson and J. Morganroth, "Spontaneous variability of complex ventricular arrhythmias detected by long-term electrocardiographic recording," Circulation **61**, 600 (1980).

[3] T. A. Denton, G. A. Diamond, R. H. Helfart, S. Khan, and H. Karagueuzian, "Fascinating rhythm: A primer on chaos theory and its application to cardiology," Am. Heart J., St. Louis **120**, 1419 (1990).

[4] A. L. Goldberger and B. J. West, "Applications of nonlinear dynamics to clinical cardiology," Ann. NY Acad. Sci. **504**, 195 (1987).

[5] A. Babloyantz and A. Destexhe, "Is the normal heart a periodic oscillator?," Biol. Cyb. **58**, 203 (1988).

[6] P. Grassberger and I. Procaccia, "Measuring the strangeness of a strange attractor," Physica D **9**, 189 (1983).

[7] H. G. Schuster, *Deterministic Chaos*, 2nd ed. (Physik-Verlag, Weinheim, 1988).

[8] P. Berge, Y. Pomeau, and C. Vidal, *Order Within Chaos* (Hermann, Paris, 1984) [and (Wiley, New York, 1986)].

[9] A. A. Tsonis, *Chaos: From Theory to Applications* (Plenum, New York, 1992).

[10] A. Provenzale, L. A. Smith, R. Vio and G. Murante, "Distinguishing low-dimensional dynamics and randomness in measured time series," Physica D **58**, 31 (1992).

[11] J. Theiler, "Spurious dimension from correlation algorithms applied to limited time-series data," Phys. Rev. A **34**, 2427 (1986).

[12] D. S. Broomhead and G. P. King, "Extracting qualitative dynamics from experimental data," Physica D **20**, 217 (1986).

[13] R. D. Berger, D. S. Rosenbaum and R. J. Cohen, "Is the power spectrum of the QRS complex related to a fractal His-Purkinje system?," Am. J. Cardiol. **71**, 430 (1993).

[14] G. A. Myers, G. J. Martin, N. M. Magin, P. S. Benett, J. W. Schaad, J. S. Weiss, M. Lesch, and D. H. Singer, "Power spectral analysis of heart rate variability in sudden cardiac death: Comparison to other methods," IEEE Trans. Biomed. Eng. **BE-33**, 1149 (1986).

[15] A. L. Goldberger, V. Bhargava, B. J. West, and A. J. Mandell, "Some observations on the question: Is verticular fibrillation "chaos"?," Physica D **19**, 282 (1986).

[16] P. S. Chen, P. D. Wolf, E. G. Dixon, N. D. Danieley, D. W. Frazier, W. M. Smith, and R. E. Ideken, "Mechanism of ventricular vulnerability to single premature stimuli in open-chest dogs," Circ. Res. **62**, 1191 (1988).

[17] A. Garfinkel, H. Karagueuzian, S. Khan, and G. Diamond, "Is the proarrhythmic effect of quinidine a chaotic phenomenon? (abstract)," J. Am. Colloid. Cardiol. A **13**, 186 (1989).

[18] S. J. Evans, S. S. Khan, A. Garfinkle, R. M. Kass, A. Aldano, and G. A. Diamond, "Is ventricular fibrillation random or chaotic? (abstract)," Circulation **80**, 11 (1989).

[19] F. Ravelli and R. Andolini, "Complex dynamics underlying the human electrocardiogram," Biol. Cyb. **67**, 57 (1992).

[20] F. Takens, "Detecting strange attractors in turbulence," in *Lecture Notes in Mathematics*, edited by D. A. Rand and L. S. Young (Springer-Verlag, Berlin, 1981), Vol. 898, pp. 366–381.

[21] M. A. Nerenberg and C. Essex, "Correlation dimension and systematic geometric effects," Phys. Rev. A **42**, 7065 (1986).

[22] A. M. Fraser and H. L. Swinney, "Independent coordinates in strange attractor from mutual information," Phys. Rev. A **33**, 1134 (1986).

[23] A. L. Goldberger, V. Bhargava, B. J. West, and A. J. Mandell, "On a mechanism of cardiac electrical stability, the fractal hypothesis," Biophys. J. **48**, 525 (1985).

[24] J. O. Valcano, H. V. Huikuri, K. E. J. Airaksinen, M. K. Linnaluoto, and J. T. Takkunen, "Changes in frequency domain measures of heart rate variability in relation of the onset of ventricular tachycardia in acutemyocardial information," Int. J. Cardiol. **38**, 177 (1985).

[25] B. Pomeranz, R. J. B. McCaulay, M. A. Candill, I. Kutz, D. Adam, D. Gordon, K. M. Kilborn, A. C. Barger, D. C. Shannon, R. J. Cohen, and H. Benson, "Assessment of autonomic function in humans by heart rate spectral analysis," Am. J. Physiol. **248**, H151 (1985).

Age-related changes in the "complexity" of cardiovascular dynamics: A potential marker of vulnerability to disease

Lewis A. Lipsitz, M.D.
Hebrew Rehabilitation Center for Aged, Beth Israel Hospital, and Harvard Medical School Division on Aging, Boston, Massachusetts 02131

(Received 16 May 1994; accepted for publication 2 August 1994)

Healthy physiologic control of cardiovascular function is a result of complex interactions between multiple regulatory processes that operate over different time scales. These include the sympathetic and parasympathetic nervous systems which regulate beat-to-beat heart rate (HR) and blood pressure (BP), as well as extravascular volume, body temperature, and sleep which influence HR and BP over the longer term. Interactions between these control systems generate highly variable fluctuations in continuous HR and BP signals. Techniques derived from nonlinear dynamics and chaos theory are now being adapted to quantify the dynamic behavior of physiologic time series and study their changes with age or disease. We have shown significant age-related changes in the $1/f^x$ relationship between the log amplitude and log frequency of the heart rate power spectrum, as well as declines in approximate dimension and approximate entropy of both heart rate and blood pressure time series. These changes in the "complexity" of cardiovascular dynamics reflect the breakdown and decoupling of integrated physiologic regulatory systems with aging, and may signal an impairment in cardiovascular ability to adapt to external and internal perturbations. Studies are currently underway to determine whether the complexity of HR or BP time series can distinguish patients with fainting spells due to benign vasovagal reactions from those due to life-threatening cardiac arrhythmias. Thus, measures of the complexity of physiologic variability may provide novel methods to monitor cardiovascular aging and test the efficacy of specific interventions to improve adaptive capacity in old age. © *1995 American Institute of Physics.*

I. INTRODUCTION

Since 1929 when Walter B. Cannon introduced the concept of "homeostasis,"[1] the study of physiology has been based on the principle that all cells, tissues, and organs maintain *static* or *constant* "steady-state" conditions in their internal environment. However, with the recent introduction of signal processing techniques that can acquire continuous time series data from physiologic processes such as heart rate, blood pressure, or nerve activity, it has become apparent that biomedical signals vary in a complex and irregular way, even during "steady-state" conditions. This observation has led to the understanding that healthy physiologic function is a result of continuous, dynamic interactions between multiple neural, hormonal, mechanical, and local subcellular biochemical control systems. These interactions generate highly variable fluctuations in the output of physiologic processes.[2]

For example, the normal resting sinus rhythm of the heart which is easily recorded on the electrocardiogram, is highly irregular, despite the widespread notion that under steady-state conditions it is monotonously regular. This irregular behavior of the heartbeat is readily apparent when heart rate is examined on a beat-to-beat basis, but is overlooked when a mean value over time is calculated (Fig. 1). Similarly, basal blood pressure varies from beat to beat, as well as over longer periods representing ultradian and circadian rhythms. These fluctuations in heart rate and blood pressure result from complex, nonlinear interactions between respiration, pressure receptors (baroreceptors), the autonomic nervous system, neuropeptides, and other factors over the short term, as well as body temperature, metabolic rate, hormones, and sleep cycles, over the long term. In concert, these multiple influences create a dynamic physiologic control system that is never truly at rest, and is certainly never static. When relatively unperturbed it remains responsive and resilient, primed and ready to react when needed.

The process of aging has a dramatic and profound impact on the complex dynamics of healthy physiologic function.[3] This is evident in many physiologic systems, but the cardiovascular system has received the most attention because of the high morbidity and mortality associated with cardiovascular disease, and the current availability of continuous noninvasive data collection and signal processing techniques to measure continuous heart rate and blood pressure. Aging impairs many of the cardiovascular mechanisms that regulate heart rate and blood pressure. As a result, there is a loss of complex variability in the dynamics of these systems. I propose that this age-related loss of dynamic range in physiologic function reduces an individual's capacity to adapt to internal and external perturbations, and thereby increases an older person's vulnerability to the development of disease.

The purpose of this paper is to illustrate the effects of normal human aging on heart rate and blood pressure dynamics, and discuss the clinical implications of these changes. I hope to stimulate future collaborations between physicists, mathematicians, and gerontologists, in order to develop new methods derived from nonlinear dynamics and chaos theory that can better quantitate physiologic aging and predict the onset of disease.

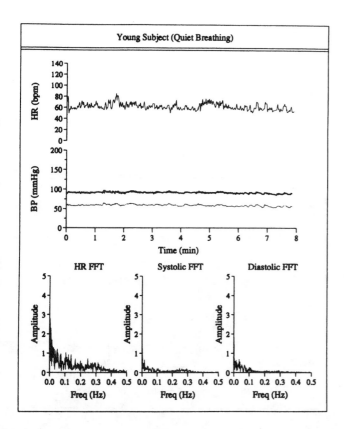
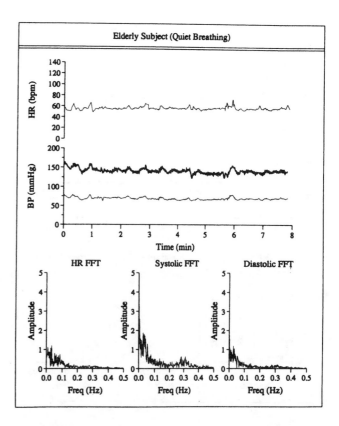

FIG. 1. Continuous heart rate time series (upper graphs), blood pressure time series (middle graphs), and fast Fourier transforms (FFT) for heart rate (HR) (left lower graphs), systolic blood pressure (middle lower graphs), and diastolic blood pressure (right lower graphs), for a healthy 22 yr old subject (left panel) and a healthy 70 yr old subject (right panel) during supine, quiet breathing conditions. Note the highly irregular, complex heart rate variability in the young subject compared to the old, despite similar mean heart rate (62 ± 5 and 57 ± 3 BPM, respectively) over 8 min of recording. In contrast, blood pressure is higher with greater variability in the old ($142/69\pm6/3$) compared to the young ($92/59\pm2/2$) subject. The fast Fourier transforms of both HR and systolic blood pressure show a broadband spectrum with low-frequency power (amplitude^2) from 0.05–0.12 Hz representing baroreflex activity, and high frequency (0.2–0.4 Hz) representing parasympathetic activity. There is greater overall HR power in the young subject, but greater overall BP power in the elderly subject.

II. HEART RATE AND BLOOD PRESSURE DYNAMICS

Previous studies of cardiovascular function and its changes with aging or disease have focused primarily on alterations in the *mean* value of physiologic variables averaged over time or in response to a stimulus. This approach ignores the dynamic nature of physiologic processes. As illustrated by the heart rate time series displayed in the top tracings of Figs. 1 and 2, the mean HR is similar between healthy young and old subjects, but the dynamics are markedly different.

This observation raises three important questions: (1) What are the underlying mechanisms of the complex dynamics illustrated in Figs. 1 and 2?; (2) Why do these dynamics change with aging?; and (3) How can we quantify the complex variability in these time series, so that we can accurately measure the effects of aging, predict the onset of disease, and test interventions to prevent cardiovascular morbidity in late life?

III. MECHANISMS OF CARDIOVASCULAR DYNAMICS IN THE HEALTHY YOUNG

The normal heartbeat originates in the sinus node of the right atrium where a small bundle of pacemaker cells spon-

taneously generate rhythmic electrical activity. This activity is conducted through specialized conduction pathways into the ventricular muscle. There it stimulates rhythmic ventricular contraction, thus generating cardiac output.

Blood pressure is determined by the product of cardiac output and systemic vascular resistance. Changes in blood pressure that may occur due to dilatation of resistance vessels or pooling of blood in various parts of the circulation (e.g., the legs and abdomen during standing) are detected by specialized pressure receptors (baroreceptors) in the large arteries or cardiac atria. These receptors send signals to the brainstem, which regulates the outflow of sympathetic and parasympathetic nervous system activity through the autonomic nervous system. Sympathetic stimulation of the heart increases heart rate, thus restoring blood pressure to normal if it falls too low. Parasympathetic stimulation slows the heart rate and lowers blood pressure if it momentarily goes too high. This feedback loop, called the baroreflex, is an important regulatory mechanism for the beat-to-beat control of blood pressure and heart rate.

The mechanics of respiration also influence the dynamical behavior of heart rate and blood pressure. During inspiration, a large negative intrathoracic pressure pulls blood into

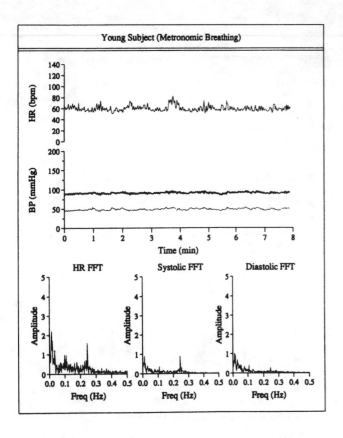

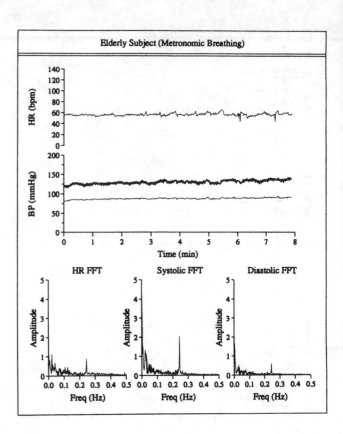

FIG. 2. Continuous heart rate time series (upper graphs), blood pressure time series (middle graphs), and fast Fourier transforms (FFT) for heart rate (HR) (left lower graphs), systolic blood pressure (middle lower graphs), and diastolic blood pressure (right lower graphs), for the same healthy young subject (left panel) and healthy elderly subject (right panel) as Fig. 1, during supine metronomic breathing at 0.25 Hz. Note the frequency spike in the FFTs at 0.25 Hz representing the respiratory influence on heart rate and blood pressure variability.

the cardiac atria and lungs where stretch receptors activate an autonomic reflex causing an increase in heart rate. Also, the transient reduction in cardiac output during inspiration reduces blood pressure, which in turn stimulates baroreceptors. A central respiratory control system in the brain may also directly entrain oscillations in the autonomic nervous system. Oscillations in heart rate associated with respiration are called the respiratory sinus arrhythmia.

Power spectral analysis of heart rate or blood pressure time series data using the fast Fourier transform has enabled physiologists to identify and quantify some of the mechanisms underlying cardiovascular dynamics.[4,5] Low-frequency oscillations with a period of approximately 10 s (0.08–0.12 Hz) in the heart rate power spectrum are attributable to baroreflex modulation of sinus node activity, while in the blood pressure power spectrum they represent baroreflex modulation of vasomotor tone.[5] The amplitude of oscillations in this frequency range increases during activities that lower blood pressure and stimulate baroreceptors, such as standing, exercise, hemorrhage, or hypotension. Higher frequency oscillations with a period of approximately 4 s (0.15–0.40 Hz), represent the respiratory influences on both heart rate and blood pressure power spectra. This is mediated predominantly by the parasympathetic nervous system along the vagus nerve. Withdrawal of parasympathetic activity by the drug atropine or the hypotensive stresses listed above, reduces the amplitude of this frequency band. Regular

breathing at a constant rate (metronomic breathing) enhances the amplitude of heart rate and blood pressure fluctuations at the frequency of respiration (Fig. 2).

The heart rate power spectrum has been shown to be highly reproducible within healthy individuals over a 3 to 65 day period.[6] The reproducibility of the blood pressure power spectrum has not been well studied, however, the standard deviation of noninvasive finger recordings is highly reproducible within subjects during stationary periods over 30 min apart.[7]

In the clinical research laboratory a postural tilt test is often used to study the effect of upright posture on baroreflex control of heart rate and blood pressure. Subjects are examined on a tilting bed that moves them from the supine position to almost standing at 60°. The results of a typical tilt study for a healthy young woman (age=21 yr) are shown in the right-hand column of Fig. 3. Note the marked variability and irregularity in the 10 min supine heart rate time series. Spectral analysis reveals a broadband power spectrum with multiple frequency components. During postural tilt, low-frequency oscillations between 0.05 and 0.1 Hz increase in amplitude. These oscillations are called Mayer waves and represent baroreflex activation. Similar dynamic behavior can be observed in the blood pressure time series (not shown) where irregular oscillations under supine conditions give rise to more organized low-frequency Mayer waves during postural tilt.

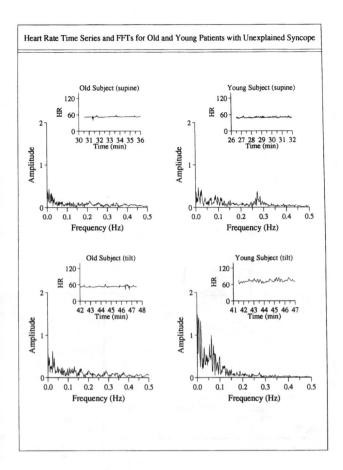

FIG. 3. Heart rate time series (upper inserts) and fast Fourier transforms for old (left side) and young (right side) patients with unexplained syncope. Data obtained while subjects were supine is shown in the upper graphs, and data during 5 min of 60° head-up tilt are shown in the lower graphs. There is less heart rate variability during both supine and tilt conditions in the old subject compared to young. Note the emergence of low-frequency Mayer waves in the heart rate time series of the young subject during upright tilt, with a corresponding increase in low frequency amplitude (0.05–0.10 Hz) in the heart rate power spectrum during upright tilt. In contrast, the old subject has no change in the heart rate power spectrum during tilt.

The parasympathetic contribution to heart rate and blood pressure variability can be demonstrated by observing the effect of metronomic breathing on the power spectrum. Note in Fig. 2 the emergence of a spike at the respiratory frequency (0.25 Hz). As respiratory frequency is lowered toward the baroreflex frequency entrainment of the two processes has been observed.[8] Based on these observations, Kitney et al. have suggested that there is nonlinear coupling between respiration and the baroreflex.[8]

The recent observation that heat rate variability demonstrates self-similarity across multiple orders of temporal magnitude, suggests that the mechanisms underlying heart rate regulation may have fractal properties. The heart rate[9–12] and blood pressure[13] power spectra have been shown to have inverse power-law $(1/f^x)$ scaling. As shown in Fig. 4, the relationship between log amplitude vs log frequency of a normal heart rate time series is linear over a broad frequency band.

Recent analyses of cardiac beat-to-beat intervals in healthy subjects over very long time intervals (up to 24 hr)

show scale-invariant long-range correlations.[14] In subjects with severe heart disease the distribution of heartbeat intervals is unchanged, but long-range correlations are lost.[14]

The $1/f$ nature of heart rate and blood pressure variability is poorly understood, but may be related to the interaction of multiple physiological control systems that operate over many different time scales. These range from seconds for autonomic nervous system control, to minutes for hormonal regulation of vascular tone (e.g., the renin–angiotensin system), to hours for changes in blood volume, to diurnal periods for temperature and circadian pacemaker influences. The regulation of heart rate and blood pressure over multiple time scales may serve to broaden the frequency response of the cardiovascular system and permit it to adapt to an unpredictable and changing environment. The breakdown of such long-range correlations may be associated with the development of disease states and an associated loss of adaptive capacity.[14]

IV. AGE-RELATED CHANGES IN CARDIOVASCULAR DYNAMICS

The process of aging in the absence of disease is known to impair many of the physiologic mechanisms that regulate heart rate and blood pressure. One of the most well-documented changes associated with normal cardiovascular aging is a reduction in baroreflex sensitivity (gain). This has been demonstrated by an attenuated heart rate response to various stimuli including medications that raise or lower blood pressure.[15–17] Healthy elderly individuals have diminished cardiac responsiveness to sympathetic stimulation.[18] Although the sympathetic neurotransmitter norepinephrine circulates in the bloodstream in larger quantities in healthy elderly compared to young subjects, the ability of beta receptors on cardiac muscle cells to respond to norepinephrine is reduced.[19] Studies are currently underway to define the receptor or intracellular signaling defect responsible for this finding. Changes in parasympathetic responsiveness have been less well studied and are poorly understood.

As a result of these changes in autonomic function, heart rate variability and its component frequencies are reduced with healthy aging. Due to a reduction in baroreflex gain, low-frequency Mayer wave oscillations are usually not seen during postural tilt in elderly subjects[20] (Fig. 3). The amplitude of the respiratory sinus arrhythmia also is greatly reduced.[21] The heat rate time series loses its complex, irregular appearance and becomes flatter and more predictable (Fig. 1).

Our previous analyses of the log-frequency vs log-amplitude $(1/f^x)$ plots of heart rate power spectra for healthy young and elderly subjects show a downward shift and more negative slope of the regression line in the elderly[12] (Fig. 4). This observation indicates that overall heart rate variability is reduced and high-frequency fluctuations are relatively more attenuated in advanced age. The slope of the regression line, which is equal to the exponent x of the $1/f^x$ relationship, can be conceptualized as the fractal dimension of the process regulating heart rate variability. The more negative slope in the elderly suggests a loss of dimensionality. This is due in

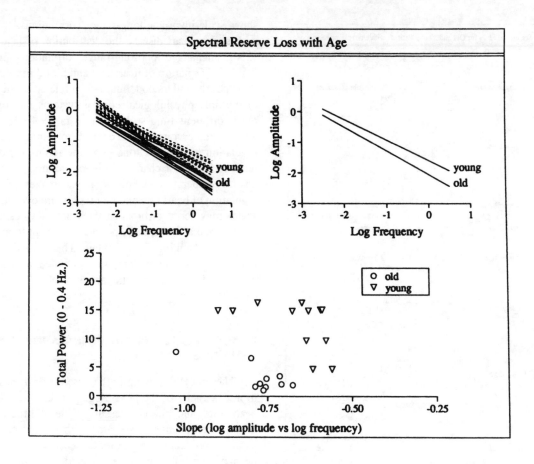

FIG. 4. Heart rate spectral distributions for young ($n=12$) and old ($n=10$) subjects, quantified by log amplitude versus log frequency ($1/f^x$) plots. *Top left panel*: individual $1/f^x$ regression lines for each subject. *Top right panel*: average regression lines for young and old subjects. Note the reduction in amplitude at all frequencies and significantly steeper slopes for old subjects compared to young. *Bottom panel*: scatter plot of total power vs slope of the $1/f^x$ plot for each subject. This plot illustrates the generalized reduction in total spectral power and relatively greater loss of high-frequency variability in old subjects compared with young. (Taken from Ref. 12 with permission from the publisher.)

part to reduced cardiac responsiveness to autonomic nervous system input.

Aging is also associated with impairment in several of the hormonal mechanisms regulating extracellular fluid volume. The production of renin, angiotensin, and atrial natriuretic peptide which regulate salt and water excretion by the kidney, decline with advancing age.[22,23] As a result, elderly individuals excrete larger quantities of salt and water, thus making them more likely to become dehydrated and hypotensive. Since fluid regulation occurs over relatively long time intervals of hours to days, age-related impairment in heart rate and blood pressure regulation is probably evident over long as well as short-range time scales. Thus, one might expect a breakdown of long-range correlations in heart rate dynamics with aging. This hypothesis remains to be tested.

The effect of aging on *blood pressure* dynamics has received much less attention, due in large part to the lack of reliable noninvasive monitoring techniques for continuous blood pressure. The recent development of an arterial tonometric device applied externally to the radial artery (Colin Electronics Co., Komaki-City, Aichi, Japan) has enabled us to analyze the dynamics of beat-to-beat systolic blood pressure in healthy young and elderly subjects.[24] Since fluctuations in heart rate buffer beat-to-beat changes in blood pres-

sure, we hypothesized that an age-related reduction in heart rate variability would be accompanied by an *increase* in blood pressure variability.

To test this hypothesis, we recorded 6 min of continuous blood pressure under supine and upright tilt conditions in 16 healthy young (age=21–35 yr) and 18 healthy elderly (age =62–90 yr) subjects. As expected, the average systolic blood pressure and its variance (standard deviation) were higher in the elderly. However, the standard deviation did not describe the complex dynamics observed in the blood pressure time series. In collaboration with Dr. Daniel Kaplan, Dr. Steven Pincus, and Dr. Ary Goldberger, we examined the "complexity" of beat-to-beat blood pressure signals from these subjects. The concept of complexity refers to the irregularity or unpredictability of a dynamic process, and can be measured by the dimension of the process, or by the amount of information needed to predict its future state. Complexity is different than variability. For example, a sine wave can be highly variable, but is not at all complex. Its dimension is one. In contrast, a random signal may be less variable, but is maximally complex, with a very large dimension.

Using two measures of complexity, "approximate dimension"[24] and "approximate entropy" (ApEn),[24–26] de-

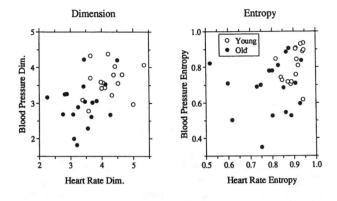

FIG. 5. Scatter plot of the approximate dimension (left plot) and approximate entropy (right plot) for 16 healthy young (open circles) and 18 healthy elderly (closed circles) subjects during supine quiet breathing. Note the reduction in both blood pressure and heart rate dimension and entropy in old subjects compared to young. [Reproduced from the *Biophysical Journal* **59**, 947 (1991) by copyright permission of the Biophysical Society.]

rived, respectively, from the correlation dimension and Kolmogorov entropy algorithms, we found that *both* heart rate and blood pressure dynamics lose complexity with age (Fig. 5). This observation has led to the theory that normal aging is associated with a generalized loss of complexity in the dynamics of the cardiovascular control system.

Pincus has proposed that greater regularity or decreased complexity of output signals from physiologic processes represents the decoupling of multinodal, integrated networks.[27] This loss of complexity results in the isolation of system components and breakdown of long-range correlations. Consequently, it limits the transmission of important physiologic information needed to respond to a changing environment. Since the breakdown of communication networks within the cardiovascular system impairs its ability to rapidly adapt to external and internal perturbations, a loss of complexity in heart rate or blood pressure signals may be an important marker of susceptibility to disease.

V. CLINICAL APPLICATIONS

Several previous observations suggest that a loss of physiologic influences responsible for complex cardiovascular dynamics, may be a generalizable mechanism for the development of cardiovascular disease states. Recent studies by us and others using spectral analysis techniques, have demonstrated that a reduction in overall heart rate variability, decrease in high-frequency (vagally mediated) heart rate fluctuations, and/or emergence of dominant low-frequency periodicities in heart rate are associated with aging,[12,20,28–30] congestive heart failure,[31–33] coronary artery disease,[32,34–36] postprandial hypotension,[37] and sudden death.[11,38,39] A decline in HR variability following a myocardial infarction is a predictor of subsequent mortality.[35,40,41] In our laboratory, Goldberger has shown that a loss of complex physiological HR variability can be seen in patients minutes to months prior to sudden death.[11] Therefore, the examination of HR dynamics can provide important physiologic and prognostic information not detected by conventional methods of analysis.

There is an accumulating body of data suggesting that the statistic approximate entropy (ApEn) may be a useful marker for aging and risk of cardiovascular disease. In a recent study of continuous heart rate in 67 healthy subjects ranging in age from 20 to 80 yr, we found an age-related linear decline in heart rate ApEn, as well as a striking difference between men and women.[42] Since women live longer and develop cardiovascular disease at a later age than men, their greater complexity in heart rate dynamics may be a marker of healthy cardiovascular control and an important clue to their longevity.

In clinical practice, the physician must often make an educated guess about the seriousness of a symptom or risk of a procedure, in order to decide whether or how aggressively to intervene. For example, fainting and associated injury due to falls is a common medical problem that increases in frequency with advancing age. Approximately 3% of medical admissions to the acute hospital are for the evaluation of this problem. This sudden loss of consciousness may be due to a serious life-threatening cardiovascular condition such as a myocardial infarction, arrhythmia, or stroke, or it may be a benign "vasovagal" faint that commonly occurs under stressful circumstances in healthy people (e.g., giving blood). Despite the expensive, highly technological procedures used to evaluate fainting spells, 40% to 50% of episodes remain unexplained. As a result, approximately one-third of patients remain at risk for recurrent events.[43]

Recent studies suggest that heart rate dynamics may differ considerably in patients with cardiovascular vs vasovagal causes of fainting. As noted above, the sinus rhythm heart rate power spectrum shows a reduction in total power and in the ratio of high- to low-frequency power in patients with heart failure, coronary artery disease, or susceptibility to life-threatening cardiac arrhythmias (sudden death). In contrast, subjects who experience typical vasovagal fainting have an exaggerated increase in low-frequency power and the emergence of Mayer wave oscillations during upright tilt[12,44] (Fig. 3). These findings suggest that statistical measures such as ApEn that can summarize complex dynamics by a single number, may have diagnostic value in distinguishing patients at risk of life-threatening cardiac disease from those with benign conditions. Such a tool would help physicians use readily available electrocardiographic data to decide which patients should be admitted to the hospital and which are safe to go home following a fainting episode.

There are numerous other potential clinical applications for complexity measures in geriatric medicine. They may provide useful tools to assess cardiovascular risk prior to anesthesia and surgery, thus enabling anesthesiologists and surgeons to take appropriate precautions during surgical procedures. Ultimately, they may prove useful as biomarkers of physiologic aging. Such indicators of physiologic fitness may facilitate investigations of interventions such as exercise, antioxidants, or treatment of hypertension or hyperlipidemia to maintain resiliency in old age, and prevent the onset of frailty.

ACKNOWLEDGMENTS

This work was supported by a Teaching Nursing Home Award (AG04390) from the National Institute on Aging. Dr. Lipsitz holds the Irving and Edyth S. Usen and Family Chair in Geriatric Medicine at the Hebrew Rehabilitation Center for Aged.

[1] W. B. Cannon, "Organization for physiological homeostasis," Physiol. Rev. **9**, 399–432 (1929).

[2] R. W. DeBoer, J. M. Karemaker, and J. Strackee, "Hemodynamic fluctuations and baroreflex sensitivity in humans: A beat-to-beat model," Am. J. Physiol. **253** (Heart Circ. Physiol. **22**), 680–689 (1987).

[3] L. A. Lipsitz and A. L. Goldberger, "Loss of complexity and aging: Potential applications of fractals and chaos theory to senescence," J. Am. Med. Assoc. **267**, 1806–1809 (1992).

[4] B. Pomeranz, R. J. B. Macaulay, M. A. Caudill, I. Kutz, D. Adam, D. Gordon, K. M. Kilborn, A. C. Barger, D. C. Shannon, R. J. Cohen, and H. Benson, "Assessment of autonomic function in humans by heart rate spectral analysis," Am. J. Physiol. **248**, (Heart Circ. Physiol. **17**), H151–H153 (1985).

[5] M. Pagani, F. Lombardi, S. Guzzetti, O. Rimoldi, R. Furlan, P. Pizzinelli, G. Sandrone, G. Malfatto, S. Dell'Orto, E. Piccaluga, M. Turiel, G. Baselli, S. Cerutii, and A. Malliani, "Power spectral analysis of heart rate and arterial pressure variabilities as a marker of sympathovagal interaction in man and conscious dog," Circ. Res. **59**, 178–193 (1986).

[6] R. E. Kleiger, J. T. Bigger, M. S. Bosner, M. K. Chung, J. R. Cook, L. M. Rolnitzky, R. Steinman, and J. L. Fleiss, "Stability over time of variables measuring heart rate variability in normal subjects," Am. J. Cardiol. **68**, 626–630 (1991).

[7] G. Pinna, M. T. La Rovere, A. Di Cesare, and A. Mortara, "Time course accuracy of the noninvasive blood pressure measurements in the assessment of the neural control of the cardiovascular system," in *Blood Pressure and Heart Rate Variability*, edited by M. Di Rienzo, G. Mancia, G. Parati, A. Pedotti, and A. Zanchetti (IOS Press, Amsterdam, 1993), pp. 109–117.

[8] R. I. Kitney, "Beat-by-beat interrelationships between heart rate, blood pressure, and respiration," in *The Beat-by-Beat Investigation of Cardiovascular Function. Measurement, analysis, and applications*, edited by R. I. Kitney and O. Rompelman (Oxford Science, London, 1987).

[9] M. Kobayashi and T. Musha, "1/f fluctuation of heartbeat period," IEEE Trans. Biomed. Eng. **BE-29**, 456–457 (1982).

[10] P. J. Saul, P. Albrecht, R. D. Berger, and R. Cohen, "Analysis of long-term heart rate variability: Methods, 1/f scaling, and implications," Comp. Cardiol. **1987**, 419–422 (1988).

[11] A. L. Goldberger, D. R. Rigney, J. Mietus, E. M. Antman, and S. Greenwald, "Nonlinear dynamics in sudden cardiac death syndrome: Heart rate oscillations and bifurcations," Experientia **44**, 983–987 (1988).

[12] L. A. Lipsitz, J. Mietus, G. B. Moody, and A. L. Goldberger, "Spectral characteristics of heart rate variability before and during postural tilt. Relations to aging and risk of syncope," Circulation **81**, 1803–1810 (1990).

[13] D. J. Marsh, J. L. Osborn, and A. W. Crowley, Jr., "1/f fluctuations in arterial pressure and regulation of renal blood flow in dogs," Am. J. Physiol. **258** (Renal Fluid Electrolyte Physiol. **27**), F1394–F1400 (1990).

[14] C. K. Peng, J. Mietus, J. M. Hausdorff, S. Havlin, H. E. Stanley, and A. L. Goldberger, "Long-range anticorrelations and non-Gaussian behavior of the heartbeat," Phys. Rev. Lett. **70**, 1343–1346 (1993).

[15] B. Gribbin, T. G. Pickering, P. Sleight, and R. Peto, "Effect of age and high blood pressure on baroreflex sensitivity in man," Circ. Res. **29**, 424–431 (1971).

[16] K. Shimada, T. Kitazumi, N. Sadakane, H. Ogura, and T. Ozawa, "Age-related changes of baroreflex sensitivity in man," Circ. Res. **29**, 424–431 (1971).

[17] K. L. Minaker, G. S. Meneilly, J. B. Young, L. Landsberg, J. S. Stoff, G. L. Robertson, and J. W. Rowe, "Blood pressure, pulse, and neurohumoral responses to nitroprusside-induced hypotension in normotensive aging men," J. Gerontol. **46**, M151–M154 (1991).

[18] J. W. Rowe and B. R. Troen, "Sympathetic nervous system and aging in man," Endocr. Rev. **1**, 167–179 (1980).

[19] R. D. Feldman, L. E. Limbird, J. Nadeau, D. Robertson, and A. J. J. Wood, "Alterations in leukocyte B-receptor affinity with aging: A potential explanation for altered B-adrenergic sensitivity in the elderly," N. Engl. J. Med. **310**, 815–819 (1984).

[20] W. R. Jarisch, J. J. Ferguson, R. P. Shannon, J. Y. Wei, and A. L. Goldberger, "Age-related disappearance of Mayer-like heart rate waves," Experientia **43**, 1207–1209 (1987).

[21] S. A. Smith, "Reduced sinus arrhythmia in diabetic autonomic neuropathy: Diagnostic value of an age-related normal range," Br. Med. J. **285**, 1599–1601 (1982).

[22] M. Epstein and N. K. Hollenberg, "Age as a determinant of renal sodium conservation in normal man," J. Lab. Clin. Med. **87**, 411–417 (1976).

[23] B. G. Haller, H. Zust, S. Shaw, M. P. Gnadinger, D. E. Uehlinger, and P. Weidmann, "Effects of posture and aging on circulating atrial natriuretic peptide levels in man," J. Hypertens. **5**, 551–556 (1987).

[24] D. T. Kaplan, M. I. Furman, S. M. Pincus, S. M. Ryan, L. A. Lipsitz, and A. L. Goldberger, "Aging and the complexity of cardiovascular dynamics," Biophys. J. **59**, 945–949 (1991).

[25] S. M. Pincus and A. L. Goldberger, "Physiologic time-series analysis: When does regularity quantify?" Am. J. Physiol. **266** (Heart Circ. Physiol. **35**), H1643–H1656 (1994).

[26] S. M. Pincus, "Approximate entropy as a measure of system complexity," Proc. Natl. Acad. Sci. USA **88**, 2297–2301 (1991).

[27] S. M. Pincus, "Greater signal regularity may indicate increased system isolation," Math Biosci. (in press).

[28] D. M. Simpson and R. Wicks, "Spectral analysis of heart rate indicates reduced baroreceptor-related heart rate variability in elderly persons," J. Geront. **43**, M21–M24 (1988).

[29] O. V. Korkushko, V. B. Shatilo, and J. K. Kaukenas, "Changes in heart rhythm power spectrum during human aging," Aging **3**, 177–179 (1991).

[30] J. B. Schwartz, W. J. Gibb, and T. Tran, "Aging effects on heart rate variation," J. Gerontol. **46**, M99–M106 (1991).

[31] J. P. Saul, Y. Arai, R. D. Berger, L. S. Lilly, W. S. Colucci, and R. J. Cohen, "Assessment of autonomic regulation in chronic congestive heart failure by heart rate spectral analysis," Am. J. Cardiol. **61**, 1292–1299 (1988).

[32] G. Casolo, E. Balli, A. Fazi, C. Gori, A. Freni, and G. Gensini, "Twenty-four hour spectral analysis of heart rate variability in congestive heart failure secondary to coronary artery disease," Am. J. Cardiol. **67**, 1154–1158 (1991).

[33] M. G. Kienzle, D. W. Ferguson, C. L. Birkett, G. A. Myers, W. J. Berg, and D. J. Mariano, "Clinical, hemodynamic and sympathetic neural correlates of heart rate variability in congestive heart failure," Am. J. Cardiol. **69**, 761–767 (1991).

[34] J. Hayano, Y. Sakakibara, M. Yamada, N. Ohte, T. Fujinami, K. Yokoyama, Y. Watanabe, and K. Takata, "Decreased magnitude of heart rate spectral components of coronary artery disease," Circulation **81**, 1217–1224 (1990).

[35] J. T. Bigger, Jr., C. A. Hoover, R. C. Steinman, L. M. Rolnitzky, J. L. Fleiss, and the Multicenter Study of Silent Myocardial Ischemia Investigators, "Autonomic nervous system activity during myocardial ischemia in man estimated by power spectral analysis of heart period variability," Am. J. Cardiol. **66**, 497–498 (1990).

[36] J. Hayano, A. Yamada, S. Mukai, Y. Sakakibara, M. Yamada, N. Ohte, T. Hashimoto, T. Fujinami, and K. Takata, "Severity of coronary atherosclerosis correlates with the respiratory component of heart rate variability," Am. Heart J. **121**, 1070–1079 (1991).

[37] S. M. Ryan, A. L. Goldberger, R. Ruthazer, J. Mietus, and L. A. Lipsitz, "Spectral analysis of heart rate dynamics in elderly persons with postprandial hypotension," Am. J. Cardiol. **69**, 201–205 (1992).

[38] G. A. Myers, G. J. Martin, N. M. Magid, P. S. Barnett, J. W. Schaad, J. S. Weiss, M. Lesch, and D. H. Singer, "Power spectral analysis of heart rate variability in sudden cardiac death: Comparison with other methods," IEEE Trans. Biomed. Eng. **BE-33**, 1149–1156 (1986).

[39] C. M. Dougherty and R. L. Burr, "Comparison of heart rate variability in survivors and nonsurvivors of sudden cardiac arrest," Am. J. Cardiol. **70**, 441–448 (1992).

[40] R. E. Kleiger, J. P. Miller, J. T. Bigger, Jr., A. J. Moss, and the Multicenter Post-infarction Research Group, "Decreased heart rate variability and its association with increased mortality after acute myocardial infarction," Am. J. Cardiol. **59**, 256–262 (1987).

[41] J. T. Bigger, J. L. Fleiss, R. C. Steinman, L. M. Rolnitzky, R. E. Kleiger, and J. N. Rottman, "Correlations among time and frequency domain measures of heart period variability two weeks after acute myocardial infarction," Am. J. Cardiol. **69**, 891–898 (1992).

[42] S. M. Ryan, A. L. Goldberger, S. M. Pincus, J. Mietus, and L. A. Lipsitz,

"Gender and age-related differences in heart rate dynamics: Are women more complex than men?" J. Am. Coll. Cardiol. (in press).

[43] P. V. Jonsson and L. A. Lipsitz, "Dizziness and syncope," in *Principles of Geriatric Medicine and Gerontology*, edited by W. R. Hazzard, R. Andres, E. L. Bierman, and J. P. Blass, 2nd ed. (McGraw Hill, New York, 1990), pp. 1062–1078.

[44] V. Lepicovska, R. Novak, and R. Nadeau, "Time-frequency dynamics in neurally mediated syncope," Clin. Auto Res. **2**, 317–326 (1992).

Approximate entropy (ApEn) as a complexity measure

Steve Pincus
990 Moose Hill Road, Guilford, Connecticut 06437

(Received 6 May 1994; accepted for publication 2 August 1994)

Approximate entropy (ApEn) is a recently developed statistic quantifying regularity and complexity, which appears to have potential application to a wide variety of relatively short (greater than 100 points) and noisy time-series data. The development of ApEn was motivated by data length constraints commonly encountered, e.g., in heart rate, EEG, and endocrine hormone secretion data sets. We describe ApEn implementation and interpretation, indicating its utility to distinguish correlated stochastic processes, and composite deterministic/ stochastic models. We discuss the key technical idea that motivates ApEn, that one need not fully reconstruct an attractor to discriminate in a statistically valid manner—marginal probability distributions often suffice for this purpose. Finally, we discuss why algorithms to compute, e.g., correlation dimension and the Kolmogorov–Sinai (KS) entropy, often work well for true dynamical systems, yet sometimes operationally confound for general models, with the aid of visual representations of reconstructed dynamics for two contrasting processes. © *1995 American Institute of Physics.*

I. INTRODUCTION

Approximate entropy (ApEn), has been recently introduced as a quantification of regularity in time-series data, motivated by applications to relatively short, noisy data sets.[1] Mathematically, ApEn is part of a general development as the *rate of entropy* for an approximating Markov chain to a process.[2] In applications to heart rate (e.g., Fig. 1), findings have discriminated groups of subjects via ApEn, in instances where classical [mean, standard deviation (SD)] statistics did not show clear group distinctions.[3-7] In applications to endocrine hormone secretion data (e.g., Fig. 2) based on as few as $N=72$ points, ApEn has provided vivid distinctions ($P<10^{-8}$) between actively diseased subjects and normals, with nearly 100% specificity and sensitivity.[8] The point of this article is to discuss ApEn, in part focusing on the technical point that motivates its definition—marginal probabilities often suffice to discriminate. We contrast reconstructed dynamics for two processes to understand why algorithms to compute correlation dimension[9] and the Kolmogorov–Sinai (KS) entropy[10] often work well for true dynamical systems, yet sometimes operationally confound for general models. This contrast indicates the need for a thematically faithful modification of a parameter such as the KS entropy for general applications so that visual intuition matches numerical results, for broad classes of stochastic processes as well as for dynamical systems.

To illustrate the distinctions we are trying to quantify, contrast Fig. 1(a) vs 1(b), Fig. 2(a) vs 2(b), and Fig. 3, taken from the MIX(p) process discussed below, for which we see time series that apparently become increasingly irregular as we proceed from (a) to (c). Historical context frames this effort. Complexity statistics developed for application to chaotic systems and relatively limited in scope recently have been commonly applied to finite, noisy and/or stochastically derived time-series, frequently with confounding and non-replicable results. This caveat is particularly germane to biologic signals, especially those taken *in vivo*, as such signals

likely represent the output of a complicated network with both stochastic and deterministic components.

II. QUANTIFICATION OF REGULARITY

Definition of ApEn: Two input parameters, m and r, must be fixed to compute ApEn—m is the "length" of compared runs, and r is effectively a filter. Given N data points $\{u(i)\}$, form vector sequences $x(1)$ through $x(N-m+1)$, defined by $x(i)=[u(i),...,u(i+m-1)]$. These vectors represent m consecutive u values, commencing with the ith point. Define the distance $d[x(i),x(j)]$ between vectors $x(i)$ and $x(j)$ as the maximum difference in their respective scalar components. Use the sequence $x(1),x(2),...,x(N-m+1)$ to construct, for each $i\leq N-m+1$, $C_i^m(r)=$(number of $j\leq N-m+1$ such that $d[x(i),x(j)]\leq r)/(N-m+1)$. The $C_i^m(r)$'s measure *within a tolerance r* the regularity, or frequency, of patterns similar to a given pattern *of window length m*. Define $\Phi^m(r)=(N-m+1)^{-1}\Sigma_{i=1}^{N-m+1}\ln C_i^m(r)$, where ln is the natural logarithm, then define the *parameter* $\text{ApEn}(m,r)=\lim_{N\to\infty}[\Phi^m(r)-\Phi^{m+1}(r)]$.

Given N data points, we estimate this parameter by defining the *statistic* $\text{ApEn}(m,r,N)=\Phi^m(r)-\Phi^{m+1}(r)$. ApEn measures the likelihood that runs of patterns that are close for m observations remain close on next incremental comparisons. Greater likelihood of remaining close, regularity, produces smaller ApEn values, and conversely. Upon unraveling definitions we deduce

$$-\text{ApEn}=\Phi^{m+1}(r)-\Phi^m(r)$$

= average over i of ln [conditional probability

that $|u(j+m)-u(i+m)|$

$\leq r$, given that $|u(j+k)-u(i+k)|\leq r$ for k

$=0,1,...,m-1]$. (1)

To develop a more intuitive, physiological understanding of this definition, a multistep description of the algorithm with figures is developed in Pincus and Goldberger.[11]

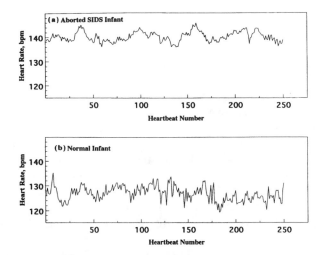

FIG. 1. Two infant quiet sleep heart rate tracings with similar variability, standard deviation (SD): (a) aborted SIDS infant, SD=2.49 beats per minute (bpm), ApEn(2, 0.15 SD, 1000)=0.826; (b) normal infant, SD=2.61 bpm, ApEn(2, 0.15 SD, 1000)=1.463. Tracing (a) appears to be more regular than tracing (b), confirmed by ApEn.

III. IMPLEMENTATION AND INTERPRETATION

The value of N, the number of input data points for ApEn computations is typically between 75 and 5000. Based on calculations that included both theoretical analysis[1,12–14] and clinical applications[3–8] we have concluded that for $m=1$ and 2, values of r between 0.1 to 0.25 SD of the $u(i)$ data produce good statistical validity of ApEn(m,r,N). For such r values, we demonstrated the theoretical utility of ApEn$(2,r,N)$ to distinguish data on the basis of regularity for both deterministic and random processes, and the clinical utility in the aforementioned applications.

ApEn is typically calculated via a short computer code (see Ref. 6, Appendix B for a FORTRAN listing). The form of ApEn provides for both *de facto* noise filtering, via choice of

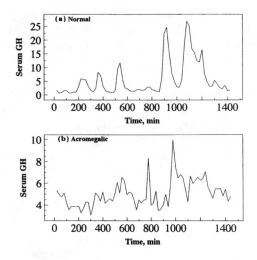

FIG. 2. Growth hormone (GH) serum concentrations, in milliunits/ml, measured at 20 minute intervals for 24 h ("fed" state) (a) normal subject, mean concentration =5.617, ApEn(1, 0.20 SD, 72)=0.783; (b) acromegalic subject, mean concentration =4.981, ApEn(1, 0.20 SD, 72)=1.420.

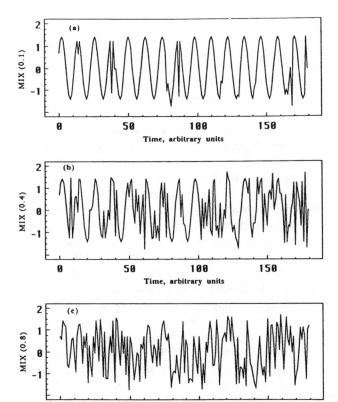

FIG. 3. MIX(p) model time-series output for three parameter values: (a) p=0.1; (b) p=0.4; (c) p=0.8. MIX(p) is a family of processes that samples a sine wave for p=0, samples independent uniform random variables for p=1, and intuitively becomes more irregular as p increases. ApEn quantifies the increasing irregularity with increasing p: for m=2, r=0.18, and N=1000, ApEn[MIX(0.1)]=0.436, ApEn [MIX(0.4)]=1.455, and ApEn[MIX(0.8)]=1.801.

"r,"[1] and artifact insensitivity,[6] useful statistical properties for practical applications. Despite algorithmic similarities, it is important to note that ApEn(m,r,N) is not intended as an approximate value of KS entropy.[1,12] It is imperative to consider ApEn(m,r,N) as a *family* of statistics; for a given application, system comparisons are intended with fixed m and r. For a given system, there usually is significant variation in ApEn(m,r,N) over the range of m and r.[5,6,12]

A significant aspect of ApEn utility is that numerical calculation generally concurs with pictorial intuition, both for theoretical and clinically derived data. ApEn confirms differences that are visually "obviously distinct," as in the comparison of (a) vs (c) in Fig. 3, and provides information in subtler comparisons, distinguishing (b) from (c) in Fig. 3. Noted below, theoretical calculations for correlation dimension and KS entropy produce confounding results for the MIX(p) model of Fig. 3, and often for general stochastic and composite models. Clinically, illustrated in Fig. 3 of a fetal heart rate study,[7] abnormally low ApEn values not only indicate the visually apparent, regular heart rate tracing of an acidotic, distressed fetus measured 1 hr before delivery, but also the less visually apparent, modestly regular tracing measured early in labor. In the endocrine hormone secretion study,[8] ApEn discerned subjects in remission as intermediate between normal and actively diseased subjects ($P<0.001$). Both these clinical results suggest the potential of a regularity statistic to not only confirm obvious findings, but to provide new diagnostic, possibly clinically predictive capability.

To enact direct comparisons of ApEn results, it is best to fix not only m and r, as indicated above, but also N (data length) and choice of coordinates (scale), as would typically be done in a set protocol. The requirement to fix N is due to the statistical bias of ApEn (similar bias occurs for other complexity statistics); if one assumes a model form, corrections could typically be made to compare ApEn results for differing data lengths. ApEn is not invariant under coordinate transformations, hence scale must be fixed; as noted below, such noninvariance is also common to the differential entropy. The choice of "r" in ApEn ensures that it will be impervious to physical device perturbations and recalibrations, important properties for laboratory applications.

The physiologic *modeling* of many complex biological systems is often very difficult; one would expect accurate models of such systems to be complicated composites, with both deterministic and stochastic components, and interconnecting network features. ApEn is a broadly applicable *statistic* in that it can distinguish many classes of systems, and can be meaningfully applied to $N>100$ data points. Via extensive Monte Carlo calculations we established that the standard deviation (SD) of ApEn(2, 0.15 SD, 1000)<0.055 for a large class of candidate models.[11–13] It is this small SD ("error bars") of ApEn, applied to 1000 points from various models, that provides its utility to practical data analysis of moderate length time series.

It seems important to determine a unifying theme suggesting greater signal regularity in diverse complicated systems. Our mechanistic hypothesis is that in a variety of systems, greater regularity corresponds to greater component and subsystem autonomy. This hypothesis has been mathematically established via analysis of several very different, representational model forms, conferring a robustness to the model form of the hypothesis.[13,15]

IV. RELATIVE CONSISTENCY—A VARIATIONAL PRINCIPLE

For many processes, ApEn(m,r,N) grows with decreasing r like $\log(2r)$, thus exhibiting infinite variation with r.[12] We typically observe that for a given time series, ApEn(2, 0.1) is quite different from ApEn(4, 0.01), so the question arises of which parameter choices (m and r) to use. The guidelines above address this, but the most important requirement is consistency. For deterministic dynamical systems, we typically see that when KS entropy(A)$\leqslant$KS entropy(B), then ApEn(m,r)(A)$\leqslant$ApEn(m,r)(B) and conversely, for a wide range of m and r. Furthermore, for both theoretically described systems[1,13] and those described by experimental data,[5,6] we have found that when ApEn(m_1,r_1)(A)$\leqslant$ApEn(m_1,r_1)(B), then ApEn($m_2 r_2$) (A)$\leqslant$ApEn(m_2,r_2)(B), and conversely. This latter property also generally holds for parametrized systems of stochastic

processes, in which KS entropy is infinite. We call this ability of ApEn to preserve order a relative property. It is key to the general and clinical utility of ApEn.

From a theoretical perspective, the interplay between meshes [(m,r) pair specifications] need not be nice, in general, in ascertaining which of (two) processes is "more" random. In general, we might like to ask: Given no noise and an infinite amount of data, can we say that process A is more regular than process B? The *flip-flop pair* of processes implies that the answer to this question is "not necessarily": in general, comparison of relative process randomness *at a prescribed level* is the best one can do.[12] Process A may appear more random than process B on many choices of partitions, but not necessarily on all partitions of suitably small diameter (r).

Fortunately, for many processes A and B, we can assert more than relative regularity, even though both A and B will typically have infinite KS entropy. For such pairs of processes, denoted a *completely consistent pair*, whenever ApEn(m,r)(A)$<$ApEn(m,r)(B) for any specific choice of m and r, then it follows that ApEn(n,s)(A)$<$ApEn(n,s)(B) for *all* choices of n and s.[12] Visually, process B appears more random than A at any level of view. We indicate elsewhere a conjecture that should be straightforward to prove, providing a sufficient condition to ensure that A and B are a completely consistent pair, and indicating the relationship of the autocorrelation function.[11]

V. RELATIONSHIP TO OTHER APPROACHES

The development of mathematics to quantify regularity has centered around various entropy measures. However, there are numerous entropy formulations, and many entropy definitions can not be related to one another.[1] KS entropy, developed by Kolmogorov and expanded upon by Sinai, classifies *deterministic* dynamical systems by rates of information generation.[10] It is this form of entropy that Grassberger and Procaccia,[16] Eckmann and Ruelle,[17] and Takens[18] estimate.

However, the KS entropy was not developed for statistical applications, and has major debits in this regard. The original, primary motivation for this entropy was to determine when two Bernoulli shifts are isomorphic. In its proper context, this form of entropy is primarily applied by ergodic theorists to well-defined theoretical transformations, for which no noise and an infinite amount of "data" are standard mathematical assumptions. Ornstein proved the important, deep result, that two dynamical systems are isomorphic if and only if they have identical KS entropy.[19] Also, for dynamical systems, positive entropy implies chaos.[17] But attempts to utilize KS entropy for practical data analysis represent out-of-context application, which often generates serious difficulties, as it does here. KS entropy is badly compromised by steady, (even very) small amounts of noise, and it generally requires a vast amount of input data to achieve convergence,[14,20] and is usually infinite for stochastic processes. All these debits are key in the present context, since most biological time series likely comprise both stochastic and deterministic components.

ApEn was constructed along thematically similar lines to the KS entropy, though with a different focus: to provide a widely applicable, statistically valid formula to distinguish data sets.[1,6] The technical point motivating ApEn is that if joint probability measures for reconstructed dynamics describing each of two systems are different, then their marginal probability distributions on a fixed partition, given by conditional probabilities as in Eq. (1), are likely different.

There exists a large literature on reconstructed dynamics for chaotic systems. Correlation dimension,[9] KS entropy, and the Lyapunov spectrum have been much studied, as have techniques to utilize related algorithms in the presence of noise and limited data.[21-23] Even more recently, prediction techniques have been developed for chaotic systems.[24-26] Most of these methods employ embedding dimensions larger than $m=2$, as is typically employed with ApEn. Thus in the purely *deterministic dynamical system* setting, they are more powerful than ApEn in that they reconstruct the probability structure of the space with greater detail. However, in the general stochastic process setting, the statistical accuracy of the aforementioned parameters and methods appears to be poor, and the prediction techniques are not always defined.

Generally, changes in ApEn agree with changes in dimension and entropy algorithms for low-dimensional, deterministic systems. The essential points here, assuring broad utility, are that (i) ApEn can potentially distinguish a wide variety of systems: low-dimensional deterministic systems, periodic and multiply periodic systems, high-dimensional chaotic systems, stochastic and mixed (stochastic and deterministic) systems, and (ii) ApEn is applicable to noisy, medium-sized data sets.[1,13] Thus ApEn can be applied to settings for which the KS entropy and correlation dimension are either undefined or infinite, with good replicability properties as discussed below.

VI. MARGINAL PROBABILITIES AND FULL RECONSTRUCTION

As noted above, full attractor (invariant measure) reconstruction is often unnecessary to distinguish processes. A primary data question is: Are data $\{X_i\}$ "atypical" (abnormal)? This is a discrimination question; the question of accurately modeling the process underlying $\{X_i\}$ is often much harder, but one that we may well be able to avoid. We think of marginal probabilities as *partial* process characterization, given by the small m and relatively coarse r in ApEn(m,r). The rationale is that we typically need orders of magnitude fewer points to accurately estimate these marginal probabilities than to accurately reconstruct the "attractor" measure defining the process. We now indicate what marginal probabilities are, and how they arise in time-series reconstruction.

A *joint probability measure* is a means of assigning probability to a region of space. Consider, e.g., all points (x,y) such that $0 \leqslant x,y \leqslant 1$ (unit square). Define the joint measure for the density $f(x,y)$: the probability of (a subset of the square) $A = \int\int_A f(x,y)dx\,dy$. Then define the *marginal density* of x, $f_X(x) = \int f(x,y)dy$ (analogously for y). An intuitive interpretation of marginal density is easiest in the finite state setting—given the joint distribution $p(x,y)$ of two variables x and y, define $p_X(x) := \Sigma_y p(x,y)$ [aggregation of

$p(x,y)$ over all values of y]. It is essential to note that marginal probabilities of two processes may be equal while the joint probabilities are quite different. *However, if two measures have distinctly different marginal probabilities, then that alone is sufficient to discriminate the measures.*

Define the *conditional probability* of $X \in A$ given (‖) $Y \in B$ as the joint probability that $X \in A$ and $Y \in B$ divided by the marginal probability that $Y \in B$; i.e., $\int_B \int_A f(x,y)dx\,dy / \int_B f_Y(y)dy$. Marginal and conditional probability definitions extend to general numbers of variables. For application to time series, we study the joint distribution for n-contiguous observations $\{X_m,...,X_{m+n-1}\}$ as the n-variable measure. Complete steady-state description is given by expressions of the form conditional probability $[u(j+m) \in A_m \| u(j+1) \in A_1,...,u(j+m-1) \in A_{m-1}]$, for all integers m and sets A_i. The question of full reconstruction (embedding dimension n) is subsumed by a broader question, is the process nth-order Markov? The general answer is not necessarily; there may be no fixed n for which the process is characterized entirely by conditioning on n previous observations. However, for fixed m, these *marginal conditional probabilities* contain a wealth of probabilistic detail about the underlying process, often allowing discrimination. Such probabilities form the building blocks of the KS entropy, correlation dimension, and ApEn, by the probabilities

$$\{|u(j+m)-u(i+m)| \leqslant r \| |u(j+k)-u(i+k)|$$

$$\leqslant r \text{ for } k=0,1,...,m-1\}. \quad (2)$$

In the KS entropy, Lyapunov spectra, and correlation dimension, $m \to \infty$ (or to full embedding) and $r \to 0$, whereas ApEn stops short via small m and coarse r, sacrificing an attempt to reconstruct the full process dynamics. The tradeoffs between the approaches to time-series reconstruction are statistical. Obviously bigger m and smaller r describe sharper parameter (probabilistic) detail. However, for each template vector $\{u(i),\ u(i+1),...,u(i+m)\}$, we estimate Eq. (2) by A/B, where $A =$ number of j such that $|u(j+k)-u(i+k)| \leqslant r$ for $k=0,1,...,$ and m, $B =$ number of j such that $|u(j+k)-u(i+k)| \leqslant r$ for $k=0,1,...,$ and $m-1$. If either m is relatively large or r is too small, then both A and (importantly) B are small numbers, thus the estimate of Eq. (2) by A/B is unreliable.

ApEn is related to a parameter in information theory, *conditional entropy*.[27] Assume a finite state space, where the entropy of a random variable X, Prob$(X=a_j)=p_j$, is $H(X) := -\Sigma p_j \log p_j$, and the entropy of a block of random variables $X_1,...,X_n = H(X_1,...,X_n) := -\Sigma\Sigma \cdots \Sigma p^n(a_{j1},...,a_{jn}) \times \log p^n(a_{j1},...,a_{jn})$. For two variables, the conditional entropy $H(Y\|X) = H(X,Y) - H(X)$; this extends naturally to n variables. Closely mimicking the proof of Theorem 3, Ref. 1, the following theorem is immediate: for $r < \min_{j \neq k} |a_j - a_k|$, ApEn($m,r$) $= H(X_{m+1} \| X_1,...,X_m)$; thus in this setting, ApEn is a conditional entropy. Observe that we do not assume that the process is mth order Markov, i.e., that we fully describe the process; we aggregate the mth-order marginal probabilities. The rate of entropy $= \lim_{n \to \infty} H(X_n \| X_1,...,X_{n-1})$ is the discrete state analog of the KS entropy. However, we cannot go from discrete to continuous state naturally as a limit; most calculations give ∞. As for differential entropy, there is no fundamental physical interpretation of conditional entropy (and no invariance, Ref. 27, p. 243) in continuous state.

VII. RECONSTRUCTED DYNAMICS—A COMPARISON OF TWO AUTOCORRELATED MAPS

General Issues: Analysis of the MIX(p) processes indicates some of the *theoretical* difficulties realized in applying correlation dimension and KS entropy statistics to general time series.[1] To define MIX(p), first fix $0 \leqslant p \leqslant 1$. For all j, define $X_j = \sqrt{2}\,\sin(2\pi j/12)$, Y_j=i.i.d. uniform random variables on $[-\sqrt{3},\sqrt{3}]$, and Z_j=i.i.d. random variables, $Z_j = 1$ with probability p, $Z_j = 0$ with probability $1-p$. Then define MIX $(p)_j = (1-Z_j)X_j + Z_j Y_j$. In conjunction with intuition, ApEn monotonically increases with increasing p (Fig. 3). In contrast, correlation dimension of MIX(p)=0 for $p<1$, and correlation dimension of MIX(1)=∞.[1,28] As well, KS entropy of MIX(p)=∞ for $p>0$, and =0 for MIX(0). Thus both of these statistics fail to quantify the evolving complexity change. Similar "confounding" results can be established for Gaussian processes, ARMA models, and more generally for weak-dependence processes, via proofs similar to that given in Ref. 1.

Nonetheless, one might still consider applying an algorithm to compute, e.g., the correlation dimension or KS entropy, and should then query what the *operational* consequences are of application to a general correlated stochastic process. To understand the statistical limitations imposed by the choice of embedding dimension m and scaling parameter r, we can think of an (m,r) choice of input parameters as partitioning the state space into uniform width boxes of width r, from which we estimate mth-order conditional probabilities. For state space, e.g., $[-A/2,A/2]$, we would have $(A/r)^{m+1}$ conditional probabilities to estimate. Specifically, divide $[-A/2,A/2]$ into A/r cells; the ith cell $C(i)$ is the half-open interval $[x,x+r)$, where $x = -(A/2)+(i-1)r$. Then define the conditional probability $p_{ivect,j}$ for all length m vectors of integers $ivect$ and integers j, $ivect = (i_1,i_2,...,i_m)$, $1 \leqslant i_k \leqslant A/r$ for all k, $1 \leqslant j \leqslant A/r$, by $p_{ivect,j}$={conditional probability that $u(k) \in C(j)$, given that $u(k-1) \in C(i_1)$, $u(k-2) \in C(i_2),...$, and $u(k-m) \in C(i_m)$}. In the very general ergodic case, these conditional probabilities are given by limits of time averages.

For general stochastic processes, many of these conditional probabilities are nonzero, so we need to accommodate reasonable estimates of the $(A/r)^{m+1}$ conditional probabilities given N data points. If m is relatively large, or if r is too small, the number of probabilities to be estimated will be unwieldy, and statistical estimates will be poor for typical data set lengths.

Probabilistic Distinction: We can now operationally see the issues in analyzing reconstructed dynamics for general stochastic processes. Compare two processes, logis(3.6), the logistic map $f(x) = 3.6x(1-x)$ and MIX(0.4) [Figs. 4(a) and 4(b)], with embedding dimension $m=2$ and a moderately coarse mesh width r that subdivides the state spaces into 20 equal-width cells [thus $r = \sqrt{3}/10$ for MIX(0.4), while $r = 0.05$ for logis(3.6)]. We want to estimate the conditional

probabilities $p_{ivect,j}$ for all length 2 vectors $ivect = (i_1,i_2)$ and integers $1 \leqslant j \leqslant 20$ for each process. For logis(3.6), the ith cell $C(i) = [0.05(i-1),\ 0.05(i-1)+0.05)$. We calculate these probabilities as $\lim_{N \to \infty} A/B$ (estimated from $N = 2\,000\,000$ points), with A =number of $k \leqslant N$ when $u(k) \in C(j)$ and $u(k-1) \in C(i_1)$ and $u(k-2) \in C(i_2)$; B =number of $k \leqslant N$ when $u(k-1) \in C(i_1)$ and $u(k-2) \in C(i_2)$. In Figs. 4(c) and 4(d), we visualize these $\{p_{ivect,j}\}$ by associating the triple $\{ivect,j\} = \{i_1,i_2,j\}$ with the three-dimensional subcube $[C(i_2) \times C(i_1) \times C(j)]$. We shade each subcube to illustrate its conditional probability $p_{ivect,j}$. The extremely different character in reconstructed dynamics between these two maps is visually apparent—logis(3.6) is extremely sparse, with only 27 nonzero subcubes of a possible 8000, whereas MIX(0.4) displays "diffuse" dynamics, with all 8000 subcubes nonzero. Furthermore, in general the conditional probabilities are not rare (nearly 0) for most nonzero cells for logis(3.6), compared to MIX(0.4), an important added distinction when considering the effects of the bias indicated below. This sparseness marks the *strong dependence*[29] of dynamical systems, and it should not be surprising that algorithms that work well for such strong-dependence processes behave entirely different for typically encountered weak-dependence (e.g., Gaussian) processes.

Primary Statistical Issues: We contrast the probabilistic distinction between logis(3.6) and MIX(0.4) with its statistical consequences, considering a "clinically sized" data set length $N = 1000$. Figs. 4(e) and 4(f) indicate the shaded subcubes of Figs. 4(c) and 4(d) for which statistical estimates based on 1000 points might be adequate. Defining A and B as in the previous paragraph, we only display subcubes for which $B > 10$; otherwise, A/B is a poor estimate of the true conditional probability as given as $N \to \infty$. The percentage of nonzero probability cells from Figs. 4(c) and 4(d) displayed in Figs. 4(e) and 4(f) thus provide a measure of how reasonably estimated the conditional probabilities (and associated statistics) are, based on $N = 1000$. As an additional indicator, in Figs. 4(e) and 4(f) darker shading corresponds to larger B, hence better estimation of the true conditional probability of the cell, given by more conditioning vectors. Note that the conditional probabilities for logis(3.6) are reasonably estimated—25/27 (93%) of the nonzero subcubes seen in Fig. 4(c) satisfy $B > 10$. In contrast, the conditional probabilities for MIX(0.4) are poorly estimated—260/8000 (3%) of nonzero subcubes satisfy $B > 10$. Furthermore, generally there are greater numbers of conditioning vectors (darker cells) for logis(3.6) than for MIX(0.4), reinforcing the superior estimation based on $N = 1000$. For example, for logis(3.6) we find that there are 108 values of $k \leqslant 1000$ for which pairs of contiguous points $(u(k-1),\ u(k-2))$ satisfy $\{u(k-1) \in C(7)$ and $u(k-2) \in C(18)\}$. Of these 108 conditioning vectors, 61 3-tuples of points $(u(k-1), u(k-1), u(k-2))$ satisfy $\{u(k) \in C(17),\ u(k-1) \in C(7),$ and $u(k-2) \in C(18)\}$; we then estimate $p_{(7,18),17} = 61/108$. A second estimate (different initial condition) based on a subsequent 1000 point sequence would likely produce a similar estimate for $p_{(7,18),17}$. It is precisely the increasing and ex-

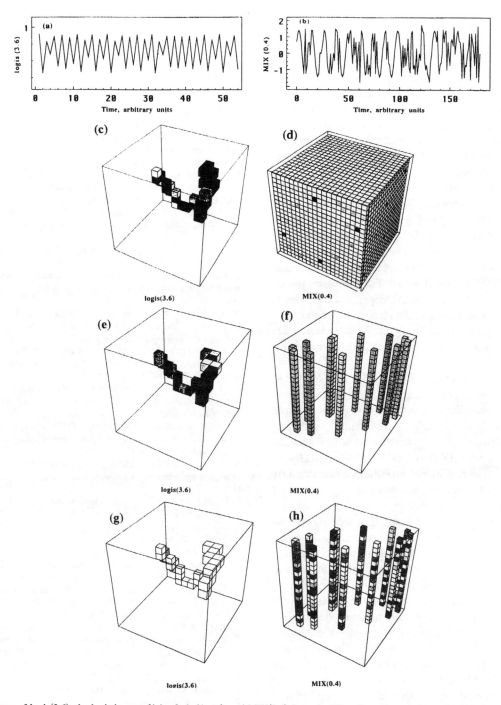

FIG. 4. Comparison of logis(3.6), the logistic map $f(x)=3.6x(1-x)$, and MIX(0.4) for embedding dimension $m=2$, mesh width $r=0.05\times$ support of state space. (a), (b) Time-series realizations; (c), (d) *probabilistic contrast*. Visualize conditional probabilities $\{p_{i\text{vect},j}\}$ for all length 2 vectors $i\text{vect}=(i_1,i_2)$, integers $1 \leq j \leq 20$ by associating triple $\{i\text{vect},j\}=\{i_1,i_2,j\}$ with three-dimensional subcube $[C(i_2) \times C(i_1) \times C(j)]$, shading each subcube per weight $p_{i\text{vect},j}$, with black indicating a conditional probability of 1, white a conditional probability of 0. Contrast the extreme sparseness of logis(3.6), with 27 nonzero subcubes, and the "diffuse" dynamics of MIX(0.4), with all 8000 subcubes nonzero. (e), (f) *Statistical contrast*, $N=1000$. Shading by subcube of adequacy of conditional probability *estimates*. We only display subcubes for which $B>10$; otherwise, A/B is a poor estimate of the true conditional probability, with darker shading corresponding to larger B (and better estimation, with more conditioning vectors). Conditional probabilities for logis(3.6) are well estimated—25/27 (93%) of nonzero subcubes in (c) satisfy $B>10$; conditional probabilities for MIX(0.4) are poorly estimated—260/8000 (3%) of nonzero subcubes satisfy $B>10$. Additionally, logis(3.6) cells are generally darker (better estimated), e.g., for logis(3.6), estimate $p_{(7,18),17}=61/108$, while for MIX(0.4), estimate $p_{(6,11),13}=1/27$. (g), (h) *Bias effects contrast*. We compare percentage error of log(conditional probability *estimate*, $N=1000$) vs log(true conditional probability), for each subcube with $B>10$, with darker shading indicating larger error. Average percentage error/subcube, given $B>10$ is 9.5% for logis(3.6), 40.5% for MIX(0.4). Virtually all "A's" for MIX(0.4) in estimates A/B were 0, 1, or 2.

treme sparseness of the set of $m+1$-tuples for which the true conditional probabilities $p_{i\text{vect},j}$ are nonzero *for true dynamical systems*, as a function of embedding dimension m and mesh width (scaling range) r, that affords large m and small

r in conditional probability statistical estimation for these processes.

Bias: There is a secondary, but oftentimes very important statistical issue in estimation of conditional probabilities such as those given by Eq. (2) by a ratio of A/B as above. The template vector $x(i)$ itself counts in the aggregation of vectors close to $x(i)$ in ApEn to ensure that calculations involving logarithms (which arise, e.g., in "correlation integrals") remain finite. This procedure ensures that ApEn is a *biased* statistic (though asymptotically unbiased for many processes), as are correlation dimension and KS entropy algorithms for similar reasons.[12,30] Operationally, the inclusion of the template vector changes a conditional probability estimate from A/B to $(A+1)/(B+1)$, adding 1 to both numerator and denominator counts.

This point is trivial, effectively irrelevant in calculations for dynamical systems—both A, B are typically much larger than 1, so that $A/B \approx (A+1)/(B+1)$. However, we aggregate expressions of the form $\log(A/B)$ in the algorithms under consideration, with $\log(A/B)$ a large negative number if A is small. In particular, $\log(A/B)$ is typically much different than $\log[(A+1)/(B+1)]$ for A small. For "diffuse" reconstructed dynamics settings [i.e., weak-dependence processes such as MIX(0.4)] with moderate data length N, frequently a nontrivial percentage of conditional probability estimates are of rare events, with $A \leq 3$, for which this issue becomes important.

We contrast the bias effects for logis(3.6) and MIX(0.4) in Figs. 4(g) and 4(h), comparing the percentage error of $\log$(conditional probability *estimate*, $N = 1000$) vs $\log$(true conditional probability), for each subcube with $B > 10$. The average percent error/subcube, given $B > 10$ is 9.5% for logis(3.6) and 40.5% for MIX(0.4). For $N = 1000$, virtually all "A's" for MIX(0.4) in conditional probability estimates A/B were 0, 1, or 2. This effect is exacerbated as m grows larger and as r shrinks.

Messages, Comparison of 2 Maps: For true dynamical (often chaotic) systems, there is extreme sparseness in reconstructed dynamics, producing well-estimated conditional probabilities for a range of embedding dimensions m and scaling ranges r, with small influence from statistical bias. Here exploit the structure by choosing large m, small r in algorithms, to estimate a fine-graded measure description. For general autocorrelated maps, one typically sees diffuse reconstructed dynamics, with many poorly estimated conditional probabilities for $m \geq 3$ and small r; further, many *rare* events produce added bias. Here, be cautious—choose small m (e.g., $m = 2$) and moderate width r to ensure replicability of a partial (dynamical) measure description.

VIII. SUMMARY AND CONCLUSION

The principal focus of this article has been the description of a recently introduced regularity statistic, ApEn. Several properties of ApEn facilitate its utility for general time-series analysis: (i) ApEn is nearly unaffected by noise of magnitude below a *de facto* specified filter level; (ii) ApEn is robust to outliers; (iii) ApEn can be applied to time series of 100 or more points, with good confidence (established by standard deviation calculations); (iv) ApEn is finite for stochastic, noisy deterministic and composite (mixed) processes, these last of which are, e.g., likely models for complicated biological systems; (v) increasing ApEn corresponds to intuitively increasing process complexity in the settings of

(iv). It thus appears that ApEn has potential widespread utility to practical data analysis, based on these five properties, and the aforementioned clinical applications.

[1] S. M. Pincus, "Approximate entropy as a measure of system complexity," Proc. Natl. Acad. Sci. USA **88**, 2297–2301 (1991).

[2] S. M. Pincus, "Approximating Markov chains," Proc. Natl. Acad. Sci. USA **89**, 4432–4436 (1992).

[3] L. A. Fleisher, S. M. Pincus, and S. H. Rosenbaum, "Approximate entropy of heart rate as a correlate of postoperative ventricular dysfunction," Anesthiology **78**, 683–692 (1993).

[4] D. T. Kaplan, M. I. Furman, S. M. Pincus, S. M. Ryan, L. A. Lipsitz, and A. L. Goldberger, "Aging and the complexity of cardiovascular dynamics," Biophys. J. **59**, 945–949 (1991).

[5] S. M. Pincus, T. R. Cummins, and G. G. Haddad, "Heart rate control in normal and aborted SIDS infants," Am. J. Physiol. **264** (Regulartory & Integrative 33), R638–R646 (1993).

[6] S. M. Pincus, I. M. Gladstone, and R. A. Ehrenkranz, "A regularity statistic for medical data analysis," J. Clin. Monit. **7**, 335–345 (1991).

[7] S. M. Pincus and R. R. Viscarello, "Approximate entropy: A regularity measure for fetal heart rate analysis," Obstet. Gynecol. **79**, 249–255 (1992).

[8] M. L. Hartman, S. M. Pincus, M. L. Johnson, D. H. Matthews, L. M. Faunt, M. L. Vance, M. O. Thorner, and J. D. Veldhuis, "Enhanced basal and disorderly growth hormone (GH) secretion distinguish acromegalic from normal pulsatile GH release," J. Clin. Invest. **94**, 1277–1288 (1994).

[9] P. Grassberger and I. Procaccia, "Measuring the strangeness of strange attractors," Physica D **9**, 189–208 (1983).

[10] A. N. Kolmogorov, "A new metric invariant of transient dynamical systems and automorphisms in Lebesgue spaces," Dokl. Akad. Nauk. SSSR **119**, 861–864 (1958).

[11] S. M. Pincus and A. L. Goldberger, "Physiological time-series analysis: what does regularity quantify?," Am. J. Physiol. **266** (Heart Circ. Physiol. 35), H1643–H1656 (1994).

[12] S. M. Pincus and W. M. Huang, "Approximate entropy: Statistical properties and applications," Commun. Statist. Theory Meth. **21**, 3061–3077 (1992).

[13] S. M. Pincus and D. L. Keefe, "Quantification of hormone pulsatility via an approximate entropy algorithm," Am. J. Physiol. **262** (Endocrinol. Metab. 25), E741–E754 (1992).

[14] A. Wolf, J. B. Swift, H. L. Swinney, and J. A. Vastano, "Determining Lyapunov exponents from a time-series," Physica D **16**, 285–317 (1985).

[15] S. M. Pincus, "Greater signal regularity may indicate increased system isolation," Math. Biosci. **122**, 161–181 (1994).

[16] P. Grassberger and I. Procaccia, "Estimation of the Kolmogorov entropy from a chaotic signal," Phys. Rev. A **28**, 2591–2593 (1983).

[17] J. P. Eckmann and D. Reulle, "Ergodic theory of chaos and strange attractors," Rev. Mod. Phys. **57**, 617–656 (1985).

[18] F. Takens, "Invariants related to dimension and entropy," in *Atas do 13.Col.Brasiliero de Matematicas* (Rio de Janeiro, 1983).

[19] D. S. Ornstein, "Bernoulli shifts with the same entropy are isomorphic," Adv. Math. **4**, 337–352 (1970).

[20] D. S. Ornstein and B. Weiss, "How sampling reveals a process," Ann. Prob. **18**, 905–930 (1990).

[21] D. S. Broomhead and G. P. King, "Extracting qualitative dynamics from experimental data," Physica D **20**, 217–236 (1986).

[22] A. M. Fraser and H. L. Swinney, "Independent coordinates for strange attractors from mutual information," Phys. Rev. A **33**, 1134–1140 (1986).

[23] G. Mayer-Kress, F. E. Yates, L. Benton, M. Keidel, W. Tirsch, S. J. Poppl, and K. Geist, "Dimensional analysis of nonlinear oscillations in brain, heart, and muscle," Math. Biosci. **90**, 155–182 (1988).

[24] M. Casdagli, "Nonlinear prediction of chaotic time series," Physica D **35**, 335–356 (1989).

[25] J. D. Farmer and J. J. Sidorowich, "Predicting chaotic time series," Phys. Rev. Lett. **59**, 845–848 (1987).

[26] G. Sugihara and R. M. May, "Nonlinear forecasting as a way of distinguishing chaos from measurement error in time series," Nature **344**, 734–741 (1990).

[27] R. E. Blahut, *Principles and Practice of Information Theory* (Addison–Wesley, Reading, MA, 1987), pp. 55–64.

[28] The reason that correlation dimension is 0, not 1 for $p < 1$ is that the sampling frequency of the sine function is commensurate with π, so that the phase space realization from the sine function is a discrete point set. If

we choose a sampling frequency incommensurate with π in the sine component of the MIX definition, the correlation dimension $=1$ almost surely for $p<1$, and the difficulty remains—the correlation dimension fails to discriminate members of this process from one another.

[29] A. N. Kolmogorov and Y. A. Rozanov, "On strong mixing conditions for stationary Gaussian processes," Theory Prob. Appl. **5**, 204–208 (1960).

[30] A family of ϵ estimators for $\text{ApEn}(m,r)$ is proposed in Ref. 11 to achieve bias reduction.

Tests for nonlinearity in short stationary time series

Taeun Chang
*Department of Neurosurgery, Children's National Medical Center and the School of Medicine,
George Washington University, Washington, D.C. 20010*

Tim Sauer
Department of Mathematics, George Mason University, Fairfax, Virginia 22030

Steven J. Schiff[a]
*Department of Neurosurgery, Children's National Medical Center and the School of Medicine,
George Washington University, Washington, D.C. 20010*

(Received 7 October 1994; accepted for publication 7 December 1994)

To compare direct tests for detecting determinism in chaotic time series, data from Hénon, Lorenz, and Mackey–Glass equations were contaminated with various levels of additive colored noise. These data were analyzed with a variety of recently developed tests for determinism, and the results compared. © *1995 American Institute of Physics.*

I. INTRODUCTION

Although it is relatively easy to generate chaotic dynamics from simple nonlinear equations, determining whether this type of nonlinear behavior is reflected in the behavior of an experimental system is a more difficult problem. Indirect measurements of deterministic properties that accompany chaotic behavior are findings of sensitivity to initial conditions (e.g., Lyapunov exponents), and fractal geometry of a reconstructed chaotic attractor (e.g., noninteger correlation dimension).

An alternative to the indirect measurements is to directly measure the degree of determinism present in a chaotic attractor. There has been much recent interest in these direct approaches, beginning with a measurement of *local flow* for continuous systems,[1] and a modification for discrete systems.[2] A recent variant of these methods is a *local dispersion* statistic.[3]

The *nonlinear prediction* tools are also direct measurements of determinism. These methods generally fit local linear maps to a chaotic attractor.[4,5] Such maps may be of arbitrary order, but we have found much predictive power in even simple "zeroth-order" (i.e., constant) maps.[6]

All of the direct approaches described above are implemented by calculating a set of numbers from experimental data, and then characterizing a measurement of central tendency of the distribution of those numbers as a discriminating statistic—a characteristic of the distribution is reduced to a single number (e.g., root mean square error). An entirely different approach would be to focus on the tail of the distribution of values from the discriminating statistic, with attention paid to *exceptional* events.[7] The theoretical advantage of such an approach is that for high dimensional systems, occasional exceptional events might be the only indication of the deterministic dynamics.

Our focus experimentally has been with biological systems, especially small neuronal ensembles. The behavior of such neuronal ensembles appears to be quite high dimensional, and any nonlinear determinism present is buried within a sea of noise. In these systems, we have employed central tendency type direct measurements of determinism,[8,9] as well as a form of local measurement, *unstable fixed point* analysis, that has been employed in several chaos control paradigms.[10–12]

It is important for the experimentalist to systematically compare the methods of detecting determinism. If different tests uncover qualitatively different properties of an attractor, then multiple tests need to be applied to novel data from systems whose dynamics are unknown. On the contrary, if multiple tests reveal the same properties of an attractor, then one would want to eliminate redundant testing, and use the test that is most sensitive. In our previous work with spinal cord reflexes[8] and circuitry from the brain,[9] we have noted that the central tendency methods of detecting determinism did not appear equally sensitive in identifying deterministic patterns in experimental data. These differential sensitivities were confirmed in a recent numerical study comparing methods of central tendency.[6] Since these findings have not been compared with the method of exceptional events, and we have not explored the limitations of these methods with interval data, the following study further explores these issues with noise-contaminated deterministic datasets.

II. METHODS

We will study univariate time series generated from known deterministic sets of equations: Hénon,[13] Lorenz,[14] and an integrate-and-fire model based on the Mackey–Glass equations.[15] These three choices allow us to study, respectively, typical discrete, continuous, and interevent interval deterministic models that produce well understood, stationary time series. For the Hénon data, the x coordinate of the iteration was recorded, resulting in a chaotic series with minimal linear autocorrelation. The x coordinate of the Lorenz equations was sampled with sampling period $\Delta t = 0.025$. At this sampling rate, the resulting series has significant autocorrelation. The Mackey–Glass delay-differential equation[15]

[a]Author to whom correspondence should be addressed.

$$\frac{dx}{dt} = \frac{ax(t-\delta)}{1+x(t-\delta)^c} - bx(t)$$

was used with parameters set at $a=0.2$, $b=0.1$, $c=10$, and $\delta=100$. For these parameters, the estimated attractor dimension is ~ 7.1. For the analysis of this study, we used a time series from the x variable of the equation as input to an integrate-and-fire model (as in Ref. 16, see also article by Sauer in this volume) to produce a series of simulated inter-event intervals. Each dataset is comprised of 1000 points.

A. Noise

For each of the deterministic systems studied both colored and Gaussian white noise were added at 5%, 25%, 50%, 75%, and 100% levels.

1. Colored noise

Colored noise was generated for a deterministic time series D_i, $i=1\ldots n$, by taking the Fourier transform of the series, randomizing the phases and then inverting the Fourier transform to get a new time series, C_i, with an identical power spectrum to the signal but with its phases randomized. Adding a constant times this noisy series to the original series

$$X_i = D_i + lC_i$$

results in a new noisy series with a level l of in-band (same frequency content) noise. This noise, by construction, cannot be separated from the original deterministic signal D_i on the basis of spectral techniques.

2. Gaussian white noise

A pseudorandom number generator was used to create a time series W_i, $i=1\ldots n$, of Gaussian-distributed random numbers with a mean of 0 and a variance of 1. The Gaussian white noise was added to the deterministic time series D_i at a level l, in the following manner

$$X_i = D_i + \epsilon W_i,$$

where

$$\epsilon = \sigma(D_i)\frac{l}{\sigma(W_i)}$$

and σ is the standard deviation.

B. Surrogate data

We make heavy use of surrogate datasets to quantitate our findings. Surrogate data refers to datasets that preserve certain linear statistical properties of the experimental data, without the nonlinear deterministic component. Such data serves to test statistically the null hypothesis that our experimental results could be accounted for by a linear stochastic process. We employ three types of surrogate data in this study: *phase randomized, Gaussian scaled, and Fourier shuffled*. A phase randomized surrogate is constructed by randomizing the phases of the Fourier transform of a signal, and

then inverting the transform. Such a surrogate has an identical power spectrum, mean, variance, and autocorrelation as the original signal, but the marginal distribution (histogram of amplitudes) is changed. The Gaussian-scaled surrogate shuffles the signal based on the assumption that the signal is a Gaussian random process that was passed through a nonlinear filter. A Gaussian-distributed random time series is shuffled in the rank order of the experimental data, phase randomized, and the amplitudes of the original data rank ordered and substituted. Because this surrogate is a shuffle of the original data, the marginal distribution is maintained. The Fourier shuffled surrogate shuffles the signal by rank ordering the original data in the rank order of a phase randomized surrogate. This surrogate in some cases more closely approximates the power spectrum than the Gaussian-scaled surrogate, still preserving the marginal distribution. Detailed descriptions of these surrogates can be found in Chang et al.,[8] and a full listing of source code to generate these surrogates can be found in Schiff et al.[17]

With a large number of comparisons to make, we initially screened data by comparing them with three separate realizations of each of the three types of surrogates. If any experimental datasets were indistinguishable from the three surrogates, further processing time would seem useless. For data that passed this initial screen, a more statistically powerful comparison was performed with 19 surrogates. This approach allows one to reject the null hypothesis that the data are linear at the 0.05 level for a 1-tailed test.[18]

C. Prediction methods

All four prediction methods directly examine the reconstructed phase space for evidence of determinism. A time delay embedding method is used to reconstruct the phase space for an embedding dimension of E and a lag time of L,

$$\mathbf{x_q} = (x_q, x_{q+L}, \ldots, x_{q+L(E-1)}),$$

where $q=1,2,\ldots,N-L$. Each method analyzes the dynamics of nearby points in phase space, assuming a certain amount of local smoothness.[19]

1. Local flow

The dynamical characteristic that the local flow method measures are local tangent vectors in the embedding space.[1] Nearby points are defined by a grid of 16^E cubes overlying the embedding space. Each grid box j contains n_j points with time indexes of $t_{j,k}$ for $k=1,2,\ldots,n_j$. For each point in embedding space, the displacement for a given translation horizon, H, was calculated,

$$\Delta\mathbf{x}_{j,k} = \mathbf{x}(t_{j,k}+H) - \mathbf{x}(t_{j,k}).$$

The average displacement of the points in each grid box yields a family of displacement magnitudes L_n^E for each embedding dimension and value of n, $n=n_j$. The expectation value of L_n^E for a stochastic process is $c_E/n_j^{1/2}$, and a more complete discussion of c_E can be found in Kaplan and

Glass.[1] The discriminating statistic is V, the average displacement for all values of n at a given embedding dimension,

$$V = \left\langle \frac{(L_n^E)^2 - [(c_E)^2/n]}{1 - (c_E)^2/n} \right\rangle,$$

where $\langle \; \rangle$ denotes the average over all grid boxes with n points.

The above method has been adapted for discrete systems[2] by applying a sine correction to the displacement vectors

$$\tilde{\Delta}\mathbf{x}_{j,k} = \left(\begin{array}{cc} \sin\left(2\pi \dfrac{x(t_{j,k}+H) - x(t_{j,k})}{\lambda}\right), & \sin\left(2\pi \dfrac{x(t_{j,k}+H+L) - x(t_{j,k}+L)}{\lambda}\right) \\ \multicolumn{2}{c}{\ldots, \sin\left(2\pi \dfrac{x[t_{j,k}+H+(E-1)L] - x[t_{j,k}+(E-1)L]}{\lambda}\right)} \end{array} \right),$$

where λ is the characteristic length of the embedded attractor.[2] This correction was designed to reduce the directional bias of trajectories from points at the edge of an attractor toward the center.

2. Local dispersion

Instead of averaging displacement vectors in embedding space for local flow, the discriminating statistic for local dispersion is the variance in displacements of selected index points and their nearest neighbors.[3] In our implementation, the first 100 points of an embedding were selected as index points x_j, and $k = 0.02N$ nearest neighbors were used. The "images" of these points for a given translation horizon into the future were denoted y_j. The vectors v_j defining the displacement between the points x_j and their images y_j is

$$v_j = y_j - x_j,$$

and the average displacement $\langle v \rangle$ is

$$\langle v \rangle = \frac{1}{k+1} \sum_{j=0}^{k} v_j.$$

The dispersion of the displacements can be defined as an error in translation, ϵ_{trans}, as

$$\epsilon_{\text{trans}} = \frac{1}{k+1} \sum_{j=0}^{k} \frac{\|v_j - \langle v \rangle\|^2}{\|\langle v \rangle\|^2},$$

where $\| \; \|$ represents the length of the vector. The median ϵ_{trans} for a given embedding dimension is the distinguishing statistic in local dispersion method.

3. Nonlinear prediction

The nonlinear prediction method compares the translation of index points in embedding space with the translation of their neighboring points. For simplicity, we choose a *zeroth-order* nonlinear predictor, fitting local constant maps to the attractor.

For each index point x_0 in embedding space, the average translation of its $k = 0.02N$ nearest neighbors for a horizon of H is

$$\langle v \rangle = \frac{1}{k} \sum_{j=1}^{k} x_{j+H}$$

while the translation of the index is x_{0+H}. The difference between the actual and average translation is the prediction error

$$\epsilon_{\text{trans}} = |x_{0+H} - \langle v \rangle|.$$

The prediction error for the mean of the time series is

$$\epsilon m_{\text{trans}} = |x_{0+H} - \text{mean}(x)|.$$

The normalized prediction error, NPE, is the distinguishing statistic for this method

$$\text{NPE} = \frac{\text{RMS}(\epsilon_{\text{trans}})}{\text{RMS}(\epsilon m_{\text{trans}})},$$

where RMS indicates root mean square.

4. Exceptional events (delta–epsilon)

This method was proposed by Kaplan,[7] and examines the trajectories of points in the embedding space for *exceptional events*. Exceptional events are points in the embedding space that track each other closely when translated. In random data, such events should be rare. These events are determined by measuring the distances δ between all pairs of points in embedding space, and comparing them with the distances between the translated images of these pairs of points ϵ. For a deterministic system, for small values of δ ($\delta \rightarrow 0$), points close together will more often track together (a smaller average ϵ) than a stochastic system. To examine ϵ values for small δ, values of δ were binned and the cumulative average of ϵ versus average δ values for each bin were plotted. *This method focuses on the values of ϵ for small δ, and thus depends on the tail of the distribution of the values of ϵ rather than a measure of central tendency.* Although it has been proposed to extrapolate the Y-intercept from a straight line fit of δ-ϵ plots,[7] we have elected to directly compare the δ-ϵ curves with their surrogate controls. This method of discrimination makes few assumptions, and helps to sort out the influence of less exceptional events (larger δ and ϵ) on the results.

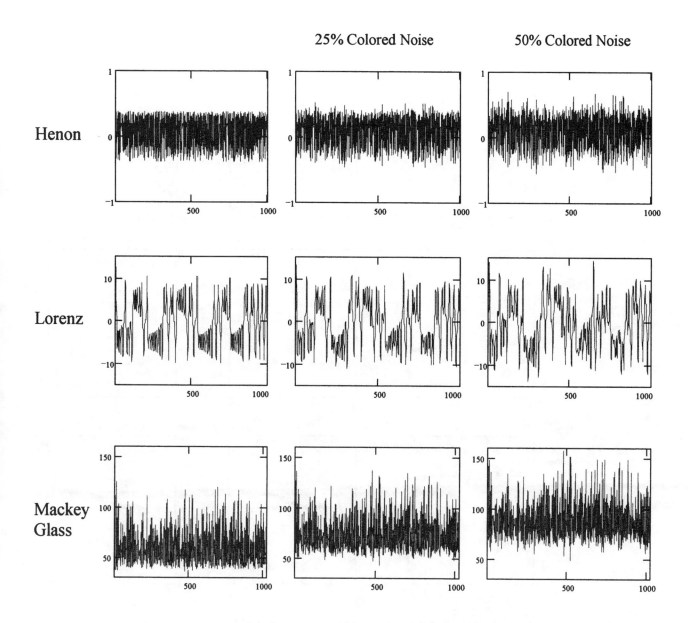

FIG. 1. Chaotic time series generated from single variables from Hénon, Lorenz, and Mackey–Glass equations. Effect of adding 25% and 50% colored noise is illustrated.

D. Prediction parameters

For the Hénon time series, the prediction parameters for discrete local flow and nonlinear prediction methods were a lag time (L) of 1, an embedding dimension (E) of 4, and translation horizons (H) of 1 to 10. For the local dispersion method, the parameters were $H=1$ and $L=1$ for $E=2-8$. For delta–epsilon method the parameters were $H=1$, $L=1$, and $E=4$.

For the Lorenz system, the continuous local flow method parameters were $E=4$ and $L=4$ for $H=6-12$, while for nonlinear prediction the translation horizon range was extended to a maximum of $H=40$. Parameters for local dispersion were $H=8$ and $L=4$ for $E=2-8$. Delta–epsilon prediction parameters were $H=8$, $L=4$, and $E=4$.

For the Mackey–Glass interevent interval series with additive Gaussian or colored noise, the parameters for nonlin-

ear prediction and delta–epsilon were $E=4$, $L=1$, and $H=1-10$ or $H=1$, respectively.

III. RESULTS

Figure 1 illustrates the effect of adding colored noise (0%, 25%, and 50%) to the three types of chaotic time series used in this report: Hénon, Lorenz, and Mackey–Glass.

Figure 2 presents a summary of determinism results for Lorenz data with 25% additive colored noise. Analyses with local flow, local dispersion, nonlinear prediction, and delta–epsilon methods are shown, compared with each of the three types of surrogates. If any of the battery of surrogates fits the experimental data well, the null hypothesis that the data could be explained by a linear stochastic process cannot be rejected. We have used only three realizations of each surrogate for this preliminary screen of these data. Note that the

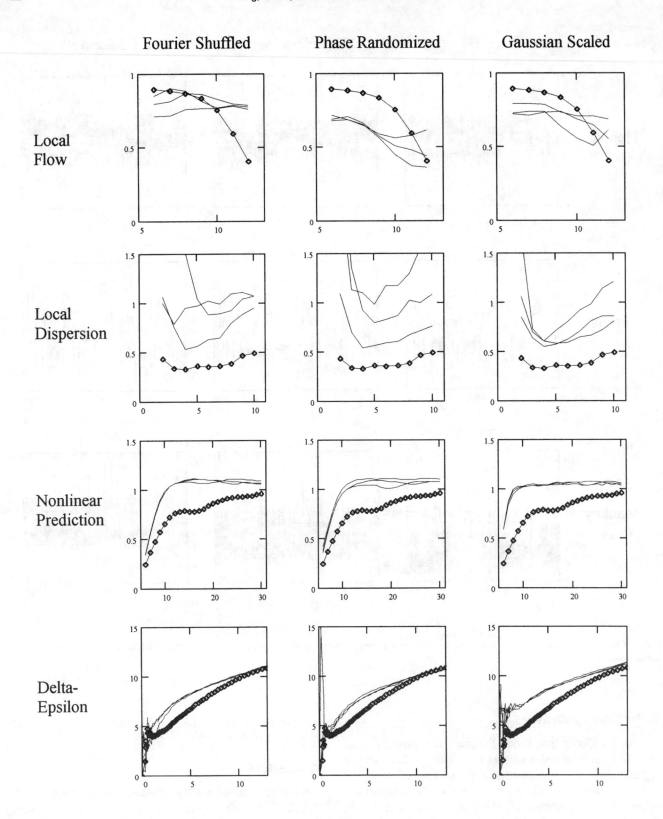

FIG. 2. Preliminary screening for determinism shown for Lorenz time series with 25% added colored noise. Experimental results shown with symbols ($\diamond$), and surrogate results shown with solid lines (———). Abscissa are translation horizon (H) for local flow and nonlinear prediction, embedding dimension (E) for local dispersion, and average delta (δ) for delta–epsilon plots. Ordinates are average displacement (V) for local flow, median dispersion (ϵ_{trans}) for local dispersion, normalized prediction error (NPE) for nonlinear prediction, and cumulative epsilon (ϵ) for delta–epsilon plots.

local flow method fails to distinguish the noisy deterministic series from its Fourier shuffled surrogates at this level of additive noise (the method clearly distinguished these data from surrogate data at lower levels of noise). The axes for

local flow represent the V statistic versus translation horizon, and for deterministic systems the values of V should be *greater than* the random surrogates. Local dispersion was able to discriminate the deterministic series from its surro-

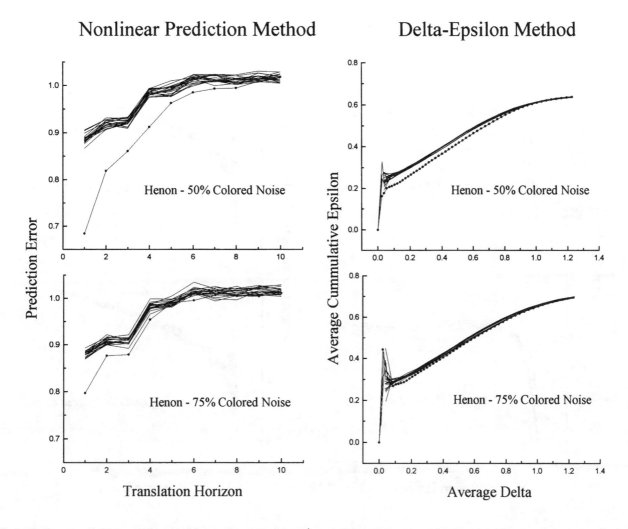

Nonlinear Prediction Method   Delta-Epsilon Method

FIG. 3. Nonlinear prediction compared with delta–epsilon method for Hénon data with 50% and 75% additive colored noise. Nineteen Gaussian scaled surrogates shown for each analysis. Experimental data: solid circles (●), surrogate data: solid lines (——).

gates at 25% added colored noise. The axes for local dispersion are median ϵ_{trans} versus embedding dimension, and the dispersion should be *less than* the random surrogates. At 50% additive noise, local dispersion failed to distinguish the noisy deterministic series from its surrogates (not shown). Nonlinear prediction was the most efficient of the three central tendency methods in detecting evidence of determinism in these noisy time series. The nonlinear prediction axes represent normalized prediction error versus translation horizon, and the values of NPE are smaller than the random surrogates for deterministic data. Note that the normalization of NPE requires that the magnitude of NPE be less than 1.0—if not, the predictions are worse than guessing the mean value of the time series for each prediction. For 25% colored noise, the separation of the experimental results from the surrogate mean (in terms of the number of standard deviations of the distribution of surrogate data about the mean—"sigmas" according to Theiler *et al.*[20]), is larger than the above two methods. Nonlinear prediction also identified determinism in these data at levels of 50% noise (not shown). The delta–epsilon method could also distinguish Lorenz with 25% added colored noise for all three surrogates; its axes are average cumulative epsilon versus average delta, and the ϵ val-

ues for deterministic data should be smaller than for surrogate data for small δ. Again, the separation between experimental results and the distribution of surrogate data is large, and this method also detected determinism in these data well at 50% noise (not shown). We note in passing that the results of the above analysis for additive white noise were quite similar to the colored noise results. Since nonlinear prediction and delta–epsilon were the most powerful of these tests in detecting determinism, we will now carry out a detailed comparison of these two methods.

We will compare nonlinear prediction and delta–epsilon methods on Hénon, Lorenz, and Mackey–Glass data. We will now employ 19 surrogate datasets for each experimental analysis, in order to apply a 1-tailed significance test at the 0.05 level (if all of the experimental results are less than the surrogate values for a given translation horizon or δ). Although we examined each of the three surrogate data types for this comparison, we will only illustrate the Gaussian scaled results in the figures that follow (the comparisons with the other surrogates were similar).

Figure 3 compares these two methods on Hénon data. The dimension of the noiseless attractor is ~1.2. Both meth-

Nonlinear Prediction Method   Delta-Epsilon Method

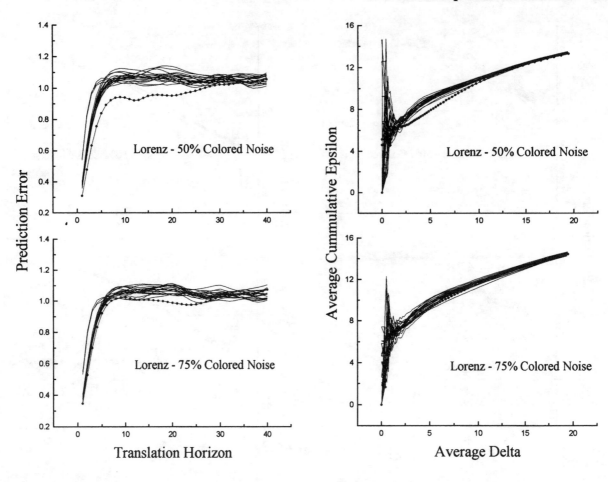

FIG. 4. Nonlinear prediction compared with delta–epsilon method for Lorenz data with 50% and 75% additive colored noise. Nineteen Gaussian scaled surrogates shown for each analysis. Experimental data: solid circles (●), surrogate data: solid lines (——).

ods are capable of distinguishing the determinism in these data at 50% and 75% additive noise.

Figure 4 compares these two methods on Lorenz data. The dimension of the noiseless attractor is ~2.1. Although both methods can distinguish the determinism at 50% additive colored noise, only nonlinear prediction detects determinism at 75% noise.

Figure 5 compares these two methods on Mackey–Glass data. The dimension of the noiseless attractor is ~7.1. Although both methods can distinguish the determinism at 25% additive colored noise, only nonlinear prediction detects determinism at 50% noise.

IV. DISCUSSION

Both nonlinear prediction and delta–epsilon methods demonstrated powerful capabilities for detecting determinism in noise-contaminated chaotic time series. Although we appeared to demonstrate an advantage with nonlinear prediction over delta–epsilon that was consistent for a range of data types (discrete map for Hénon, continuous for Lorenz, and integrate-and-fire for Mackey–Glass) and attractor dimensions (1.2–7.1), the comparison is rather unfair. Since there are numerous parameters that were fixed for these com-

parisons (see Sec. II D), and the parameter selection is both in part arbitrary and controversial, our lack of an exhaustive optimization of parameters renders our conclusions tentative.

Of more importance is the fact that these two very different approaches, a nonlinear predictor examining central tendency (root mean square of predictions), and delta–epsilon (examining the tail of the distribution of epsilons), were both robust in their abilities to detect determinism in the face of significant levels of additive noise. Since an arbitrary experimental dataset may contain traces of determinism better suited for one over the other of these methods, a screen for determinism in such data might logically employ both independent methods.

Unfortunately, the lack of an adequate surrogate data fit to one's data is necessary but insufficient to prove that the data are nonlinear or chaotic. Our use of a battery of surrogate data will reduce our chances for spurious identification of determinism, but the impossibility of performing an exhaustive surrogate analysis (the varieties of such surrogates are infinite) is problematic for data that appears deterministic with these methods. Although we would prefer to analyze experimental data without such surrogate techniques, the power of the technique is difficult to supplant at this time.

Nonlinear Prediction Method   Delta-Epsilon Method

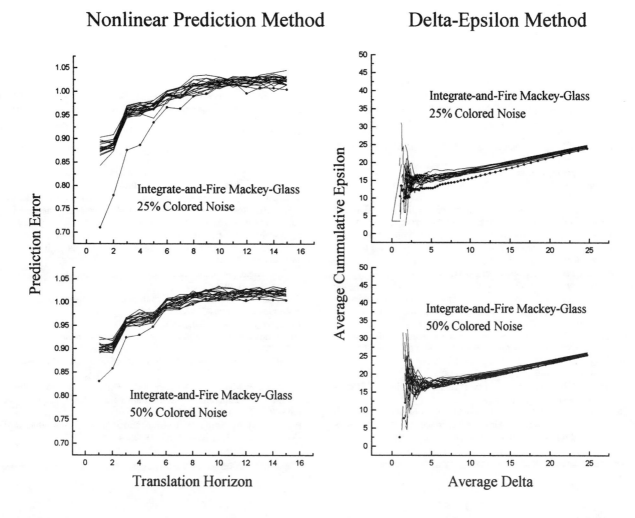

FIG. 5. Nonlinear prediction compared with delta–epsilon method for Mackey–Glass data with 25% and 50% additive colored noise. Nineteen Gaussian scaled surrogates shown for each analysis. Experimental data: solid circles (●), surrogate data: solid lines (——).

One of our interests is in applying these methods to biological data, especially neuronal. Although traditional time series can be recorded from neuronal networks, often by applying repetitive stimuli at fixed frequency,[8,9] the natural functioning nervous system is autonomous and not subjected to such stobing with stimuli. When discrete events can be identified from autonomously functioning neural tissue (e.g., EEG spikes), an event sequence of such intervals provides dynamical data.[9] With the recent demonstration that attractor reconstruction using delay coordinate embeddings of such event series is possible,[16] the application of the above techniques to such data is reasonable (see also article by Sauer[16] in this volume). The use of the high dimensional Mackey–Glass equations in an integrate-and-fire model in this report was specifically intended to simulate autonomous neuronal data (although the similarity to heartbeat data has not escaped us).

There are several critical questions that need to be addressed for better utilization of these methods. First is the issue to nonstationarity in biological data. Most neuronal data is characteristically nonstationary in both the strong and weak senses of the statistician. Since the surrogates we employ tend to be far more stationary than the original data, the above analysis for nonstationary data is flawed as it stands. We have applied simple methods of removing linear trends from our neuronal data (see Ref. 9), but have been hesitant to apply more sophisticated methods of removing linear structure from our data such as "bleaching."[21] A test for determinism could in principle deal with some nonstationarities if it could track the evolving dynamics of a system as the attractor translated through phase space. We have no means of implementing such tracking at this time.

Second is the issue of the simplicity of our nonlinear predictor. We have not compared our results with higher-order nonlinear predictors,[4] and such more complex methods might improve our detection of determinism.

Last, we note that the delta–epsilon method may predict properties of a chaotic system similar to an analysis of unstable orbits or *fixed points*. Such unstable orbit analysis has been used to implement recent chaos control experiments in physical,[11,22] and biological systems.[12,23] Nevertheless, the relationship between the detection of determinism with unstable orbit analysis, the delta–epsilon method, and nonlinear prediction is unknown at this time.

ACKNOWLEDGMENTS

T.C. received support from the Children's Research Institute. T.S. receives support from the National Science Foundation Computational Mathematics program and the U.S. Department of Energy. S.J.S. receives support from the Children's Research Institute, and from the National Institutes of Mental Health, Grant No. 1-R29-MH50006-03.

[1] D. T. Kaplan and L. Glass, "Direct test for determinism in a time series," Phys. Rev. Lett. **68**, 427–430 (1992).

[2] D. T. Kaplan, "Evaluating deterministic structure in maps deduced from discrete-time measurements," Int. J. Bifurcations Chaos **3**, 617–623 (1993).

[3] R. Wayland, D. Bromley, D. Pickett, and A. Passamante, "Recognizing determinism in a time series," Phys. Rev. Lett. **70**, 580–582 (1993).

[4] J. D. Farmer and J. J. Sidorowich, "Exploiting chaos to predict the future and reduce noise," in *Evolution, Learning, and Cognition*, edited by Y. C. Lee (World Scientific, Singapore, 1988).

[5] T. Sauer, "Time series prediction using delay coordinate embedding," in *Time Series Prediction: Forecasting the Future and Understanding the Past*, SFI Studies in the Sciences of Complexity, edited by A. S. Wiegend and N. A. Gershenfeld (Addison–Wesley, Reading, MA, 1993), Vol. XV, pp. 175 and 193.

[6] T. Chang, S. J. Schiff, and T. Sauer, "Tests for deterministic chaos in noisy time series," in *Proceedings of the Second Experimental Chaos Conference*, edited by W. Ditto, L. Pecora, M. Shlesinger, M. Spano, and S. Vohra (World Scientific, Singapore, in press).

[7] D. T. Kaplan, "Exceptional events as evidence for determinism," Physica D **73**, 38–48 (1994).

[8] T. Chang, S. J. Schiff, T. Sauer, J.-P. Gossard, and R. E. Burke, "Stochastic versus deterministic variability in simple neuronal circuits I. Monosynaptic spinal cord reflexes," Biophys. J. **67**, 671–683 (1994).

[9] S. J. Schiff, K. Jerger, T. Chang, T. Sauer, and P. G. Aitken, "Stochastic versus deterministic variability in simple neuronal circuits II. Hippocampal slice," Biophys. J. **67**, 684–691 (1994).

[10] E. Ott, C. Grebogi, and J. A. Yorke, "Controlling chaos," Phys. Rev. Lett. **64**, 1196–1199 (1990).

[11] W. L. Ditto, S. N. Rauseo, and M. L. Spano, "Experimental control of chaos," Phys. Rev. Lett. **65**, 3211–3214 (1990).

[12] S. J. Schiff, K. Jerger, D. H. Duong, T. Chang, M. L. Spano, and W. L. Ditto, "Controlling chaos in the brain," Nature **370**, 615–620 (1994).

[13] M. Hénon, "Two dimensional mapping with a strange attractor," Comm. Math. Phys. **50**, 69–77 (1976).

[14] E. N. Lorenz, "Deterministic nonperiodic flow," J. Atmos. Sci. **20**, 130–141 (1963).

[15] M. C. Mackey and L. Glass, "Oscillation and chaos in physiological control systems," Science **197**, 197–287 (1977).

[16] T. Sauer, "Reconstruction of dynamical systems from interspike intervals," Phys. Rev. Lett. **72**, 3811–3814 (1994); "Interspike interval embedding of chaotic signals," Chaos **5**, 127–132 (1995).

[17] S. J. Schiff, T. Sauer, and T. Chang, "Discriminating deterministic versus stochastic dynamics in neuronal activity," Integrative Physiol. Behav. Sci. **29**, 246–261 (1994).

[18] A. C. A. Hope, "A simplified Monte Carlo significance test procedure," J. R. Stat. Soc. B **30**, 582–598 (1968).

[19] L. W. Salvino and R. Cawley, "Statistical test for smooth dynamics in embedded time-series," Phys. Rev. Lett. **73**, 1091–1094 (1994).

[20] J. Theiler, S. Eubank, A. Longtin, B. Galdrikian, and J. D. Farmer, "Testing for nonlinearity in time series: the method of surrogate data," Physica D **58**, 77–94 (1992).

[21] J. Theiler and S. Eubank, "Don't bleach chaotic data," Chaos **4**, 1–12 (1993).

[22] R. Roy, T. W. Murphy, T. D. Maier, and Z. Gills, "Dynamical control of a chaotic laser: Experimental stabilization of a globally coupled system," Phys. Rev. Lett. **68**, 1259–1262 (1992).

[23] A. Garfinkel, M. Spano, W. L. Ditto, and J. Weiss, "Controlling cardiac chaos," Science **257**, 1230–1235 (1992).

Interspike interval embedding of chaotic signals

Tim Sauer
Department of Mathematical Sciences, George Mason University, Fairfax, Virginia 22030

(Received 27 May 1994; accepted for publication 24 October 1994)

According to a theorem of Takens [*Lecture Notes in Mathematics* (Springer-Verlag, Berlin, 1981), Vol. 898], dynamical state information can be reproduced from a time series of amplitude measurements. In this paper we investigate whether the same information can be reproduced from interspike interval (ISI) measurements. Assuming an integrate-and-fire model coupling the dynamical system to the spike train, there is a one-to-one correspondence between the system states and interspike interval vectors of sufficiently large dimension. The correspondence implies in particular that a data series of interspike intervals, formed in this manner, can be forecast from past history. This capability is demonstrated using a nonlinear prediction algorithm, and is found to be robust to noise. A set of interspike intervals measured from a simple neuronal circuit is studied for deterministic structure using a prediction error statistic. © *1995 American Institute of Physics.*

I. INTRODUCTION

The impact of the discovery of chaos lies in the realization that nonlinear systems with few degrees of freedom, while deterministic in principle, can create output signals that look complex, and mimic stochastic signals from the point of view of conventional time series analysis. The exponential separation rate of chaotic trajectories causes chaotic systems in the laboratory to exhibit much of the same medium to long-term behavior as stochastic systems. On the other hand, short-term correlation of trajectories is not ruled out for chaotic systems, if there are a reasonably low number of active degrees of freedom. This leaves open the possibility of analysis and exploitation of these correlations using deterministic models.

A key element in such an analysis is provided by embedding theory. In typical situations, points on the dynamical attractor in the full system phase space have a one-to-one correspondence with vectors of time-delayed amplitude measurements of a generic system variable. System analysis of this type is suggested in Ref. 1 and an embedding theorem due to Takens[2] (later extended in Ref. 3) established its validity.

The fact that the current system state can be identified using a vector of time series measurements leads to a number of applications, owing to the fact that analysis of the topology and sometimes the geometry of the chaotic attractor underlying the time series can be performed in the state-space reproduced from the delay-coordinate vectors. Applications include noise-filtering and prediction of chaotic time series, and control of unstable periodic orbits solely from a time series record.[4]

Increased attention is being paid to the dynamic properties of physiological systems, and particularly to the nonlinear aspects of the systems. Given the nonlinearity of subsystems, it is often expressed that the existence of deterministic chaotic behavior in physiological systems is likely—after all, although irregular signals are being produced, useful information is being passed through the system. However, little direct evidence for chaos exists within the research literature at present, possibly due to the high noise level present and the high-dimensionality of the dynamics, paired with the difficulty of collecting relevant data and the primitive state of our statistical methods.

An interesting feature of dynamical processing in physiological systems is the capacity of information to change in form while being passed between individual units. In some cases amplitude and frequency data are important; in others, amplitudes may be of minimal importance. It is hypothesized, for example, that some information-passing in nervous systems depends primarily on spike trains, or temporal patterns of firing of action potentials, and is largely independent of the amplitudes of the potentials. A wide spectrum of modes of information may be helpful for accomplishing the variety of tasks necessary in a large interconnected system.

In this paper we touch on a small part of a much larger issue: the diversity of types of information that may exist in dynamical systems, and on the conversion between them. We restrict our study to the following question: Can amplitude time series data be converted to spike trains with no loss of information content? In Sec. II, we answer this question affirmatively by showing that under a certain hypothesis for spike generation, the current state of a deterministic system can be reflected solely through its interspike interval history. In Sec. III we demonstrate a practical consequence: that spike trains of moderate length are predictable. Section IV deals with the effects of noise in the process of converting amplitude data to spike trains, and Sec. V contains an analysis of interspike interval data from a neurobiological system. Section VI discusses the limitations of this study and directions for further work.

II. DETERMINISTIC INTERSPIKE INTERVALS

A statistical process in which the dynamical information is carried by a series of event timings is called a *point process*. See Ref. 5 for an introduction to the statistical literature on this subject. The main question of this paper is the following: If a point process is the manifestation of an underlying deterministic system, can the states of the deterministic system be identified from the information provided by the point process? Previous work on this question can be found in Refs. 6 and 7.

In particular, neurobiological systems are often marked by measurable pulses corresponding to a cell reaching a threshold potential, which triggers rapid depolarization, followed by repolarization, which restarts the cycle. The times of these discrete pulses can be recorded. This type of data differs from a time series of an observable measured at regular time intervals. Many hypotheses and models for the description of the time variability of these pulses have been proposed.[8]

Our approach is meant to be a simple paradigm that shares qualitative characteristics with real systems, and that demonstrates feasible ways in which complicated information about system states can be communicated and transformed in type. In particular, we will focus on the linkage between continuous dynamics and the interspike intervals (ISI's) produced by them, rather than modeling the detailed mechanism of any single system.

For concreteness, we make a simple hypothesis connecting an underlying continuous dynamical system to the point process. The time series from the dynamical system is integrated with respect to time; when it reaches a preset threshold, a spike is generated, after which the integration is restarted. This integrate-and-fire model is chosen for its simplicity and potential wide applicability. In our simulations we hypothesize that the input to be integrated is a low-dimensional chaotic attractor. We use the Mackey–Glass equation and the Lorenz equations as simple representative examples.

Let $S(t)$ denote the signal produced by a time-varying observable of a finite-dimensional dynamical system. Assume that the trajectories of the dynamical system are asymptotic to a compact attractor X. Let θ be a positive number which represents the firing threshold. After fixing a starting time T_0, a series of "firing times" $T_1 < T_2 < T_3 < ...$ can be recursively defined by the equation

$$\int_{T_i}^{T_{i+1}} S(t)dt = \theta. \qquad (1)$$

From the firing times T_i, the interspike intervals can be defined as $t_i = T_i - T_{i-1}$.

Figure 1 shows a time trace of the Mackey–Glass[9] delay differential equation

$$\dot{x}(t) = -0.1x(t) + \frac{0.2x(t-\Delta)}{1+x(t-\Delta)^{10}}, \qquad (2)$$

where $\Delta = 100$, together with spiking times generated by (1) where the threshold was set at $\theta = 50$. In this paper we will study behavior of this example dynamical system for two parameter settings. When $\Delta = 30$, the attractor for this system has dimension around 3.5, according to numerical estimation. For $\Delta = 100$, as in Figure 1, the correlation dimension is approximately 7.1 (see Ref. 10).

It turns out that if the interspike intervals are finite, and under certain genericity conditions on the underlying dynamics, signal and threshold, the series $\{t_i\}$ of ISI's can be used to reconstruct the attractor X. In other words, there is a one-

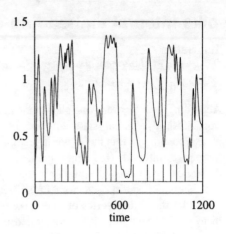

FIG. 1. The upper trace is a solution of the Mackey–Glass equation ($\Delta = 100$) graphed as a function of time. The lower trace shows the times at which spikes are generated according to Eq. (1), with $S(t) = x(t)$ and $\theta = 50$.

to-one correspondence between m-tuples of ISI's and attractor states, which associates each vector $(t_i, t_{i-1}, ..., t_{i-m+1})$ of ISI's with the corresponding point $x(T_i)$ on the attractor. In analogy with the original Takens' theorem[2] and its generalization,[3] the condition $m > 2D_0$ is sufficient, where D_0 is the box-counting dimension of the attractor X. As with Takens' theorem, smaller m may be sufficient in particular cases.

Figure 2 shows a delay plot of interspike intervals produced by the x-coordinate of the Lorenz attractor,[11] governed by the equations $\dot{x} = \sigma(y-x), \dot{y} = \rho x - y - xz, \dot{z} = -\beta z + xy,$

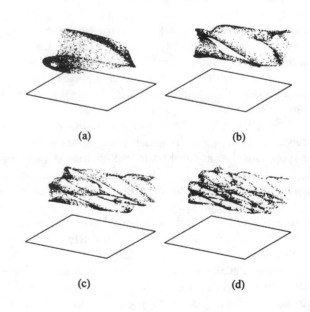

(a)   (b)

(c)   (d)

FIG. 2. The Lorenz attractor reconstructed from interspike intervals. Each of these representations is a three-dimensional projection of a reconstruction which in five dimensions is topologically equivalent to the Lorenz attractor. The signal used to create spikes was $S(t) = x(t) + 25$, using the x-coordinate of the Lorenz equations, with thresholds (a) $\theta = 2$, (b) $\theta = 12$, (c) $\theta = 20$, (d) $\theta = 28$.

where the parameters are set at the standard values $\sigma=10$, $\rho=28$, $\beta=8/3$. The signal $S(t)=x(t)+25$ is used with four different thresholds θ in Equation (1) to generate the interspike interval delay plot shown.

Recall that the box-counting dimension of the Lorenz attractor is about 2.1. The theorem stated above says that generic reconstructions in $m=5$ dimensions are topologically equivalent to the original Lorenz attractor, although its orientation in five-dimensional Euclidean space could be rather twisted. Each part of Figure 2 can be viewed as a projection from five-dimensional space to three-dimensional space of this topologically equivalent attractor.

III. SHORT-TERM PREDICTION

One practical consequence of such a theorem is that the ISI vectors $(t_i,...,t_{i-m+1})$ can be used to reconstruct the attractor X sufficiently to make measurements of dynamical invariants of X possible, and to do short-term prediction on the series $\{t_i\}$. Thus the possibility exists of predicting future interspike intervals from past history, which has practical applications. To explain the meaning of short-term, it is instructive to recall the time series case. For chaotic time series, the length of time horizon for which prediction is effective depends on the separation time of nearby trajectories, and so inversely on the largest Lyapunov exponent. For ISI series, the horizon depends both on the Lyapunov exponents of the underlying process and on the threshold θ. As θ increases, the predictability decreases.[12]

We will apply a simple version of a nearest-neighbor prediction algorithm (see, for example, Ref. 13). The simple version used here is sufficient to measure the level of determinism in the series. In order to quantify the predictability of the series of ISI's we will use the concept of surrogate data[14] to produce statistical controls.

The prediction algorithm works as follows. Given an ISI vector $V_0=(t_{i_0},...,t_{i_0-m+1})$, the 1% of other reconstructed vectors V_k that are nearest to V_0 are collected. The values of the ISI for some number h of steps into the future are averaged for all k to make a prediction. That is, the average $p_{i_0}=\langle t_{i_k+h}\rangle_k$ is used to approximate the future interval t_{i_0+h}. The difference $p-t_{i_0+h}$ is the h-step prediction error at step i_0. We could instead use the series mean m to predict at each step; this h-step prediction error is $m-t_{i_0+h}$. The ratio of the root mean square errors of the two possibilities (the nonlinear prediction algorithm and the constant prediction of the mean) gives the normalized prediction error (NPE)

$$\text{NPE}=\frac{\langle(p_{i_0}-t_{i_0+h})^2\rangle^{1/2}}{\langle(m-t_{i_0+h})^2\rangle^{1/2}}, \tag{3}$$

where the averages are taken over the entire series. The normalized prediction error is a measure of the (out-of-sample) predictability of the ISI series. A value of NPE less than 1 means that there is linear or nonlinear predictability in the series beyond the baseline prediction of the series mean.

Our goal in predicting ISI's is to verify that the nonlinear deterministic structure of the dynamics that produced the in-

tervals is preserved in the ISI's. Linear autocorrelation in the time series, present for example in correlated noise, can cause NPE to be less than 1. In order to control for this effect, we calculate the NPE for the original series of ISI's as well as for stochastic series of the same length, called surrogate data, which share the same linear statistical properties with the original series.

We use two types of surrogate data in our analysis. The first, called a random phase (RP) surrogate, is a series with the same power spectrum as the original series, but is the realization of a stochastic process. The autocorrelation of the original series is preserved in the surrogate series, while the nonlinear deterministic structure is eliminated. If the predictability of the original can be shown to be statistically different from the predictability of such surrogates, the null hypothesis that the original series was produced by a stochastic process can be rejected, which is evidence that the nonlinear structure of the underlying dynamical system is present in the interspike intervals. The second type of surrogate, called a Gaussian-scaled shuffle (GS) surrogate,[14] is a shuffle (rearrangement) of the original series. The GS surrogate (called an amplitude-adjusted surrogate in Ref. 14) corresponds to the null hypothesis that the series is a monotonically-scaled version of amplitudes produced by a Gaussian random process with similar autocorrelation.

The result of applying the prediction algorithm to interspike intervals from the Mackey–Glass equation is shown in Figure 3. Part (a) of the figure deals with the low-dimensional ($D\approx3.5$) attractor, for parameter setting $\Delta=30$, and part (b) the higher-dimensional ($D\approx7$) version, where $\Delta=100$. In both cases 1024 spikes were generated according to (1) with $\theta=50$ and $S(t)=x(t)$ from the delay-differential equation (2). For these calculations we fixed the embedding dimension $m=3$, and predicted one step ahead ($h=1$). Ten surrogate series of each of the two types were generated. Prediction results for the original ISI series and the 10 Gaussian-scaled surrogates are shown in Figure 3; results for the RP surrogates are similar to those of the GS surrogates and are not shown. For low prediction horizons there is a statistically significant difference between the original series and its surrogates, for both parameter settings $\Delta=30$ and $\Delta=100$. The conclusion is that there is predictability in the ISI series caused by the underlying deterministic dynamics. (More precisely, there is predictability not explained by any of the null hypotheses controlled for by the surrogate data.)

This example shows that there is measurable nonlinear predictability in reasonably short spike trains generated deterministically according to ansatz (1), even when the generator is moderately high-dimensional. The theory referred to above implies predictability, but gives no estimate for the length of spike train necessary to detect it. Our findings indicate that data sets of lengths accessible in physiological settings can be sufficient in principle.

The fact that NPE <1 for the stochastic surrogates for small prediction horizons in Figure 3 is a reflection of the nontrivial linear autocorrelation in the ISI series. For example, the mean NPE of the 10 Gaussian-scaled surrogates for the case $\Delta=30$, $h=1$ was 0.73 ± 0.03. The fact that the NPE of 0.47 for the original ISI series is significantly differ-

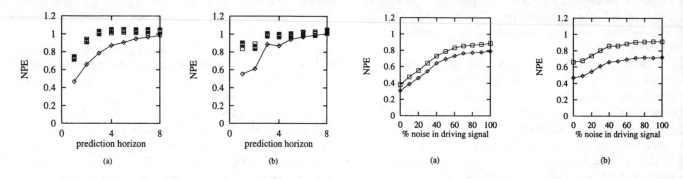

FIG. 3. One-step-ahead prediction for deterministic interspike intervals (designated by diamonds) versus 10 Gaussian-scaled surrogates (squares) for (a) $\Delta=30$ and (b) $\Delta=100$. In both cases, a threshold of $\theta=50$ was used.

FIG. 4. Normalized prediction error for ISI series produced from noisy Mackey–Glass time series. (a) $\Delta=30$ in Eq. (2), threshold $\theta=25$ in Eq. (1). The lower curve (diamonds) is NPE for horizon $h=1$, the upper curve (squares) for $h=2$. (b) Same as (a), except $\theta=50$.

ent means that there is nonlinear deterministic dynamics beyond what is explained by the stochastic hypothesis.

An amplitude time series of length approximately 60K in natural time units for the Mackey–Glass equation is required to generate the 1K interspike intervals used for the results of Figure 3 (for either $\Delta=30$ and $\Delta=100$). A relevant question (which we have not answered here) is to study the level of interchangeability of modes of information by comparing predictability of the original amplitude time series and the (much shorter) ISI series derived from it.

IV. INTERSPIKE INTERVALS DRIVEN BY NOISY DYNAMICS

The previous section showed that deterministically-generated interspike intervals can be predicted from relatively short histories, at least well enough to be distinguished from stochastic processes. We show next that this result is robust in the presence of a significant amount of noise in the time series generating the spikes.

The following numerical experiment was carried out. A time series was obtained by integrating the Mackey–Glass equation (2) for $2^{16} \approx 64$ K time units. In-band noise (noise with the same power spectrum as the original series) was added to the time series. A series of 1024 interspike intervals was generated using (1), and normalized prediction error was calculated from (3). Figure 4 quantifies the predictability of ISI series formed from the noisy time series. In Figure 4(a), a threshold of $\theta=25$ was used, and in Figure 4(b), $\theta=50$. In each diagram, the lower curve represents NPE for prediction horizon $h=1$ (one interspike interval ahead), and the upper curve represents $h=2$.

Figure 4 shows that for moderate amounts of additive noise in the driving signal, deterministic structure as measured by prediction error can be detected. At the right-hand side of the figures, where the deterministic driving signal is swamped by noise, the NPE reaches an asymptotic limit due to the predictive power of the linear autocorrelation alone. For example, in Figure 4(b), the high-noise limit NPE for horizon $h=1$ is approximately 0.73, matching the value shown in Figure 3(a) for the stochastic surrogates with the corresponding horizon ($h=1$).

Adding noise to the generating time series also changes the distribution of interspike intervals (where time order is ignored). Figure 5(a) shows the probability distribution of ISI generated from a Mackey–Glass time series with parameter $\Delta=30$, with no added noise. The histogram has two distinct peaks, corresponding to preferred firing intervals. As higher levels of noise are added, the peaks gradually merge, forming a unimodal distribution in the limit that the deterministic dynamics are swamped with noise. The role of ISI histograms in the detection of determinism is an intriguing question.

V. INTERSPIKE INTERVALS FROM NEURONAL CIRCUITS

A set of experimental data from a mammalian neuronal circuit was analyzed from the point of view of recognizing deterministic nonlinear dynamics solely from an interspike interval series. This data was collected and previously analyzed by the authors of Ref. 15. In this experiment, a hippocampal slice from a rat was suffused with a high concentration potassium solution, eliciting spontaneous population response burst firing in CA3 pyramidal cells. The time intervals between bursts were recorded at CA1 for analysis. Some of the preparations produced interburst interval series that could be distinguished from linear stochastic models by our statistical methods, as reported in Ref. 15. Here we report in detail on an interesting case that could not be explained by simple stochastic models.

We will measure the significance of nonlinearity following the methodology of Prichard and Theiler in Ref. 16 applied to nonlinear prediction error. For a section of the interval series of length 1024 (the intervals between 1025 events) we created 39 Gauss-scaled (amplitude-adjusted) surrogate series. Each of the 39 series consists of the same 1024 time intervals rearranged in an order which is designed to be random up to keeping the power spectrum approximately unchanged. The experimental interval series and a typical surrogate are displayed in Figure 6.

We compare the relevant statistic (normalized prediction error, as above) for the original data series with the same statistic computed from the 39 surrogates. If the statistic from the original experimental series lies outside the distri-

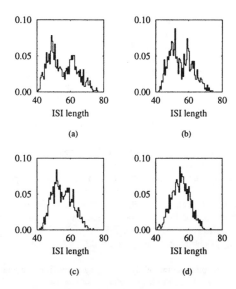

(a)

(b)

(c)

(d)

FIG. 5. Sample probability distribution histograms for noisy interspike intervals from the Mackey–Glass equation with $\Delta = 30$. Spikes are generated according to Eq. (1) where $S(t)$ is a time series from Eq. (2) with added in-band noise of level (a) 0%, (b) 20%, (c) 40%, (d) 100%.

bution of the 39 values measured from the surrogates, the null hypothesis that the experimental series can be explained by the surrogates is rejected at a 95% confidence level.

Figure 7 shows the results in computing the normalized prediction error as described in Sec. III. The prediction horizon is one step, i.e., the length of the next interval is predicted on the basis of the previous history of intervals. We computed the NPE for the original series of Figure 6(a) and for 39 surrogates of GS type. The NPE for the experimental data was well outside the range of the NPE for the 39 surrogates for all 5 embedding dimensions used. We conclude that a linear stochastic process, even with amplitudes adjusted to match those of the experimental series, is a statistically unlikely generator for the data.

After making Figure 7, we repeated the statistical tests separately for the first and second half of the experimental series. Our motivation was the hypothesis that the findings of nonlinearity could be partially caused by a slight nonstationarity in the series. [A visual inspection of Figure 6(a) may

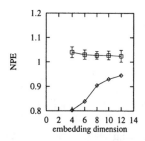

FIG. 7. Normalized one-step-ahead prediction error. The lower curve is the NPE for the experimental data; the upper curve is the mean of the NPE for 39 surrogates. The error bars denote 2 standard deviations.

suggest this to the reader.] We cut the experimental series into two equal parts, and for each of the two length 512 sequences, we created 39 surrogates and did a separate analysis. Figure 8 shows typical surrogates for the first half and second half, respectively. The results from computing the nonlinear prediction error statistic for the two sequences and their surrogates were quite similar to the results for the full sequence, with larger uncertainty because of the smaller amount of data. Once again, the null hypothesis was rejected for both halves of the series individually at the 95% confidence level.

VI. DISCUSSION

We have attempted to suggest methods of studying interspike interval series recorded from experiment in a model-free manner. If they are generated according to hypothesis (1), there is theory to say that ISI vectors can be used to represent states of the underlying attractor in a similar manner as delay coordinate vectors from amplitude time series. Although (1) was chosen to be as free of assumptions as possible, we caution that it is a hypothesis, and that the primary features of any particular physiological system may not be well represented by this hypothesis. This study is there-

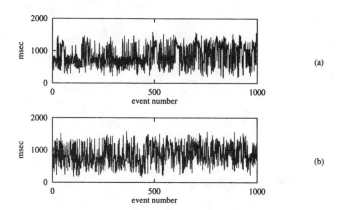

(a)

(b)

FIG. 6. (a) Interevent intervals from experiment; (b) typical Gauss-scaled surrogate.

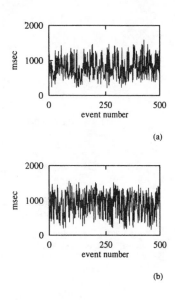

(a)

(b)

FIG. 8. (a) Gauss-scaled surrogate from first 512 points; (b) from second 512 points.

fore a kind of feasibility study. Further work with more re-alistic integrate-and-fire models for specific contexts is needed.

Our main conclusion under hypothesis (1) is that there need be no loss of information in principle when converting from dynamical amplitude information to spike trains. Along with the conventional statistical modeling of interspike intervals as point processes, there is the possibility of deterministic modeling, which can lead to richer understanding for model-building and prediction purposes.

ACKNOWLEDGMENTS

I express appreciation to S. J. Schiff, K. Jerger, T. Chang, and P. G. Aitken for making the hippocampus data available. This research was supported in part by the National Science Foundation (Computational Mathematics) and the U.S. Department of Energy.

[1] N. Packard, J. Crutchfield, J. D. Farmer, and R. Shaw, "Geometry from a time series," Phys. Rev. Lett. **45**, 712 (1980).

[2] F. Takens, "Detecting strange attractors in turbulence," *Lecture Notes in Mathematics* (Springer-Verlag, Berlin, 1981), Vol. 898.

[3] T. Sauer, J. A. Yorke, and M. Casdagli, "Embedology," J. Stat. Phys. **65**, 579 (1991).

[4] *Coping with Chaos: Analysis of Chaotic Data and the Exploitation of Chaotic Systems*, edited by E. Ott, T. Sauer, and J. A. Yorke (Wiley-Interscience, New York, 1994), 418 pp.

[5] M. Miller and D. Snyder, *Random Point Processes in Time and Space* (Springer-Verlag, New York, 1991); P. A. W. Lewis (editor), *Stochastic Point Processes: Statistical Analysis, Theory, and Applications* (Wiley-Interscience, New York 1972).

[6] H. Preissl, A. Aertsen, and G. Palm, in *Parallel Processing in Neural Systems and Computers*, edited by R. Eckmiller, G. Hartmann, and G. Hauske (Elsevier, North-Holland, Amsterdam, 1990), p. 83.

[7] A. Longtin, "Nonlinear forecasting of spike trains from sensory neurons," Int. J. Bifurcation Chaos **3**, 651 (1993); A. Longtin, A. Bulsara, and F. Moss, "Time-interval sequences in bistable systems and the noise-induced transmission of information by sensory neurons," Phys. Rev. Lett. **67**, 656 (1991).

[8] H. Tuckwell, *Introduction to Theoretical Neurobiology* (Cambridge University Press, Cambridge, 1988), Vols. 1 and 2.

[9] M. C. Mackey and L. Glass, "Oscillations and chaos in physiological control systems," Science **197**, 287 (1977).

[10] M. Ding, C. Grebogi, E. Ott, T. Sauer, and J. A. Yorke, "Estimating correlation dimension from a chaotic time series: When does plateau onset occur?" Physica D **69**, 404 (1993).

[11] E. Lorenz, "Deterministic nonperiodic flow," J. Atmos. Sci. **20**, 130 (1963).

[12] T. Sauer, "Reconstruction of dynamical systems from interspike intervals," Phys. Rev. Lett. **72**, 3811 (1994).

[13] G. Sugihara and R. M. May, "Nonlinear forecasting as a way of distinguishing chaos from measurement error in time series," Nature **344**, 734 (1990).

[14] J. Theiler, S. Eubank, A. Longtin, B. Galdrakian, and J. D. Farmer, "Testing for nonlinearity in time series: the method of surrogate data," Physica D **58**, 77 (1992).

[15] S. J. Schiff, K. Jerger, T. Chang, T. Sauer, and P. G. Aitken, "Stochastic versus deterministic variability in simple neuronal circuits. II. Hippocampal slice," Biophys. J. **67**, 684 (1994).

[16] D. Prichard and J. Theiler, "Generating surrogate data for time series with several simultaneously measured variables," Phys. Rev. Lett. **73**, 951 (1994).

Noise in chaotic data: Diagnosis and treatment

Thomas Schreiber and Holger Kantz
Department of Physics, University of Wuppertal, D-42097 Wuppertal, Germany

(Received 8 June 1994; accepted for publication 21 September 1994)

A prominent limiting factor in the analysis of chaotic time series are measurement errors in the data. We show that this influence can be quite severe, depending on the nature of the noise, the complexity of the signal, and on the application one has in mind. Theoretical considerations yield general upper bounds on the tolerable noise level for dimension, entropy and Lyapunov estimates. We discuss methods to detect and analyze the noise present in a measured data set. We show how the situation can be improved by nonlinear noise reduction. © *1995 American Institute of Physics.*

I. INTRODUCTION

Most characteristic quantities of living beings change with time. Observing this time evolution can provide better understanding of the processes at work. Qualitative changes in the dynamics can provide information about the state a subject is in, e.g. if it is healthy or suffers from some disease.

Time records of biological or medical phenomena typically show some irregularity; they are neither constant nor strictly periodic. The classical approach of time series analysis would try to identify the irregular part as random fluctuations and the correlations as resulting from some linear process. However, this approach often leaves part of the structure of the data unexplained.

The paradigm of deterministic chaos suggests a fundamentally different interpretation: nonlinear deterministic systems can exhibit very irregular dynamical behavior autonomously, without random inputs. Since the theory of such systems has been well studied in the last few years, it seems quite natural to try to observe chaotic behavior in experiments and in real world data. However, some difficulties occur when turning theoretical concepts from deterministic chaos into analyzing tools for real time series. This paper will concentrate on the problems which occur as a consequence of measurement error present in the data.

The evolution of a low dimensional dynamical system can be expressed either as a set of ordinary differential equations or as a discrete time mapping. Although most real systems evolve continuously in time, data are always sampled discretely. Since furthermore the results we will present assume a simpler form, without loss of generality, we will concentrate on discrete time maps in what follows. Thus, a trajectory of the underlying system can be obtained by iterating $\mathbf{y}_{n+1} = \mathbf{F}(\mathbf{y}_n)$ starting from some initial condition $\mathbf{y}_0$. Thus the state of the system at any time n is a vector $\mathbf{y}_n$ in some m-dimensional space. A very long trajectory eventually will settle onto an attracting set (provided it does not run away to infinity, a case not considered here). This attracting set, or rather the invariant measure defined on it by the average visitation frequency of a typical trajectory, is the natural object to study from the point of view of nonlinear dynamics.

Reality deviates from this description in several respects. First we usually cannot obtain $\mathbf{y}_n$ directly, instead we measure some function $g(\mathbf{y})$ of it, in many cases yielding only scalar values. [Even in cases where multiprobe measurements are available, like multichannel EEG, the set of measurement functions $\{g_k(\mathbf{y})\}$ is presumably not sufficient to reconstruct $\mathbf{y}$ uniquely.] Second, this measurement is always subject to some error, either due to random fluctuations or due to the discretization. Further, the data represent only a finite, often short, piece of a trajectory, which may or may not explore most of the attractor, or may not even reach the attractor at all. Finally, at each moment the state $\mathbf{y}_n$ of the system may be perturbed by a stochastic process or by fluctuations in the control parameters.

In order to focus the discussion in this paper on the influence of the measurement noise, we will assume throughout that the data are otherwise well behaved. By this we mean that the signal would be to some extent predictable by exploiting an underlying stationary deterministic rule—were it not for the noise. This is the case for data sets which can be embedded in a low dimensional phase space, which are stationary and which are not too short. Violation of each one of these requirements leads to further complications which will not be addressed here. (However, we are aware of the fact that clinical data almost never fulfill these requirements to a satisfactory degree.)

For all of the methods of data processing described below we have to reconstruct a higher dimensional trajectory $\{\mathbf{x}_n\}$ which is in some sense equivalent to $\{\mathbf{y}_n\}$, knowing only noisy scalar measurements $\{x_n\}$. Without noise, this is successfully achieved using a time delay embedding.[1] In the presence of noise, state space reconstruction becomes a very intricate problem. However, we will cut the discussion short by assuming that a delay embedding of sufficiently high dimension forms a proper reconstruction and our data yield trajectories deterministic up to the noise. For the reconstruction problem we refer the reader to the literature, in particular to a paper by Casdagli *et al.*[2] A review of nonlinear time series analysis in general can be found in Ref. 3.

II. MEASUREMENT ERROR AND DYNAMICAL NOISE

Measurement noise refers to the corruption of observations by errors which are independent of the dynamics. The dynamics satisfies $\mathbf{y}_i = \mathbf{f}(\mathbf{y}_{i-1})$, but we measure scalars $x_i = g(\mathbf{y}_i) + \eta_i$, where g is a smooth function that maps points on the attractor to real numbers, and the η_i are independent and identically distributed (iid) random variables.

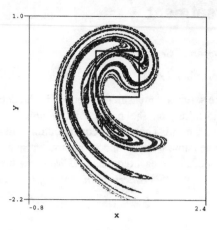 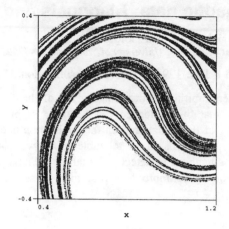

FIG. 1. A set of points on the Ikeda attractor,[6] $z_{n+1} = 1 + 0.9z_n \exp[0.4i - 6i/(1 + |z_n|^2)]$, together with an enlargement by a linear factor of 4. On smaller length scales, more and more structure becomes visible. Although we do not expect exact self-similarity, the line structure repeats itself. The region shown in each picture contains about 50 000 points.

(Even in multichannel measurements, generally $y_n + \eta_n$ is not recorded, but different scalar variables corresponding to different measurement functions g_j.)

Dynamical noise, in contrast, is a feedback process wherein the system is perturbed by a small random amount at each time step:

$$\mathbf{x}_i = \mathbf{f}(\mathbf{x}_{i-1} + \boldsymbol{\eta}_{i-1}). \qquad (1)$$

Dynamical and measurement noise are two notions of the error that may not be distinguishable *a posteriori* based on the data only. Both descriptions can be consistent to some extent with the same signal. (For strongly chaotic systems which are everywhere hyperbolic, more precisely, for *Axiom A* systems, measurement and dynamical noise can be mapped onto each other.[4])

Generally, dynamical noise induces much greater problems in data processing than measurement noise, since in the latter case a nearby clean trajectory of the underlying deterministic system exists and can indeed be found to some degree of accuracy by a proper noise reduction procedure. Furthermore, what one interprets to be dynamical noise sometimes may be a higher dimensional deterministic part of the dynamics with small amplitude. Even if this is not the case, dynamical noise may be essential for the observed dynamics. Consider a situation, where the system possesses a weakly attracting periodic orbit and a chaotic repeller, for example the logistic equation $x_{n+1} = a - x_n^2$ with $a = 1.9408$.[5] A typical noise-free trajectory will eventually settle down to a period three orbit. Now, if we let Gaussian noise interact with the dynamics, there is a finite probability that the noise kicks the trajectory off the periodic orbit onto the repeller. The signal in such a case will consist of chaotic bursts with exponentially distributed durations, embedded in intervals of periodic motion. Any attempt to model this behavior without noise will presumably fail. We do not want to enter such intricate problems, but this example should serve as a warning that dynamical noise may have more severe effects than simply smearing out some small-scale deterministic structures.

III. NOISE AND SCALING

The complicated dynamics of chaotic systems results in a nontrivial geometrical structure of the attracting set in state space (see Fig. 1). The typical self-similarity, or *fractal* geometry, of these *strange attractors* can be quantified by scaling properties of the distribution of probabilities that a trajectory visits a certain point in space, and of the transition probabilities.

In order to observe scaling of an attractor, as opposed to the shape of a particular trajectory, we have to require stationarity of the process. This means on the one hand that the governing dynamical laws remain the same when time goes on, but on the other hand that the probabilities mentioned above are time invariant. Every attempt has to be made to detect if nonstationarity is present in a data set. Unresolved nonstationarity can lead to spurious results when methods defined for stationary processes are applied nevertheless. Particular problems with the correlation dimension are discussed in Ref. 7.

Obviously, the range of scales accessible from the data is limited from above by the overall size of the attractor and from below by the noise amplitude (see Fig. 2). We want to study this limiting effect of measurement noise in this section.

A. Dimensions

There are several concepts quantifying scaling properties and self-similarity of a set, most of them use dimension-like quantities. In practice, the most useful probe for scaling is the correlation integral $C(\epsilon)$ introduced by Grassberger and Procaccia[8] in order to compute the correlation dimension of a strange set. Let

$$C_N(\epsilon) = \frac{2}{N(N-1)} \sum_{i,j} \Theta(\epsilon - \|\mathbf{x}_i - \mathbf{x}_j\|), \qquad (2)$$

denote the fraction of pairs of points on the attractor whose distance apart is less than ϵ. In the limit as $\epsilon \to 0$ and

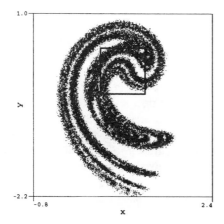 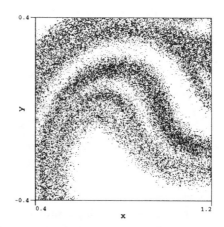

FIG. 2. Same as Fig. 1. Now 2% Gaussian measurement noise has been added to the data. Obviously we can no longer observe the self-similar structure found before.

$N \to \infty$, and in the absence of noise, we have $C(\epsilon) \sim \epsilon^d$, where d is the correlation dimension of the attractor. This can also be written as

$$d = \lim_{\epsilon \to 0} \lim_{N \to \infty} d(\epsilon), \quad d(\epsilon) = \frac{d}{d \log \epsilon} \log C_N(\epsilon), \quad (3)$$

which is a more useful definition in practice.

Typically, one reconstructs the attractor in a suitable space of dimension m and computes $C(\epsilon)$ and its slope $d(\epsilon)$ as functions of ϵ. When interested in the correlation dimension d, one would look for a range of ϵ values where $d(\epsilon)$ is relatively constant. In practice one can often distinguish four different types of behavior of $d_m(\epsilon)$ for different regions of length scales ϵ (see Fig. 3). For small ϵ (region I) the lack of data points is the dominant feature. Therefore, the values of $d_m(\epsilon)$ are subject to large statistical fluctuations. On the other hand, if ϵ is of the order of the size of the entire attractor (region IV), no scale invariance can be expected.

In between, we can distinguish two regions. Region II is dominated by the noise in the data: the reconstructed points are not restricted to the fractal structure of the attractor but fill the whole phase space available, thus we expect $d_m(\epsilon) \approx m$, the dimension of phase space. Between regions II and IV we have region III, where the proper scaling behavior of the attractor may be observed: $d_m(\epsilon) \sim d$.

For higher values of m, regions II and III will be very distinct: we will see a crossover between $d_m(\epsilon) \approx m$ below and $d_m(\epsilon) \approx d$ above the noise level. In Ref. 9 a formula describing this crossover is derived analytically for the case of Gaussian measurement noise. Here we only give the result.

Let us consider a signal which can already be faithfully reconstructed in m dimensional space. If we reconstruct the same signal in $m+1$ dimensions, the effective dimensions $d_{m+1}(\epsilon)$ in $m+1$ space are related to those in m space by the formula

$$d_{m+1}(\epsilon) = d_m(\epsilon) + \frac{\epsilon \exp[-(\epsilon/2\sigma)^2]}{\sigma \sqrt{\pi} \operatorname{erf}(\epsilon/2\sigma)}. \quad (4)$$

An important consequence of this analytical result for the shape of the correlation integral is that already a small amount of noise conceals possible scaling behavior: even at $\epsilon = 3\sigma$ the effective dimension increases visibly with the embedding dimension, namely by an amount of 0.2 per additional dimension. That means, since even in the best case scaling can be expected up to about one-fourth of the attractor extent and down to three times the noise level, a data set with 2% noise can give at most a tiny scaling region of two octaves. For noises with tails, very unevenly distributed data and for short data sets, the situation can be much worse.

The data in Fig. 3 consist of a time series of 40 000 values from a laser experiment by Flepp, Simonet, and Brun.[10] The curves illustrate attempts to estimate the correlation dimension of the data before and after a nonlinear noise reduction method[11] was applied. The region labeled III on each curve corresponds to an approximate power law relationship between the correlation $C(\epsilon)$ defined in Eq. (2) and the ball size ϵ. Before noise reduction (represented by diamonds), a scaling region is difficult to discern, because the noise obscures the fine scale structure up to 1/16 of the

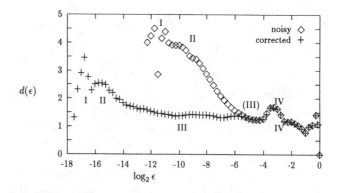

FIG. 3. A typical plot of the correlation dimension as a function of the range of distances ϵ used to estimate the scaling exponent. Noise obscures the fine scale structure up to 1/6 of the attractor extent, making an accurate estimate of the attractor dimension impossible. Data from the NMR-laser experiment by Flepp, Simonet, and Brun,[10] about the noise reduction (see Ref. 11).

attractor extent. We would hesitate to conclude from this plot that the data set represents a low dimensional attractor or even give a dimension. Even small levels of noise significantly complicate estimates of the dimension.

The shape of the effective dimension curves can be used to gain knowledge about the noise present in the data. The characteristic shape, Eq. (4), is a signature of Gaussian noise, in which case we can estimate the noise level from a function fit. See Ref. 9 for details.

B. Entropies

While dimensions characterize the scaling properties of the invariant measure which is the probability distribution of the data in state space, entropies do the same for transition probabilities from one part of the state space to another. If the dynamics is regular, all points inside a small ball in the state space will be mapped into another small ball, such that all but one of the transition probabilities are almost zero. Conversely, if we regard a pure noise process, the future of such a set of points is almost undetermined by its present state. Chaotic systems are somewhere in between. Thus entropies measure the loss of information about the state of the system due to the time evolution. However, as in the case of dimensions, a reasonable definition has to involve infinitely small scales and, furthermore, infinite times.

The correlation entropy K_2 can be determined numerically quite easily[12]; one computes the correlation sum Eq. (2), but this time one does not investigate its dependence on ϵ but on the embedding dimension m. Then for ideal data one finds

$$C(\epsilon,m) := \lim_{N\to\infty} C_N(\epsilon,m) \propto \epsilon^d \exp(-mK_2), \qquad (5)$$

and numerically,

$$K_2(\epsilon,m) = \ln \frac{C_N(\epsilon,m)}{C_N(\epsilon,m+1)} \qquad (6)$$

should approximate K_2 for a reasonable range of m and ϵ. The discussion about the proper range of ϵ carried out in the last subsection applies here as well. An increase of the scaling exponents $d(\epsilon)$ with the embedding dimension, as it is typical of region II, corresponds to an overestimation of $K_2(m)$. More precisely, for Gaussian iid noise one finds:

$$K_2(\epsilon,m) = K_2 - \frac{\epsilon \exp[-(\epsilon/2\sigma)^2]}{\sigma\sqrt{\pi}\,\mathrm{erf}(\epsilon/2\sigma)} \ln \epsilon. \qquad (7)$$

In particular, for ϵ smaller than the noise level the estimate of the entropy is $K_2 - \ln \epsilon$, which diverges for $\epsilon \to 0$ as expected. Thus again the variance of the noise has to be sufficiently small compared to the overall size of the attractor, such that there remains a window of ϵ where $K_2(m)$ becomes independent of ϵ and thus represents the correct value. Note that noise does not destroy the scaling properties of $C_N(\epsilon,m)$ in m, but primarily results in an overestimation of K_2.

From the point of view of physics the Kolmogorov-Sinai entropy K_1 is more interesting than the correlation entropy. Only the case $q=1$ of the order q "entropies" K_q formally

yields an entropy, i.e. an extensive, additive quantity. The Kolmogorov-Sinai entropy differs from K_2 in the way averages are performed; it assigns larger weights to small probabilities. This makes it more sensitive to lack of neighbors (small ϵ), to saturation effects (large ϵ) and to statistical fluctuations. It is in general much harder to estimate from a time series than K_2. See Ref. 13 for an algorithm.

The Kolmogorov-Sinai entropy is related to the Lyapunov exponents, which will be discussed later. On a generic attractor, K_1 is simply the sum of all positive Lyapunov exponents. Thus the fact that K_2 is a lower bound to K_1 can be used as a consistency check if both, K_2 and the Lyapunov exponents are computed.

IV. DYNAMICS FROM A TIME SERIES

In many situations one wants to reconstruct the dynamical evolution from the data. If there is already some theoretical understanding of the underlying system one might try to extract the parameters for a specific model. In the absence of a model one could still be interested in predictions of future measurements. Moreover, several algorithms for the determination of Lyapunov exponents and nonlinear noise reduction methods are based on an explicit approximation of the dynamical laws from the data.

A. Estimating the dynamics

The realistic case that the dynamical evolution $\mathbf{F}$ has to be estimated from the data is hard to study in general. (However, some interesting material can be found in Ref. 14.) Only some simple cases can be understood theoretically, more realistic examples can be evaluated numerically. Let us investigate the ideal case first and say we know what $\mathbf{F}$ looks like (i.e., we have a reliable model), but need to fit some coefficient(s).

A nontrivial example which can still be studied analytically and which yields quite unexpected results is the Hénon map. Given a long but noisy Hénon trajectory, let us assume that we know the functional form of the equations, $y_{n+1} = 1 - ay_n^2 + by_{n-1}$, but we do not know the actual values of a and b which have been used to create the trajectory. An ordinary least squares fit, minimizing the one step prediction error

$$\sigma^2 = \sum_{n=3}^{N} [x_{n+1} - (1 - ax_n^2 + bx_{n-1})]^2 \qquad (8)$$

produces systematically wrong estimates $\hat{a}$ and $\hat{b}$. One can after some algebra derive analytical expressions for $\hat{a}$ and $\hat{b}$ as a function of the true parameters a and b and the noise level, under the assumption of infinitely many input data. In Fig. 4 we show the results as a function of the relative noise level $\sqrt{\langle \eta_n^2 \rangle / \langle y_n^2 \rangle}$ for uniformly distributed and for Gaussian noise respectively. The deviation from the correct value $a=1.4$ and $b=0.3$ is tremendous for larger noise amplitudes and is a systematic, not statistical error. The bias is introduced by the fact that a fit like Eq. (8) implicitly assumes that the independent variables are noise free. The map with the estimated parameter indeed yields the best one-step pre-

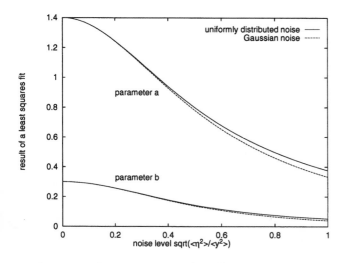

FIG. 4. The analytical results of the least squares fit for the Hénon parameters a and b, Eq. (8). We show the fitted parameters $\hat{a}$ and b as a function of the noise level, using trajectories generated with $a=1.4$, $b=0.3$.

diction but we will fail to reproduce the attractor when we iterate the biased map, and using it for the computation of Lyapunov exponents will yield wrong results.

Let us mention that there are ways to largely avoid biased fits in the presence of noise. A forthcoming paper by Kantz[15] will report on work on this problem.

The bias due to the "errors-in-variables" problem is not the only way noise enters the estimation of the dynamics from the data. The values of the fit parameters are also affected by statistical fluctuations. How severe this influence is depends on the kind of model one wants to fit. In a generic situation we know little about the expected functional form of the dynamics and thus we have to approximate $\mathbf{F}$ by a model which is general enough to reproduce essential features of $\mathbf{F}$. Two distinct approaches have been studied in the literature, local (or piecewise) linear and global nonlinear function fits.

The main idea of locally linear models[16,17] is to assume that $\mathbf{F}$ is at least piecewise differentiable and smooth enough such that the local tangent maps are reasonable approximations to $\mathbf{F}$. In delay coordinates all components of the image of a vector $\mathbf{x}_n = (x_n, x_{n-1}, ..., x_{n-m+1})$ are trivially known except the first one, x_{n+1}, which in an appropriate embedding is a function of only the present delay vector. Thus one has to determine $x_{n+1} = f(\mathbf{x}_n)$, which in linear approximation reads $x_{n+1} = \mathbf{a}x + b$. The parameters $\mathbf{a}$ and b can be easily determined by a least squares fit, using as input all delay vectors from a small neighborhood $\mathscr{U}$ of $\mathbf{x}_n$ and their images.

This procedure is able to approximate very general functional forms, which makes it very attractive. It has some weak points, though. Obviously, dynamically correct linear fits can only be obtained when the size of the neighborhoods $\mathscr{U}$ is larger than the noise level. Since larger neighborhoods yield poorer linear approximations due to the nonlinearity of $\mathbf{F}$, errors in the dynamics increase with the noise level. Note that increasing the amount of data does not improve the situ-

ation as long as no explicit noise reduction step is performed. In Refs. 18 and 19 nonlinearity was taken into account by adding a bilinear term to the RHS of Eq. (12), but it is our experience that for noisy data these fits become rather unstable.

Currently, global fits are quite popular[17,20–23] and in many cases quite successful. In delay coordinates, the task is again to fit a scalar function f in an m-dimensional space. Thus the ansatz can in principle be any reasonable set of basis functions, examples include higher order polynomials, radial basis functions, or neural networks. In the first two cases the determination of the parameters still is a linear minimization problem, in the latter case it is nonlinear and therefore more troublesome. Neural nets have the potential of astonishingly good performance, but one must not forget that the theory and application of neural nets is a field of research in itself, often leaving the inexperienced user disappointed.

Since global fits are obtained using all the available data they show less statistical fluctuations than local models, in particular for small data sets. Like local linear fits they react to noise by smoothing out nonlinearities. It is however hard to predict how severe this effect will be for a given global ansatz.

A problem specific for global fits is that the basis may be too small to capture essential features of the surface. A systematic bias is introduced through the choice of basis functions.

V. NOISE AND LYAPUNOV EXPONENTS

An important concept of characterizing chaotic behavior are the Lyapunov exponents. In chaotic systems, the states of two copies of the same system, started with very similar initial conditions separate on average exponentially with time. The leading contribution to the rate of this separation is given by the largest exponent, the next to leading contribution by the second, etc. These quantities are obtained in a relatively easy way from dynamical equations using information from the dynamics in tangent space, while their estimation from a data series poses some difficulties. This is not the place to review the theory of Lyapunov exponents or methods to obtain them from a time series in detail. (The interested reader is referred to the original literature[24–27] and to recent treatments of this topic.[19,23,28–30]) We rather want to concentrate on limitations to the current algorithms induced by noise in the data.

A. Methods in real space

The most straightforward computation of Lyapunov exponents consists in tracing the exponential divergence of nearby tarjectories. In the presence of noise, however, the deterministic divergence is concealed by the noise process on the small scales. For uncorrelated noise distances between trajectories follow a random walk on small scales, such that in total the time dependence of distances δ between initially nearby trajectories is given by

$$\delta(n) \approx \alpha\sigma\sqrt{n} + \beta e^{\lambda_+ n}. \tag{9}$$

Thus for small n one would find a diverging effective exponent, which would lead to an estimate of the Lyapunov exponent which is substantially too large. Only for trajectories whose initial separation is larger than the noise level would the pure exponential increase be observed.[27] However, as soon as the distance becomes of the order of the attractor size, due to saturation and folding processes it will not increase any more with an exponential law, such that the maximum distance should be of the order of 1/5 (assuming normalized data). If the maximal Lyapunov exponent of the clean dynamics is λ_+, on average the distance will grow by a factor of e^{λ_+} in each time step. If we optimistically assume that the diffusive regime is left at twice the noise level, the acceptable noise amplitude is

$$2\sigma < 1/5 e^{-\lambda_+ n}, \tag{10}$$

if we require n time steps between successive searches for new neighbors. To obtain a reasonable estimate for example of λ_+ for the Henon map one would require at least $n>5$ to make sure we do not leave the unstable manifold. With $\lambda_+ = 0.4169$ this means $\sigma_{max} < 0.012$, i.e., less than 1.2%.

One method to exploit this divergence in real space was proposed in the well known paper by Wolf et al.[27] However, their method is not very robust and difficult to apply. Recently, considerable progress was made independently in Refs. 28 and 29. The main idea is to record explicitly the time dependence of distances between nearby trajectories in order to be able to select the appropriate length scale and range of times from the output. In the original Wolf algorithm this dependence was absorbed in a single number with the problem that parameters had to be chosen in advance.

To determine the Lyapunov exponents, one has to compute[28]

$$S(\Delta n) = \frac{1}{N-m} \sum_{n=m+1}^{N} \log \left(\frac{1}{|\mathcal{U}_n|} \sum_{\mathbf{x}_{n'} \in \mathcal{U}_n} |x_{n'+\Delta n} - x_{n+\Delta n}| \right) \tag{11}$$

for different embedding dimensions m and neighborhoods of different sizes ϵ. Here, $\mathbf{x}_n = (x_n, x_{n-1}, ..., x_{n-m+1})$ is a delay vector of dimension m, and $\mathcal{U}_n$ is the set of all other delay vectors in an ϵ-neighborhood of $\mathbf{x}_n$. $|\mathcal{U}_n|$ is the number of elements in $\mathcal{U}_n$. If $S(\Delta n)$ as a function of Δn shows a linear regime, the slope can be interpreted as the maximal Lyapunov exponent. This is illustrated in Fig. 5 for a normalized Hénon time series with 1% measurement noise: Only on scales between the noise level, $\log \epsilon_{min} \approx -5.33$, and $\epsilon_{max} \approx e^{-2} = 0.135$ the expected linear behavior can be found, yielding an average slope of all the shown curves of 0.41 ± 0.015, which is a very good estimate of the maximal Lyapunov exponent $\lambda_+ = 0.4169 \pm 0.0001$.

Furthermore, Fig. 5 shows impressively that neighbors closer than the noise level yield very large effective exponents (observe the two lower bundles of curves). Due to the linear averaging in Eq. (11), scaling extends down to the noise level resulting in an admissible noise amplitude *twice* as large as the estimate Eq. (10), i.e., 2.5% for the Hénon example.

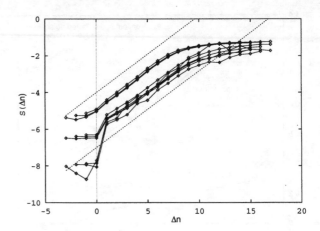

FIG. 5. The function $S(\Delta n)$, Eq. (11), for a Hénon time series of length 5000 with 1% additive noise. The three bundles of curves correspond to neighborhood sizes $\epsilon = 0.001$, 0.004, and 0.016 from below to top, and each bundle consists of curves with embedding dimension from 2 to 4. The coordinates used to determine the neighborhoods are denoted by $\Delta n = 0,...,1-m$. The slopes of two dashed lines are the accurate values for λ_+.

B. Exploiting the dynamics in tangent space

Another class of methods obtains the momentary expansion rates from the dynamics in tangent space, in close analogy to the methods for known dynamical equations.[24] This approach not only yields the largest Lyapunov exponent, but m exponents for an m dimensional embedding. Since the dimensionality of the underlying dynamical system generally is unknown, many of the negative exponents may be spurious. For a discussion of this problem see Refs. 23, 25, and 30.

The Lyapunov exponents are determined by the logarithms of the eigenvalues of the product of the Jacobians of **F** along the trajectory. Thus one has to know the local Jacobians with sufficient accuracy. The problem of fitting the dynamics from data has been discussed above.

The original works[25,26] perform linear fits of the local dynamics (as described above) in small volumes of phase space. This process immediately yields the corresponding local Jacobian:

$$\mathbf{x}_{n+1} = A^{(n)} \mathbf{x}_n + \mathbf{b}^{(n)}, \quad J^{(n)} = A^{(n)}. \tag{12}$$

In delay coordinates, the first row of the matrix $A^{(n)}$ is the previously introduced vector **a**. All other entries are zero apart from the lower off-diagonal, which is filled by 1's. Alternatively, one can compute the local Jacobians from global nonlinear fits. The advantages and disadvantages of either method have already been discussed. The accuracy of the resulting Lyapunov exponents is limited by the quality of the fitted dynamics.

No matter what kind of model is used, the resulting approximation is subject to the bias induced by the errors in the independent variables. From Fig. 4 it is obvious that for large noise levels the Lyapunov exponents computed by the Jacobians of this fitted map are systematically wrong. This is shown in Fig. 6. The two broken curves represent the positive and negative Lyapunov exponent obtained by the local

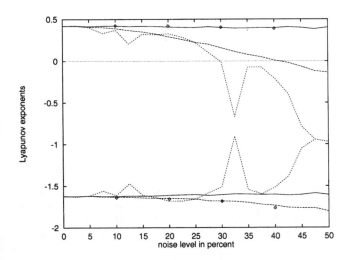

FIG. 6. Lyapunov exponents obtained from the local Jacobians for noisy Hénon trajectories. The continuous curves show the values obtained from the exact Jacobians along the noisy trajectories. For the dashed curves, the fitted parameters from Fig. 4 were used. The dotted curves are obtained from surrogate trajectories generated by the fitted dynamics. The diamonds represent the results when a noise reduced trajectory is used to fit the parameters but the Jacobians are multiplied along the original data.

Jacobians with the parameters from Fig. 4 on a noisy trajectory of length 10 000 with the indicated noise level. For comparison, the continuous lines are the corresponding values obtained with the correct Jacobians on the same noisy trajectories. One clearly observes that the additive noise on the trajectory is relatively harmless as long as the correct dynamics is known.

Some authors (e.g., Ref. 31) suggested to fit the dynamics underlying a given noisy time series and to generate a new trajectory by iterating the fitted dynamics. This "bootstrapping" yields a clean trajectory of arbitrary length which is then used for further analysis. The dotted curves in Fig. 6 show the resulting exponents of such a procedure. Obviously, for large noise levels the fitted dynamics creates a completely different attractor, which is no more compatible with the original noisy time series. Note that for more than 30% noise the surrogate attractor is a periodic orbit.

Thus we have shown that one can recover the correct Lyapunov exponents with good accuracy even for high noise levels if one has a faithful estimate of the underlying deterministic dynamics. The latter could be obtained by an unbiased fit, to which problem a forthcoming paper will be devoted. An alternative solution is to apply nonlinear noise reduction and afterwards perform a usual fit. The success of such a procedure[32] is shown by the diamonds in Fig. 6, which represent the Lyapunov exponents obtained from the noisy data sets after noise reduction.

To finish this section we want to recall the Kaplan-Yorke conjecture, which states that

$$D_{KY} = l + \frac{\sum_{i=1}^{l} \lambda_i}{|\lambda_{l+1}|}, \qquad (13)$$

where l is chosen such that $\sum_{i=1}^{l} \lambda_i \geq 0$ and $\sum_{i=1}^{l+1} \lambda_i < 0$, is

equal to the information dimension D_1 of the attractor. Since D_2 is a lower bound of the latter, one should check for consistency whether $D_{KY} \geq D_2$.

VI. NONLINEAR NOISE REDUCTION

Traditionally, noise in time series is reduced by Fourier based filtering techniques. For data with mainly linear features they are quite successful, since the Fourier spectrum often allows for a clear distinction between signal and noise. However, since data from nonlinear sources generally possess a broadband spectrum by itself, such a distinction fails. Only for chaotic flows recorded with a very small sampling time (compared to the internal time scale) a low pass filter may be applicable. Unfortunately, certain recursive filters used as real-time filters in experiments may change the dimension of the systems attractor.[33]

Several noise reduction methods based on ideas from nonlinear dynamics have been suggested. (See Ref. 34 for a review.) They all make use of the fact that data points subsequent in time are dynamically related and that for continuous dynamics points in the same region of the state space have to behave similarly. Methods which are most apt for scalar time series without any *a priori* knowledge of the dynamics make use of projections onto a reconstructed local manifold containing the attractor.[35–37,32] (An alternative formulation of the same idea is to fit the dynamics with a locally linear model and adjust the series to be more consistent with this model dynamics.[35,38]) These algorithms can be applied with a reasonable effort and yield stable results when being applied to physical laboratory data.[11] Furthermore, for long trajectories with high noise levels a very simple but robust variant of nonlinear noise reduction is applicable.[39] Before we lose the reader when entering into technicalities let us comment on the usefulness of noise reduction on physiological data. They are definitely subject to dynamical noise, which is not random but a very high dimensional part of the signal, reflecting the coupling between the investigated subsystem (e.g. heart) and the rest of the organism. In such a case a nonlinear noise reduction algorithm still projects onto a low dimensional component of the signal, *if it can be identified*, i.e., if the relative amplitude of the low dimensional part is large enough. Thus the signal one is interested in can be isolated to some extent.

Let us outline the main steps of one noise reduction scheme[32] which can be seen as a synthesis of two other recent methods Refs. 35, and 36 and 37. More details and its theoretical background are given in Ref. 32 where also its relation to other methods[35–37] is discussed. Our approach to nonlinear noise reduction is to assume that the unknown *true* signal y_i is generated by a deterministic dynamics, whereas the noise η_i is random, i.e. one measures the noisy signal $x_i = y_i + \eta_i$. (This is referred to as measurement noise, see above.) We expect the noise to be independent of the signal, have zero average, δ-(or fast decaying) correlation and some fixed probability distribution. The deterministic time evolution may be discrete or continuous in time.

In delay coordinates of dimension m, the noise free dynamics is described by $y_i = f(y_{i-1}, ..., y_{i-m})$. Rewriting this relation in an implicit form

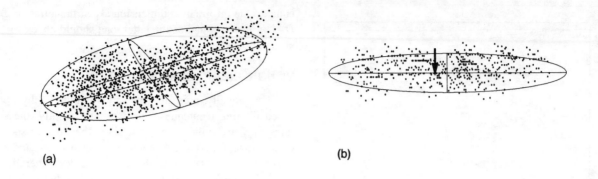

(a)   (b)

FIG. 7. Schematic diagram of the noise reduction process. Consider a cluster of points on a two-dimensional surface which are corrupted by noise. The noise spreads the points above and below the surface so that in three-space they form a three-dimensional object of small but finite thickness [panel (a)]. We can identify the direction of the smallest extent and project the points onto the plane orthogonal to it. Panel (b) illustrates this (arrow), showing a slice through the ellipsoid of panel (a).

$$\tilde{f}(y_i, y_{i-1}, ..., y_{i-m}) = 0 \qquad (14)$$

shows that in an $m+1$ dimensional delay coordinate space the noise free dynamics is constrained to an m dimensional hypersurface. For the measured values x_i this is not true, but the extension of the cloud of data points perpendicular to this hypersurface is of the size of the noise level. Therefore one can hope to identify this direction and to correct the x_i by simply projecting them onto the subspace spanned by the clean data. Before this, one has to reconstruct this surface from the noisy data. These are the two main ingredients, which are processed as follows.

In an embedding space of dimension $m+1$ we compute the covariance matrix of all state vectors in a small neighborhood of a given point which we want to correct. The eigenvectors of this matrix are the semiaxes of the best approximating ellipsoid of this cloud of points (see Fig. 7). Now the important assumption is that the clean signal lives on a smooth manifold with dimension $d < m+1$ and the variance of the noise is smaller than the signal. Then for the noisy data the covariance matrix has large eigenvalues corresponding to the directions of the attractor and small eigenvalues in all other directions. Therefore we project the vector under consideration onto the subspace of large eigenvectors to get rid of the noisy components. Our fit of the assumed deterministic dynamics thus is a local and linear one, being implicitly contained in the construction of the linear subspace. In Ref. 32 it is shown that this intuitive recipe can be derived from a minimization problem, and precise formulas for the computation of the corrections are given.

Here we do not want to go into these details but only mention a few fundamental aspects. The scheme sketched above yields a correction vector for each embedding vector, such that we end up with a set of corrected vectors in embedding space. Since each element of the scalar time series occurs in $m+1$ different embedding vectors, we finally have as many different suggested corrections, of which we simply take the average. Therefore in embedding space the corrected vectors do not precisely lie on the local subspaces but are only moved towards them. Furthermore, all points in the neighborhood change a bit such that the local hyperplane

also changes. Thus one has to repeat the correction procedure several times to find convergence.

The embedding dimension, the dimension of the subspace and the sizes of the neighborhoods are important parameters which have to be chosen appropriate to the data. This is in general not difficult, since due to the robustness of the algorithm some estimate is good enough. A thorough discussion of the setting of the parameters can be found in Ref. 11. In addition, we recommend to compute the amplitude of the noise before and after noise reduction by the method sketched in Sec. III A. More details on this method can be found in Ref. 9. See the review[34] for material on alternative possibilities to verify the success of nonlinear noise reduction.

We have shown in Fig. 3 the improvement of dimension estimates applying this method to experimental data, and in Fig. 6 we show improved Lyapunov exponents. In some cases the improvement of the data quality is visible even in phase portraits as in Fig. 8.

VII. CONCLUSIONS AND PERSPECTIVES

First the bad news: Noise degrades the whole field of nonlinear time series analysis so strongly that many algorithms are rendered useless already by a few percent of noise. Since many nonlinear phenomena are observed in nonlaboratory systems (in the atmosphere, ocean, human body, at Wall Street) and thus the dynamical noise cannot be controlled, one could think that the most interesting data cannot be processed. However, we do not assume this pessimistic attitude.

Fortunately, there is good news as well: First, the influence of noise in many instances is well understood. This helps to identify noise, to estimate its strength and to see how much of the deterministic structure still is visible. Second, in many situations nonlinear noise reduction works satisfactorily. Many experiments yield data which are at the edge of being processable by nonlinear tools, and after nonlinear noise reduction one can successfully treat them. Third, there are still some things that can be done also in the presence of strong noise. Global fits are statistically quite stable

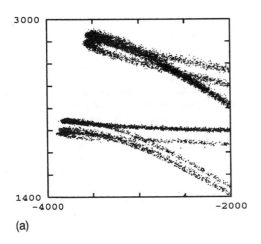
(a)

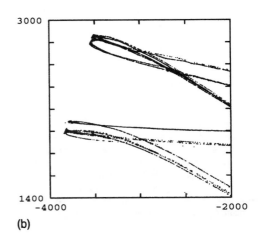
(b)

FIG. 8. Enlargements of phase portraits of the NMR laser data taken by Flepp, Simonet, and Brun.[10] Panel (a) shows about one quarter of the linear extent of the whole phase space, panel (b) the same area after nonlinear noise reduction was applied.

against noise. The errors-in-variables problem seems to be tractable, such that we hope to perform unbiased fits of the dynamics in the future.[15] This being done, one could in fact produce a new noise free trajectory. A test whether these synthetic data are compatible with the original noisy ones exists,[40] such that erroneous results like those presented in Fig. 6 for the naive "bootstrapping" can be ruled out. Thus work is in progress which makes us optimistic about the problem of noise in data.

There are other hard problems which remain, like too short observation times, nonstationarity, and the problem of spatiotemporal chaos. In the latter case, data do not represent a low dimensional attractor, but rather a process where characteristic quantities like dimensions and Lyapunov exponents become intensive quantities. How can we reconstruct the corresponding state space? Although some theoretical results are already available, they are far from being applicable to time series. Thus for many realistic systems we are only on the second step of a long staircase towards satisfactory data analysis with predictive power.

ACKNOWLEDGMENTS

We thank the organizers for giving us the opportunity to participate in this very stimulating meeting and the sponsors of the conference for funding. H.K. is supported by Deutsche Forschungsgemeinschaft, SFB 237, T.S. received a European Communities grant within the framework of the SCIENCE programme, Contract No. B/SCI*-900557.

[1] T. Sauer, J. A. Yorke, and M. Casdagli, "Embedology," J. Stat. Phys. 65, 579 (1991).
[2] M. Casdagli, S. Eubank, J. D. Farmer, and J. Gibson, "State space reconstruction in the presence of noise," Physica D 51, 52 (1991).
[3] P. Grassberger, T. Schreiber, and C. Schaffrath, "Nonlinear time-sequence analysis," Int. J. Bifurcation Chaos 1, 521 (1991).
[4] J. P. Eckmann and D. Ruelle, "Ergodic theory of chaos and strange attractors," Rev. Mod. Phys. 57, 617 (1986).
[5] H. Kantz and P. Grassberger, "Repellers and long-lived chaotic transients," Physica D 17, 75 (1985).
[6] K. Ikeda, "Multiple valued stationary state and its instability of the transmitted light by a ring cavity system," Opt. Commun. 30, 257 (1979).
[7] H. Kantz and T. Schreiber, "Dimension estimates and physiological data," Chaos 5, 143 (1995).
[8] P. Grassberger and I. Procaccia, "Characterization of strange attractors," Phys. Rev. Lett. 50, 346 (1983).
[9] T. Schreiber, Determination of the noise level of chaotic time series," Phys. Rev. E 48, R13 (1993).
[10] L. Flepp, R. Holzner, E. Brun, M. Finardi, and R. Badii, "Model identification by periodic-orbit analysis for NMR-laser chaos," Phys. Rev. Lett. 67, 2244 (1991); M. Finardi, L. Flepp, J. Parisi, R. Holzner, R. Badii, and E. Brun, "Topological and metric analysis of heteroclinic crises in laser chaos," Phys. Rev. Lett. 68, 2989 (1992).
[11] H. Kantz, T. Schreiber, I. Hoffmann, T. Buzug, G. Pfister, L. G. Flepp, J. Simonet, R. Badii, and E. Brun, "Nonlinear noise reduction: A case study on experimental data," Phys. Rev. E 48, 1529 (1993).
[12] P. Grassberger and I. Procaccia, "Estimation of the Kolmogorov entropy from a chaotic signal," Phys. Rev. A 28, 2591 (1983).
[13] A. Cohen and I. Procaccia, "Computing the Kolmogorov entropy from time signals of dissipative and conservative dynamical systems," Phys. Rev. A 31, 1872 (1985).
[14] E. J. Kostelich, "Problems in estimating dynamics from data," Physica D 58, 138 (1992).
[15] H. Kantz, in preparation (1994).
[16] J. D. Farmer and J. J. Sidorowich, "Predicting chaotic time series," Phys. Rev. Lett. 59, 845 (1987).
[17] M. Casdagli, "Nonlinear prediction of chaotic time series," Physica D 35, 335 (1989).
[18] H. D. I. Abarbanel, "Local and global Lyapunov exponents on a strange attractor," in Nonlinear Modeling and Forecasting, edited by M. Casdagli and S. Eubank, Santa Fe Studies in the Science of Complexity (Addison-Wesley, Reading, MA, 1992), Vol. XII.
[19] R. Brown, P. Bryant, and H. D. I. Abarbanel, "Computing the Lyapunov spectrum of a dynamical system from an observed time series," Phys. Rev. A 43, 2787 (1991).
[20] D. Broomhead and D. Lowe, "Multivariable function interpolation and adaptive networks," Complex Systems 2, 321 (1988).
[21] L. A. Smith, "Identification and prediction of low-dimensional dynamics," Physica D 58, 50 (1992).
[22] J. Holzfuss and J. B. Kadtke, "Global nonlinear noise reduction using radial basis functions," Int. J. Bifurcation Chaos 3, 589 (1993).
[23] R. Gencay and W. D. Dechert, "An algorithm for the n Lyapunov exponents of an n-dimensional unknown dynamical system," Physica D 59, 142 (1992).
[24] G. Benettin, L. Galgani, A. Giorgilli, and J.-M. Strelcyn, "Lyapunov characteristic exponents for smooth dynamical systems and for Hamiltonian systems: A method for computing all of them," Meccanica 15, 9 (1980).
[25] J.-P. Eckmann, S. Oliffson Kamphorst, D. Ruelle, and S. Ciliberto, "Lyapunov exponents from a time series," Phys. Rev. A 34, 4971 (1986).

[26] M. Sano and Y. Sawada, "Measurement of the Lyapunov spectrum from a chaotic time series," Phys. Rev. Lett. **55**, 1082 (1985).

[27] A. Wolf, J. B. Swift, H. L. Swinney, and J. A. Vastano, "Determining Lyapunov exponents from a time series," Physica D **16**, 285 (1985).

[28] H. Kantz, "A robust method to estimate the maximal Lyapunov exponent of a time series," Phys. Lett. A **185**, (1994) 77 (1994).

[29] M. T. Rosenstein, J. J. Collins, and C. J. De Luca, "A practical method for calculating largest Lyapunov exponents from small data sets," Physica D **65**, 257 (1993).

[30] U. Parlitz, "Identification of true and spurious Lyapunov exponents from time series," Int. J. Bifurcation Chaos **2**, 155 (1992).

[31] J. D. Farmer and J. J. Sidorowich, "Exploiting chaos to predict the future and reduce noise," in *Evolution, Learning and Cognition*, edited by Y. C. Lin (World Scientific, Singapore, 1988).

[32] P. Grassberger, R. Hegger, H. Kantz, C. Schaffrath, and T. Schreiber, "On noise reduction methods for chaotic data," Chaos **3**, 127 (1993).

[33] R. Badii, G. Broggi, B. Derighetti, M. Ravani, S. Ciliberto, A. Politi, and M. A. Rubio, "Dimension increase in filtered chaotic signals," Phys. Rev. Lett. **60**, 979 (1988).

[34] E.J. Kostelich and T. Schreiber, "Noise reduction in chaotic time-series data: A survey of common methods," Phys. Rev. E **48**, 1752 (1993).

[35] T. Schreiber and P. Grassberger, "A simple noise-reduction method for real data," Phys. Lett. A **160**, 411 (1991).

[36] R. Cawley and G.-H. Hsu, "Local-geometric-projection method for noise reduction in chaotic maps and flows," Phys. Rev. A **46**, 3057 (1992).

[37] T. Sauer, "A noise reduction method for signals from nonlinear systems," Physica D **58**, 193 (1992).

[38] E. J. Kostelich and J. A. Yorke, "Noise reduction in dynamical systems," Phys. Rev. A **38**, 1649 (1988).

[39] T. Schreiber, "Extremely simple nonlinear noise reduction method," Phys. Rev. E **47**, 2401 (1993).

[40] H. Kantz, "Quantifying the distance between fractal measures," Phys. Rev. E **49**, 5091 (1994).

Dimension estimates and physiological data

Holger Kantz[a)] and Thomas Schreiber[b)]

Fachbereich Physik, Universität Wuppertal, D-42097 Wuppertal, Germany

(Received 5 July 1994; accepted for publication 21 September 1994)

Dimension estimates for data from physiological systems are notoriously difficult since the data are far from ideal in the sense of deterministic dynamical systems. Possible pitfalls and necessary precautions are pointed out and a recipe is given which is viable for those researchers who want to use the Grassberger–Procaccia algorithm but who are not familiar with the vast existing literature on dimension estimates. The relevance of dimension estimates for the characterization of physiological data is discussed, where both the cases of finding and not finding a low dimension are considered. © *1995 American Institute of Physics.*

I. INTRODUCTION

It is commonplace that physiological systems, like most complicated systems, are nonlinear. Consequently, the analysis of data from physiology could profit from the tools and concepts developed within the framework of nonlinear dynamics. However, most recent nonlinear methods of time series analysis are based on the paradigm of deterministic chaos. Obviously, the human body is not deterministic. Thus despite of the underlying nonlinearity, physiological data are different from low dimensional chaos and the chaos concepts are used outside of their domain.

The theory of dynamical systems deals with closed systems whereas physiological systems interact with the rest of the world. They must be considered as open systems coupled to an infinite "heat bath" of unobserved degrees of freedom. Usually, one hopes that this background can be interpreted as noise and effectively decouples from the signal. However, this "noise" has very inconvenient statistical properties. Changes of the environment occur on all time scales, including those which are of the order of the duration of the experiment, which leads to nonstationarity. Furthermore, there is no clear limitation of the influence such changes may have. This can mean that the environment at each moment disturbs the current state by a small amount, but it can also mean that the parameters change erratically.

In his talk, Kaplan[1] showed a diagram measuring the degree of nonlinearity and of stochasticity on its two axes. In this setting most physiological data have to be put somewhere far from the axes, being nonlinear and to some degree stochastic. Depending on the application in mind, this means they can be quite far from deterministic low dimensional chaos.

As a paradigmatic example for what happens to a concept from deterministic chaos when brought to the hostile environment of real world data we want to discuss in this paper the estimation of the attractor dimension by the Grassberger–Procaccia algorithm[2] which, in spite of many objections, is the dimension algorithm most suitable for time series analysis. We briefly recall the definition of the algorithm in Sec. II, and describe its limitations with respect to shortcomings in the database in Sec. III. Prominent pitfalls, and, if available, their fixes will be discussed in more detail, mainly reporting the work of other people (Sec. IV). By a series of examples we shall illustrate the major items and discuss the peculiarities of physiological data under these aspects. The result will be a recipe for how to avoid spurious dimension estimates. One of our conclusions is that for a number of problems the only meaningful solution will be not to report a dimension at all. The last section is devoted to the question of what one has learned about the time series in case one has found a low (or a high) correlation dimension.

II. THE CORRELATION DIMENSION: AN ALGORITHM TO CHARACTERIZE LOW DIMENSIONAL DATA

In this section we want to recall the basic definition of the algorithm and discuss its behavior in the situation it was invented for: for the quantification of self-similarity of low dimensional fractal sets given through a time series.

Before applying any phase space algorithm, the scalar time series $\{s_i\}$, $i=1,..,N$ has to be embedded in a higher dimensional space where the attractor is unfolded. Generally, one uses *delay coordinates,*[3] i.e., forms vectors $\mathbf{x}_i=(s_i,s_{i-\tau},...,s_{i-(m-1)\tau})$ as elements of the $\mathbf{R}^m$, where m is the embedding dimension and the (integer) τ is the time lag. It has been proven[4] that if the original attractor has a fractal dimension D_f, then the correlation dimension is preserved through the process of scalar measurement and subsequent delay reconstruction, as soon as $m>D_f$. The choice of an appropriate lag τ is relevant for the quality of the reconstruction, but will not be discussed here. As a guideline we suggest to compute the first zero of the autocorrelation function of the signal.

Chaotic attractors generally are fractals, i.e., sets or measures which are characterized by noninteger dimensions. Most generalizations from integer dimensions of smooth manifolds to fractals rely on some self-similarity of the set, or, in other words, on scale invariance of statistical quantities. The details are specific for the different definitions of dimensions. One class, the order-q Renyi dimensions, is widely used to characterize strange attractors.[5] A partition $\mathscr{P}_\epsilon$ has to be introduced, i.e., a countable disjoint covering of

[a)]E-mail: kantz@wpts0.physik.uni-wuppertal.de
[b)]E-mail: schreibe@wpts0.physik.uni-wuppertal.de

the attractor with sets of diameter $\leq \epsilon$. Denote by p_i the probability that the trajectory visits the ith element of the partition. Then the dimensions are found by

$$D_q = \lim_{\epsilon \to 0} \frac{1}{q-1} \frac{\ln \Sigma_{\mathscr{P}_\epsilon} p_i^q}{\ln \epsilon}. \quad (2.1)$$

Setting $q=0$, D_0 is called the fractal dimension and in general is identical to the capacity and the Hausdorff dimension. D_1 is found by the application of the rule of l'Hospital and is called *information dimension* of the attractor. Finally, D_2 is the *correlation dimension*. One possibility to compute the D_q is *box-counting*,[6] i.e., defining an m-dimensional lattice and counting how often the trajectory visits each box of this lattice. Thus, $p_i = n_i/N$, if N is the length of the time series and n_i the number of passages through the ith box. This has to be done for several box sizes ϵ in order to evaluate Eq. (2.1). Unfortunately, this intuitive approach has several drawbacks[7] and cannot be recommended. The *fixed-mass* approach[8] is based on similar ideas as the algorithm we present in the following, such that we will not enter this. Finally, we should mention the *local intrinsic dimensions*,[9] which usually are computed by local principal component analysis. Since these dimensions do not rely on scaling properties of the data, they are not an estimate of the fractal dimension of the attractor, but might offer an alternative for noisy data.

In 1983, Grassberger and Procaccia[2] presented an algorithm for the computation of the correlation dimension (and which can be easily extended to D_q for $q \neq 2$). The basic idea is that instead of sampling the state space uniformly as in the case of box-counting one introduces an *importance sampling*. One computes the *correlation sum*

$$C_2(\epsilon) = \frac{2}{(N-m)(N-m-1)} \sum_{i=m+1}^{N} \sum_{j=i+1}^{N} \Theta(\epsilon - |\mathbf{x}_i - \mathbf{x}_j|), \quad (2.2)$$

where Θ is the Heaviside step function [$\Theta(x)=0$ if $x \leq 0$ and $\Theta(x)=1$ for $x>0$], such that $C_2(\epsilon)$ is the number of pairs of points with distance less than ϵ among the points on the attractor. For an infinite amount of data and for small ϵ, we expect $C_2 \propto \epsilon^{D_2}$ and obtain the correlation dimension D_2 by

$$d(N,\epsilon) = \frac{\partial \log C_2(\epsilon,N)}{\partial \log \epsilon},$$

$$D_2 = \lim_{N \to \infty, \epsilon \to 0} d(N,\epsilon), \quad (2.3)$$

for sufficiently large embedding dimension m. Numerically, one can expect only some intermediate range of ϵ where $d(m,N,\epsilon) \approx$ const and independent of N and m.

The power law decay of $C_2(\epsilon)$ cannot be observed on small scales because points become sparse. Whereas for generalized dimensions the finiteness of the input trajectory induces systematic errors on the small scales, Eq. (2.2) only suffers from statistical errors, provided the pairs $i=j$ are discarded from the summation.[10]

A straightforward implementation of the Grassberger–Procaccia algorithm on a computer will be quite time con-

suming for data sets of more than moderate sizes; counting all pairs of points needs a time proportional to N^2. However, on the large scales already a small fraction of the pairs yield sufficient statistics and we need to compute *all* pairs only for $\epsilon < \epsilon_0 \approx 1/8$ or even smaller. Algorithmically, this amounts to search for close neighbors of the "reference points" [the first sum in Eq. (2.2)]. Theiler[11] was the first (to our knowledge) to introduce an optimized neighbor-search algorithm for dimension calculations. By now, a number of very efficient algorithms exist, like K-d-trees[12] or box-assisted methods.[13] For a tutorial see Ref. 14. In both cases the data are arranged in a suitable structure so that afterwards only a small portion of all points has to be checked to determine a certain neighborhood.

Unlike other dimension algorithms, the correlation integral does not require an *a priori* estimate of the embedding dimension m. One can easily implement the algorithm in such a way that in the same run one computes $C_2(\epsilon)$ for all m in the range of 2 to, say, 15, with marginal extra cost for each additional value of m.

To illustrate the typical output of the correlation algorithm for a (simulated) experimental sample of a low dimensional dynamical system, we plot in Fig. 1 the correlation sums and their local slopes of a low dimensional attractor with additive noise for a range of embedding dimensions m. One can clearly distinguish four different regions (from large to small scales):

Macroscopic regime: Scaling means self-similarity, which is obviously destroyed on large scales by the finite size of the attractor. For large ϵ (here: $\epsilon > 1/5$) the correlation sum does not exhibit scaling since the macroscopic structures of the attractor determine its value.

Scaling range: Below this in length scale, the true scaling behavior may be found. In the scaling range the local scaling exponent is constant and the same for all embedding dimensions larger than $m_{\min} > D$. This scaling exponent is the estimate of the correlation dimension of the fractal set.

Noise regime: If the data are noisy, then below a length scale of a few multiples of the noise level the method detects that data points are not confined to the fractal structure but smeared out in the whole available state space. Thus the local scaling exponents increase and at the noise level they reach the value of the embedding dimension.

Lacking neighbors: On even smaller length scales the lack of neighbors within the ϵ-balls becomes the dominant effect and the curves start to fluctuate tremendously. This scale is smaller than the average interpoint distance in embedding space (which is $N^{-1/m}$ in the noise regime) and is characterized by the fact that less than, say, 100 pairs contribute to $C_2(\epsilon)$.

Noise and the lack of neighbors can conceal the true scaling regime, and parts of the macroscopic regime may be misinterpreted as scaling. The discussion of this and other possible misinterpretations will be taken up in Sec. IV. Several authors[15–17] report improvements in the estimate of D_2 from a given correlation sum when applying a maximum likelihood method instead of fitting the slope in a log–log plot. This reduces statistical errors in the presence of fluctuations in the correlation sums.

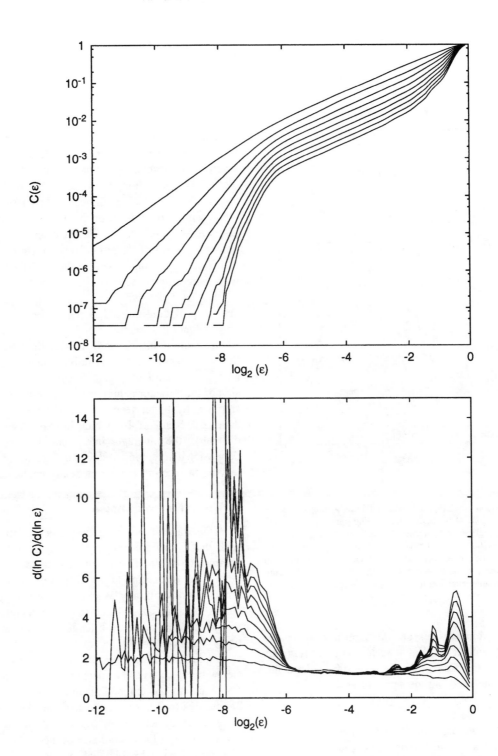

FIG. 1. A typical plot of the correlation sums C_2 and their local scaling exponents $\partial \ln C_2(\epsilon)/\partial \ln \epsilon$ for different embedding dimensions m. The data are a trajectory of the Hénon system (Ref. 37), $x_{t+1} = 1 - 1.4x_t^2 + 0.3x_{t-1}$, of length 20000 with 1.5% additive uniform noise, $M=1500$ reference points were used in Eq. (2.2), such that there are 3×10^7 potential pairs.

III. LIMITATIONS FOR REAL DATA

A. Limitations due to the finite amount of data

If the data set is too small compared to its dimension, any estimate of the value D_2 becomes very unsafe or even wrong. Several authors[18-21] give upper bounds for the dimension an attractor may have such that it can be determined with some confidence from a trajectory with a given number of points. The argument is that in order to clearly identify the scaling range in a plot like Fig. 1 it should extend over at least one octave. Experience shows that the macroscopic structures affect the correlation sum above one-fifth of the attractor extension. For attractors with very intricate structures this may even be too optimistic. As we demonstrated by Fig. 1 the scaling is destroyed on the small scales if less than

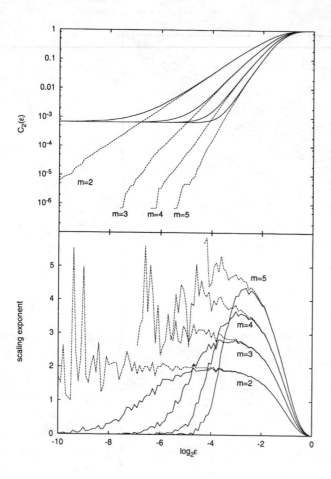

FIG. 2. The correlation sums (upper panel) and local scaling exponents (lower panel) as functions of the scale ϵ (embedding dimensions m). The underlying data are independently identically distributed Gaussian noise with a width of $\sigma=0.166$, 2000 scalar data. The dashed lines represent the values obtained with the correct method, the continuous lines result when including the self-pairs $i=j$ in the sum in Eq. (2.2). Since the input is pure noise, the accurate scaling exponent for small ϵ is $d(m,\epsilon)=m$.

about 100 pairs remain. This should happen only below $\epsilon_{min}\approx1/10$. The number of pairs at scale ϵ is roughly given by $n(\epsilon)\approx(N^2/2)\ \epsilon^D$. Requiring $n(\epsilon_{min})\approx100$ leads to the conclusion that one needs a time series of at least

$$N_{min}\approx10^{(D+2)/2} \tag{3.1}$$

points, or, in other words, the maximal dimension to be determined from a time series of length N is $D_{max}\approx2\ \log_{10}N-2$.

Several papers[15,22,23] give the impression that the above reasoning is too pessimistic. However, the positive results concerning high dimensions with few data have poor practical relevance: The authors of Refs. 22 and 23 are able to resolve a scaling range with the correct scaling exponent for examples where the correlation dimension is known. Thus it is only confirmed that among other structures there is some range with the correct exponent, but it is most unclear whether one would recognize it without prior knowledge. Similarly, the theoretical result of Gershenfeld[15] is obtained for an idealized situation. He proves that the statistical fluctuations do not increase explicitly with the attractor dimension provided the number of pairs within the scaling regime

remains constant. Unfortunately, as Gershenfeld himself points out, the macroscopic structures become more and more relevant with higher attractor dimensions, leaving less and less points inside the scaling region. As an illustration, we show in Fig. 2 the correlation sums for Gaussian white noise (dashed lines), which in an m dimensional space has correlation dimension m. For ϵ larger than the noise level the local scaling exponents smoothly decay to zero. Thus the macroscopic structures in this example start at $\epsilon\approx2^{-3}$. The plot of the correlation sums clearly shows that the larger m the smaller is $C_2(2^{-3})$, indicating that less pairs are inside the scaling region. (For white noise this is trivial: $C_2(\epsilon,m)=C_2(\epsilon,1)^m$. For Gaussian distributed noise in particular $C_2(\epsilon,m)=[\sqrt{2}\ \mathrm{erf}(\epsilon/2\sigma)]^m$.) Thus due to the upper cutoff of the scaling in reality the statistical errors do grow with increasing attractor dimension and fixed N.

Let us make two more remarks concerning the usefulness of providing more data points. First of all, the scaling range cannot be directly extended below the noise regime by adding more points. Thus if noise delimits the scaling range then only explicit nonlinear noise reduction can make use of an excessive amount of data. Second, if the supposed dimension of the attractor is high (say, 10) more points do not yield significantly better results: if one increases the amount of data by a factor of 10 (which in experiments may be very difficult), the average interpoint distance on the ten-dimensional attractor is reduced by a factor of about 0.8, thus leaving the scaling range practically unchanged.

B. The influence of noise

Noise as a random process has an infinite dimension, such that below a length scale related to the noise level a completely different scaling behavior occurs, as we already pointed out discussing Fig. 1. If the remaining "true" scaling range is too small, any estimate of the scaling exponent becomes rather unsafe. The correlation integral starts to mirror the presence of noise on a length scale which is about two times the noise amplitude for uniformly distributed noise[24] and more than three times the variance of Gaussian noise.[25] Below these scales $C_2(\epsilon)$ decays faster and faster, reaching a rate equal to the embedding dimension at the noise level. Taking this together with the fact that the large scale structures of the attractor allow for scaling only on scales below, say, one-fifth of the overall size of the attractor, a noise level of at most 2% can be tolerated. A more detailed investigation of the influence of noise on nonlinear analyzing methods can be found in Ref. 24.

IV. INTERPRETING CORRELATION INTEGRALS OF PHYSIOLOGICAL DATA

As pointed out before, in physiology we would not expect any system to be strictly deterministic. But for some phenomena the determinism might be a dominant feature and low dimensional chaos might be the most plausible effective description of the data, such that one would like to test for this by computation of the correlation dimension. Applying the algorithm in a too naive way will presumably lead to wrong conclusions. In the following we will discuss some known sources of misleading results. In many cases they do not pose serious problems if the data is examined carefully *before* applying any nonlinear algorithm.

A. General precautions

Before we discuss some pitfalls particular to dimension calculations let us make a general remark concerning the stationarity of a time series. To gain maximal insight we have to try to isolate a situation where the basic dynamical properties—deterministic or stochastic—remain approximately constant during the period of observation. To achieve this, it is neither necessary nor sufficient to artificially "pin down" the subject or isolate some phenomenon physically. Ultimately, it has to be decided *from the data* if the observation represents a stationary situation or some transient phenomenon. Both can be interesting but the algorithm considered here can only be used in the former case.

B. Finite dimension versus dynamical correlations

Dynamical correlations between the data are the most relevant origin of spuriously small dimensions.

The pairs $i=j$ are not included in the sum Eq. (2.2). If they were, any point on the attractor had at least itself as a neighbor, and in the limit of small scales the correlation sum would converge towards a constant, $C_2(\epsilon \rightarrow 0) \rightarrow 1/N$. Thus the local slope approaches zero, saying nothing but that the dimension of this finite collection of points is zero which is of course true for all finite sets. This is not what we wanted to learn. We rather want to interpret the set as a finite sample of an infinite set, the strange attractor under study. This is why we look at the scaling behavior for intermediate ranges of ϵ, where the finiteness of the set is not yet visible for the algorithm. In order to extend this scaling region as far as possible towards the small scales, one has to discard the "self-pairs." The difference between accepting or discarding the self-pairs is illustrated in Fig. 2. Including them, the curves of the correlation sums versus ϵ are $\int$-shaped, such that the scaling range with the "correct" exponent is reduced or, as in Fig. 2 for $m=4$ and 5, completely destroyed. For

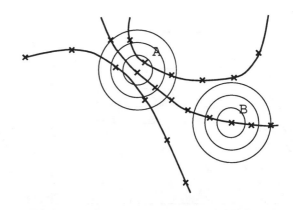

FIG. 3. A typical situation for the computation of C_2 for a flow: Whereas for point A there are still some neighboring points lying on dynamically uncorrelated parts of the data (in this enlargement shown as different trajectories), all neighbors of point B are direct images and pre-images of B and thus simulate a dimension of one. To avoid this one has to ignore all neighbors in time [i.e., $|i-j| > t_{min}$ in Eq. (2.2), if t_{min} is some correlation time], although this reduces the numbers of pairs on small scales.

high enough embedding dimension the slopes around the inflection point even seem to saturate, the attractor thus looking finite dimensional. The data underlying this figure are white Gaussian noise, such that the true scaling exponent equals the embedding dimension for $\epsilon < \sigma$, the width of the Gaussian (which is $\sigma = 0.166$).

The above considerations may appear to be trivial but they are worth understanding since the "self-pairs" are the limiting case of dynamical correlations in general, which are present in densely sampled flow data. (*Flow* data, as opposed to map-like data, is data taken from a system evolving continuously in time.) A typical autocorrelation function of a flow decays slowly, indicating that points successive in time also tend to be close in space. If the sampling time is small, then the closest neighbors of a given point will be its immediate images and pre-images, as illustrated in Fig. 3. They also have to be discarded in the correlation sum. If not, in the limit of small scales the attractor looks one dimensional since the (discretized version of the) continuous trajectory is

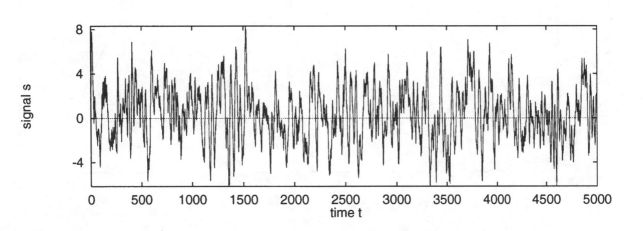

FIG. 4. Colored noise generated by a moving average filter.

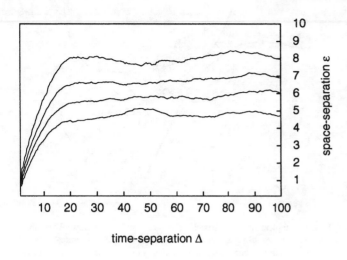

FIG. 5. Space-time-separation plot for moving average data.

resolved. Again, the correlation sums will be $\int$-shaped, only that now the small scale limit looks slightly different.

The remedy is very simple.[26] When computing the correlation sum Eq. (2.2) one discards all pairs with $|i-j| < t_{min}$. The corresponding time t_{min} may be estimated with generosity, since the loss of potential pairs is negligible. A simple method to detect dynamical correlations and determine a good value for t_{min} is to compute space-time-separation plots as described in Provenzale et al.[27] In the absence of dynamical correlations, the distribution of the distances of pairs of points i,j should not depend on their distance in time $\Delta = |i-j|$. This property can be tested for by computing a histogram of the number of pairs over the Δ-ϵ

plane. For flow data one usually finds that for short separations in time Δ, more close neighbors are found. The separation in time for which the fraction of neighbors closer than a given ϵ approaches a constant is a good estimate for t_{min}. (In some cases, stable oscillations around a constant are seen.)

We use a time series containing colored noise to demonstrate the effect of dynamical correlations. We generate the correlations by applying the moving average filter $x_t = \sum_{j=1}^{20} \sqrt{j(21-j)}\, \eta_{t-j}$ to the white input noise η_t. The signal is shown in Fig. 4. The corresponding space-time-separation plot is shown in Fig. 5. Contour lines $\epsilon(\Delta)$ are drawn so that a fixed fraction of the pairs with a time separation Δ are spatially closer than ϵ. During the correlation time of 20 iterations many pairs are close in space because they are close in time. For longer time-separations the contour lines are approximately constant indicating that now the correlations are of geometrical nature.

In Fig. 6, we show the correlation sums and local scaling exponents for an $m=10$ dimensional embedding, where in one case all pairs with $i \neq j$ are included in the correlation sum, in the other only those with $|i-j| > 21$. Unless the pairs close in time are discarded, the range in ϵ on which the attractor looks almost one dimensional increases with the embedding dimension m.

As an extreme but not uncommon case, all data points in the series can be dynamically correlated. In order to interpret the data as a random sample representing the underlying invariant measure we have to assume that the whole attractor is sampled and the distribution we see is in fact invariant under time evolution. If on the contrary the trajectory has not yet explored the whole attractor and is thus effectively nonstationary, one can often find signatures of a finite dimension.

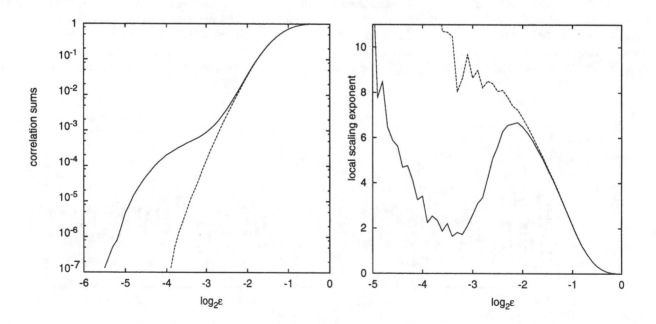

FIG. 6. The effect of dynamical correlations: $C_2(\epsilon)$ and local scaling exponents for correlated noise with a correlation time 20 are shown, for fixed $m=10$. The continuous curve results from counting all pairs with $i \neq j$, the broken line from omitting pairs with $|i-j| < 22$.

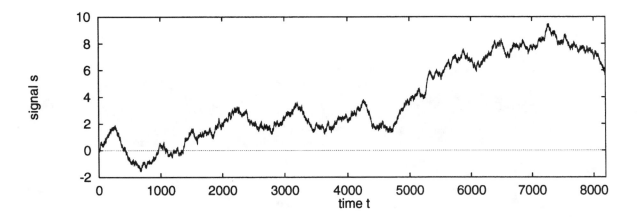

FIG. 7. Simulated path of a particle undergoing Brownian motion.

(Remember that we have to impose a notion of stationarity which is stronger than keeping the accessible parameters of the experiment constant. We have to justify the assumption that the data set is a representative sample of a phenomenon with well defined dynamical properties.) In fact, such data may lie on a low dimensional object since the process at work may have filled only a lower dimensional subset of the attractor, which itself could be even infinite dimensional. A typical example is $f^{-\alpha}$ noise (Osborne and Provenzale;[28] Theiler[29]). Some indication whether the data are "stationary enough" to represent an invariant measure can be obtained from the power spectrum. If there is much power in the low frequencies, then a finite scaling exponent presumably does not represent the dimension of the invariant measure. The most direct and safe indication however comes from the space-time-separation plots discussed above.

The correlation sum for one trajectory of a particle undergoing Brownian motion (Fig. 7) is presented in Fig. 8. Brownian motion is known to be nonrecurrent in more than two dimensions, but in any dimension the average end-to-end distances of a path of length T increases like $T^{1/2}$. Thus any finite path on average looks like a two-dimensional object.[30] The resulting local exponents from the Grassberger–Procaccia algorithm are in agreement with this fact.

Our Brownian path is an accumulation of Gaussian white noise. Its power spectrum (panel A) is clearly $1/f^2$ and for our purpose the process must be regarded as nonstationary. The scalar data are embedded in 2 to 10 dimensions. Because of the strong correlations, a delay of 300 was used. The resulting local scaling exponents (panel B) show a clear saturation for some range of ϵ in the sense that they are

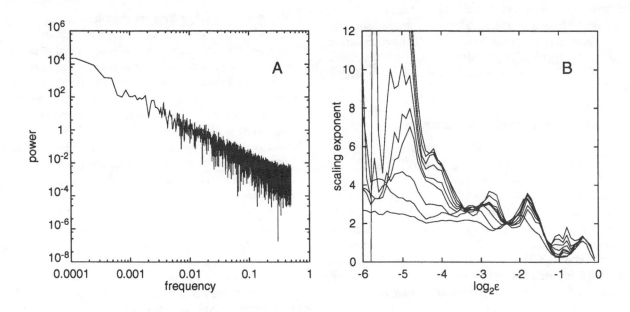

FIG. 8. The spectrum (panel A) and the local scaling exponents (panel B) of a Brownian path.

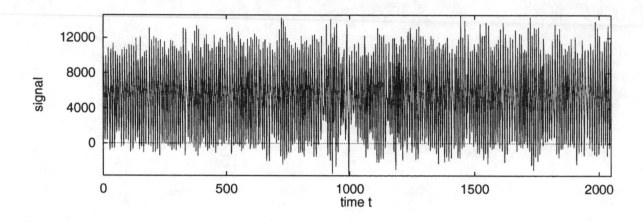

FIG. 9. A time series of 2048 successive measurements of the air flow through the nose of a human. The data are a subset (starting at $t=12750$) of data set B2 of the SFI time series competition (Ref. 38) supplied by A. Goldberger.

independent of the embedding dimension. This could be misinterpreted as a finite dimension. Note however that there is no true scaling behavior because of the fluctuations in ϵ. Thus is some sense all what we see above $\epsilon \approx 1/64$ are macroscopic structures.

The estimated dimension would increase toward the correct value given by the embedding dimension if we could get rid of the dynamical correlations. Unfortunately, as evidenced by, the power spectrum evidenced by, all the data are correlated (since the lowest frequency is dominant) and the remedy applied before cannot be used. To render a data set stationary one can apply an explicit detrending, or one could replace the original data by its numerical derivative $(x_t \mapsto x_t' = x_{t+1} - x_t)$. Unfortunately, this worsens the signal-to-noise ratio, especially for flows, where the deterministic part of two successive values x_t and x_{t+1} is highly correlated.

The possible pitfalls mentioned here are not limited to the correlation algorithm. They have in common that they either obscure the true scaling behavior or pretend some fake scaling behavior, which will be seen by all algorithms testing for scaling properties. The problems arise due to deficiencies in the data which do not properly represent the underlying invariant measure.

C. No scaling but structures: Surrogate data

Generally, in physiological data one will not find a true scaling region in the sense of Fig. 1, since, as already discussed, the system under consideration may be so strongly perturbed by the rest of the world. Is there still something we can learn from the correlation integral in such a case? It many cases it contains structures which might reflect some nonlinearity. In Fig. 9 a record of the respiration rate of a human is shown. In Fig. 10(A) we present the corresponding correlation integral. No scaling region can be discerned, but it seems unlikely that such a correlation sum is created by white noise.

This is the starting point for the method of *surrogate data*.[31] The goal is to make a more reliable statement as to

how unlikely the null hypothesis of white or possibly colored noise is. For this purpose an ensemble of "surrogate" data sets is created which by construction has the same linear properties as the data to be analyzed. (An interesting suggestion of Paluš[32] is not to rely on the construction but to explicitly test for the linear properties as well. In particular for short data sets this yields a much better idea about the statistical deviations within the sample.) This usually means that the power spectrum has to be the same. Then some nonlinear statistic (like the correlation sum) is computed for each set. This gives an indication how probable it is that the original data are generated by a random process with this spectrum: when the nonlinear statistic yields a significant difference between the surrogates and the original data, there might be something more than the particular linear model to it. Technically, surrogates are created by first rendering the distribution of the original data Gaussian. Then one computes the Fourier transform and changes all the phases to random numbers. For each realization of the random phases the back-transform yields one surrogate data set.

Rendering the distribution of the original data Gaussian is a delicate operation, since nowhere is it a smooth rescaling of the data. In practice, one orders both the data and a set of Gaussian random numbers in magnitude, and maps the ith largest data item to the ith largest random number. It is not guaranteed at all that the dimension (and thus the structures in the correlation sum) remain the same under this operation. In contrast to this, structures in data sets generated by Gaussian noises are conserved on the average, since they are only due to statistical fluctuations.

A more refined technique avoids rescaling of the signal.[33] Let us start with a set of random numbers, adjust their distribution to the one of the original data, and enforce their spectrum to become identical to that of the original data by applying a Wiener filter. Since filtering does not preserve the distribution, and changing the distribution does not preserve the spectrum, these two steps have to be repeated many times. Empirically, convergence is found, such that one ends up with a data set consisting of random numbers with both

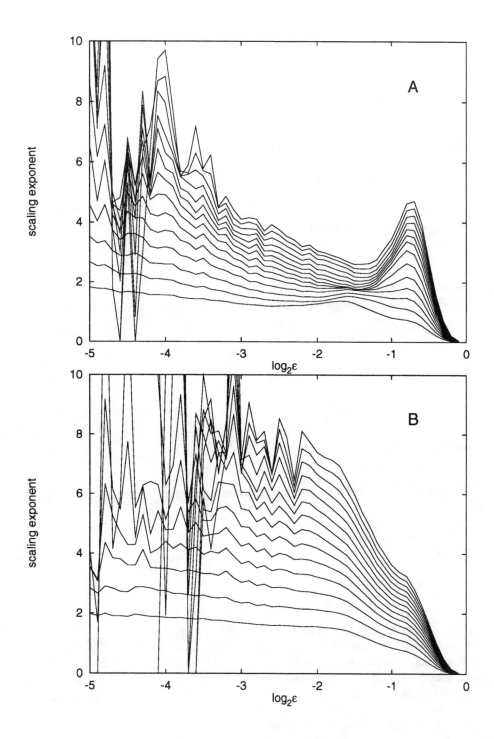

FIG. 10. Panel A shows the local scaling exponents for $m=2$ to 15 for the data of Fig. 9. Panel B shows results for typical surrogates of this set.

the correct distribution and the correct spectrum. Again one creates a whole ensemble of sets and compares the properties of the original data with respect to the average behavior of the ensemble.

In the case of the data underlying Fig. 8(B) the method of surrogates would lead to the result that similar structures occur in almost all surrogate samples, although the details are different. The reason can be found looking at the spectrum: Its clear $1/f^2$ behavior indicates that the time series is nonstationary. Therefore, the structures found in $C_2(\epsilon)$ for the original data have nothing to do with low dimensionality.

Thus one possible origin of structures in the correlation sum is nonstationarity. If this were always the case, the method of surrogate data would be obsolete since knowning (from the spectrum) that the time series is nonstationary one can immediately conclude that structures in the correlation sum cannot be interpreted in the sense of low dimensionality.

Figure 10 demonstrates that a different situation may be encountered as well. From a physiological time series of length 30000 we selected a part which looks most stationary to the eye. In this case typical surrogates yield clearly different local scaling exponents as shown in the figure. Thus the null hypothesis of colored Gaussian noise can be rejected. Now, what can be the origin of this signature and how can it be interpreted?

Generally, since the noise amplitudes in physiological data are large, no fractal structure would remain, even if the attractor were low dimensional. However, on the large scales the global geometry of the attractor might still be apparent. Such a situation is shown in Fig. 11 for a numerical example. In panel A we show the local scaling exponents of a noise free attractor, which has correlation dimension 1.21. By construction, it is very wrinkled, such that the global structures influence the correlation integral down to scales of $\epsilon \approx 2^{-4}$. Now, adding Gaussian white noise, (panel B), the scaling range is completely wiped out, but the structures on large scales remain almost unchanged. Applying the methods of surrogate data in this situation yields a positive answer. The local scaling exponents for the clean data, the noisy data, and one typical set of surrogates (using Schreiber's method) are shown in Fig. 11. Obviously, the structures disappear when randomizing the data. Thus in fact one can conclude that they are related to the shape of the geometrical object represented by the data, although in no way can it serve to extract the true dimension of the clean data.

D. A recipe for dimension estimates

Summarizing the above aspects, we want to give a recipe to avoid wrong dimension estimates. Wrong generally means too small, first since all the known pitfalls result in lowering the number one extracts, and second because it is peculiar to the human nature to see what one is looking for. In practice, the only way the observed "dimension" can be raised is by noise which hides the fractal structures of an attractor.

Before computing any correlation sum one should carefully inspect the data and use conventional techniques to extract as much information as possible. In particular one should compute the autocorrelation function of the signal and its power spectrum. Sometimes, nonstationarity in the data is reflected by a divergence of the power spectrum towards the low frequencies. Other cases of nonstationarity may be detected by comparing pictures and statistical tests for different sections of the data. For the particular case of the correlation integral we highly recommend computing space-time-separation plots as discussed above. In any case, data which do not represent the invariant measure of the underlying process are not apt for dimension estimates. Other quantities for their description have to be used. For example, to characterize a random walk, one could measure the scaling exponent of the end-to-end distance rather than the dimension.[34]

For a stationary time series, one has to choose the correlation time to exclude dynamically correlated pairs. The correlation sums and local scaling exponents are then computed for different choices of the delay time τ. If self-similarity is found consistently, a numerical value of the correlation dimension may be determined. In order to make the result transparent one should always show the local exponents versus ϵ for some range of m. Claiming to find a finite

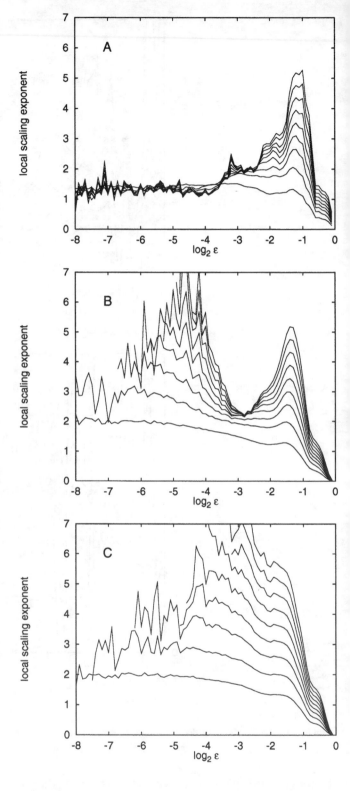

FIG. 11. Data from an attractor whose geometry destroys the scaling in the correlation sum on scales larger than 2^{-4} (panel A for clean data). Adding noise of sufficient amplitude in such a case leaves structures but no scaling range in the correlation sums (panel B). A typical surrogate data set with the same distribution and same power spectrum as the noisy data lacks these structures (panel C), indicating that they are related to determinism.

dimension of more than $\approx 2 \log_{10} N - 2$ needs additional justification, e.g., by a much finer sampling of ϵ inside the scaling region and by showing that the result is robust under changes in parameters like the delay time.

Fluctuations of the local scaling exponent around a mean value inside the scaling regime are anticorrelated. Therefore, to determine a statistical error of D_2 one should rather fit a straight line to the log–log data than averaging over the local exponents. To detect the scaling regime, however, this is not the method of choice, since it cannot distinguish between systematic and statistical deviations from the scaling law. Thus, one should first determine the beginning and end of the scaling range by the local scaling exponents, and afterwards use the log–log data to determine the numerical value of D_2. It is also possible to use a maximum likelihood estimator[16] for the estimation of D_2. (See however Ref. 35 for some critical issues.)

V. WHY DIMENSION ESTIMATES FOR PHYSIOLOGICAL DATA?

Physiological data generally are aperiodic. Since Lorenz' famous work it is known that deterministic dynamics can cause aperiodic signals. Furthermore, it is very likely that the dynamics in physiological systems is nonlinear, thus allowing for chaotic motion. Low dimensional strange attractors are one possible signature of deterministic chaos. Therefore, if one could demonstrate the existence of such an object in a particular system one has gained a lot.

The system under investigation is (i) effectively deterministic, (ii) it is nonlinear, (iii) it can be characterized by only a very few degrees of freedom, although the true phase space may possess a very high dimension, and (iv) it can in principle be described by simple models. The numerical value of the correlation dimension gives an estimate for the number of active degrees of freedom. This collection of information is difficult to obtain from other quantities.

Unfortunately, most physiological time series do not exhibit clear scaling, and positive evidence for a low dimensional attractor is lacking. In the best case one finds structures which disappear for surrogate data, such that one still can conclude to have an effectively low dimensional object, but loses almost all other information listed above.

Finally, what should be the conclusion when no signature of low dimensionality is found, but the data seem to be stationary? We think the correct answer is either the noise part of the data is comparable or larger than the deterministic component (if there is any), or the attractor's dimension is too large to be recognized, i.e., much above $2 \log_{10} N - 2$, or even infinite. The crucial point is that nonlinear dynamical systems with a huge phase space are not forced to exhibit an attractor which is really low dimensional. There is generally no upper limit for the dimension of an attractor below D, the dimension of the phase space. Especially with delay equations one can very easily construct dissipative systems with high attractor dimensions,[36] and feedbacks in physiology generally are delayed. Thus, to summarize, finding a low dimensional attractor is a sufficient condition for deterministic chaos, but not a necessary one, and data may well be highly deterministic on an invariant object we are not able to reconstruct from the data. However, if this is the case, it is obvious that such a dynamics cannot be modeled by simple equations with few degrees of freedom.

Let us also repeat that dimension estimates for nonstationary data are ill-defined since the data do not represent the attractor. If at all possible, one has to render the data stationary (e.g., by differentiating or detrending), or one has to apply other statistical methods.

In a nutshell, if a data set indeed is low dimensional, the correlation algorithm yields strong results, but the probability that a given physiological data set has this property is small. We still think that for each data set some information can be gained by applying the method, but one should not expect that the outcome is positive, and moreover, one should not try to characterize every data set by a number called dimension.

ACKNOWLEDGMENTS

We thank the organizers for giving us the opportunity to attend the Dynamical Diseases conference. We appreciated very much the stimulating atmosphere and discussions. We owe particular thanks to P. Grassberger for carefully reading the manuscript.

[1] D. Kaplan, Conference talk, 1994.

[2] P. Grassberger and I. Procaccia, "Characterization of strange attractors," Phys. Rev. Lett. **50**, 346–349 (1983); "Measuring the strangeness of strange attractors," Physica D **9**, 189–208 (1983).

[3] F. Takens, "Detecting strange attractors in turbulence," in *Dynamical Systems and Turbulence*, Lecture Notes in Mathematics, edited by D. A. Rand and L.-S. Young (Springer-Verlag, Berlin, 1981), Vol. 898, pp. 366–381.

[4] T. Sauer and J. A. Yorke, "How many delay coordinates do you need?," Int. J. Bifurcation Chaos **3**, 737–745 (1993).

[5] P. Grassberger, "Generalizations of the Hausdorff dimension of fractal measures," Phys. Lett. A **107**, 101–105 (1985).

[6] D. A. Russell, J. D. Hanson, and E. Ott, "Dimension of strange attractors," Phys. Rev. Lett. **45**, 1175–1178 (1980).

[7] H. S. Greenside, A. Wolf, J. Swift, and T. Pignataro, "Impracticality of a box-counting algorithm for calculating the dimensionality of strange attractors, Phys. Rev. A **25**, 3453–3456 (1982).

[8] Y. Termonia and Z. Alexandrowicz, "Fractal dimension of strange attractors from radius versus size of arbitrary clusters," Phys. Rev. Lett. **51**, 1265–1268 (1983); R. Badii and A. Politi, "Statistical description of chaotic attractors: the dimension function," J. Stat. Phys. **40**, 725–750 (1988).

[9] D. S. Broomhead, R. Jones, and G. P. King, "Topological dimension and local coordinates from time series data," J. Phys. A **20**, L563–L569 (1987); T. Hediger, A. Passamante, and M. E. Farrell, "Characterizing attractors using local intrinsic dimensions calculated by singular-value decomposition and information-theoretic criteria," Phys. Rev. A **41**, 5325–5332 (1990).

[10] P. Grassberger, "Finite sample corrections to entropy and dimension estimates," Phys. Lett. A **128**, 369–373 (1988).

[11] J. Theiler, "Efficient algorithm for estimating the correlation dimension from a set of discrete points," Phys. Rev. A **36**, 4456–4462 (1987).

[12] S. Bingham and M. Kot, "Multidimensional trees, range searching, and a correlation dimension algorithm of reduced complexity," Phys. Lett. A **140**, 327–330 (1989).

[13] P. Grassberger, "An optimized box-assisted algorithm for fractal dimensions," Phys. Lett. A **148**, 63–68 (1990).

[14] T. Schreiber, "Efficient neighbor searching in nonlinear time series analysis" to appear in Int. J. Bifurcation Chaos.

[15] N. A. Gershenfeld, "Dimension measurements on high-dimensional systems," Physica D **55**, 135–154 (1992).

[16] F. Takens, "On the numerical determination of the dimension of an attractor," in *Dynamical Systems and Bifurcations*, Lecture Notes in Mathematics, edited by B. L. J. Braaksma, H. W. Broer, and F. Takens (Springer-Verlag, Berlin, 1985), Vol. 1125.

[17] J. Theiler, "Statistical precision of dimension estimators," Phys. Rev. A **41**, 3038–3041 (1990).

[18] J. Holzfuss and G. Mayer-Kress, "An approach to error-estimation in the application of dimension algorithms," in *Dimensions and Entropies in*

Chaotic Systems, edited by G. Mayer-Kress (Springer-Verlag, Berlin, 1986).

[19] I. Procaccia, "Weather systems: Complex or just complicated?," Nature **333**, 498–499 (1988).

[20] L. A. Smith, "Intrinsic limits on dimension calculations," Phys. Lett. A **133**, 283–288 (1988).

[21] J.-P. Eckmann and D. Ruelle, "Fundamental limitations for estimating dimensions and Lyapunov exponents in dynamical systems," Physica D **56**, 185–187 (1992).

[22] J. W. Havstad and C. L. Ehlers, "Attractor dimension of nonstationary dynamical systems from small data sets," Phys. Rev. A **39**, 845–853 (1989).

[23] N. B. Abraham, A. M. Albano, B. Das, G. De Guzman, S. Yong, R. S Gioggia, G. P. Puccioni, and J. R. Tredicce, "Calculating the dimension of attractors from small data sets," Phys. Lett. A **114**, 217–221 (1986).

[24] T. Schreiber and H. Kantz, "Noise in chaotic data: diagnosis and treatment," Chaos **5**, 133–142 (1995).

[25] T. Schreiber, "Determination of the noise level of chaotic time series," Phys. Rev. E **48**, R13–R16 (1993).

[26] J. Theiler, "Spurious dimension from correlation algorithms applied to limited time-series data," Phys. Rev. A **34**, 2427–2432 (1986).

[27] A. Provenzale, L. A. Smith, R. Vio, and G. Murante, "Distinguishing between low-dimensional dynamics and randomness in measured time series," Physica D **58**, 31–49 (1992).

[28] A. R. Osborne and A. Provenzale, "Finite correlation dimension for systems with power law spectra," Physica D **35**, 357–381 (1989).

[29] J. Theiler, "Some comments on the correlation dimension of $1/f^\alpha$ noise," Phys. Lett. A **155**, 480–493 (1991).

[30] B. B. Mandelbrot, *The Fractal Geometry of Nature* (Freeman, San Francisco, 1982).

[31] J. Theiler, S. Eubank, A. Longtin, B. Galdrikian, and J. D. Farmer, "Testing for Nonlinearity in time series: The method of surrogate data," Physica D **58**, 77–94 (1992).

[32] M. Paluš, "Testing for Nonlinearity Using Redundancies: Quantitative and Qualitative Aspects," Santa Fe Institute preprint 93-12-076 (1993).

[33] T. Schreiber (unpublished).

[34] J. Collins and C. J. DeLuca, "Upright, correlated random walks: A statistical-biomechanics approach to the human postural control system," Chaos **5**, 57–63 (1995).

[35] J. Theiler, "Lacunarity in a best estimator of fractal dimension," Phys. Lett. A **133**, 195–200 (1988).

[36] G. Baier and M. Klein, "Maximum hyperchaos in generalized Hénon maps," Phys. Lett. A **151**, 281–284 (1990).

[37] M. Hénon, "A two-dimensional mapping with a strange attractor," Commun. Math. Phys. **50**, 69–77 (1976).

[38] *Time Series Prediction: Forecasting the Future and Understanding the Past*, edited by A. S. Weigend and N. A. Gershenfeld, SFI Studies in the Sciences of Complexity (Addison–Wesley, Reading, MA, 1993), Vol. XV.

A basic mathematical model of the immune response

H. Mayer
Institute of Immunology and Institute of Mathematics, University of Witten/Herdecke, Stockumer Strasse 10, D-58448 Witten, Germany

K. S. Zaenker
Institute of Immunology, University of Witten/Herdecke, Stockumer Strasse 10, D-58448 Witten, Germany

U. an der Heiden
Institute of Mathematics, University of Witten/Herdecke, Stockumer Strasse 10, D-58448 Witten, Germany

(Received 3 June 1994; accepted for publication 21 September 1994)

Interaction of the immune system with a target population of, e.g., bacteria, viruses, antigens, or tumor cells must be considered as a dynamic process. We describe this process by a system of two ordinary differential equations. Although the model is strongly idealized it demonstrates how the combination of a few proposed nonlinear interaction rules between the immune system and its targets are able to generate a considerable variety of different kinds of immune responses, many of which are observed both experimentally and clinically. In particular, solutions of the model equations correspond to states described by immunologists as "virgin state," "immune state" and "state of tolerance." The model successfully replicates the so-called primary and secondary response. Moreover, it predicts the existence of a threshold level for the amount of pathogen germs or of transplanted tumor cells below which the host is able to eliminate the infectious organism or to reject the tumor graft. We also find a long time coexistence of targets and immune competent cells including damped and undamped oscillations of both. Plausibly the model explains that if the number of transformed cells or pathogens exeeds definable values (poor antigenicity, high reproduction rate) the immune system fails to keep the disease under control. On the other hand, the model predicts apparently paradoxical situations including an increased chance of target survival despite enhanced immune activity or therapeutically achieved target reduction. A further obviously paradoxical behavior consists of a positive effect for the patient up to a complete cure by adding an additional target challenge where the benefit of the additional targets depends strongly on the time point and on their amount. Under periodically pulsed stimulation the model may show a chaotic time behavior of both target growth and immune response. © *1995 American Institute of Physics.*

I. INTRODUCTION, THE MODEL

Like the nervous system the immune system has a very high degree of complexity, even if its connection to the nervous system[1] is not taken into account. Therefore it is impossible to develop a nearly completely realistic mathematical model for every situation of host defense. Increasingly complicated mathematical models have been developed, for a few examples see Refs. 2–9. However, despite their complexity there is still incomplete understanding of the mechanisms of how the immune system really works, even though there is an enormous amount of "isolated" data.[2] In high-dimensional models often problems arise with parameter estimations[4,5,8] and lack of insight into the model itself.

The model presented here follows a different strategy. It demonstrates that a considerable plurality of immunological phenomena can be the result of very few and simple basic interactive mechanisms. This approach is motivated by the modern theory of nonlinear dynamical systems[10] implying that the behavior of a system may be far richer than its internal structure from which this behavior results. To find an interactive structure as simple as possible is a contribution to the question of how complex the immune system at least has to be in order to produce its observed responses.

We consider the relationship between the target and the immune system as a feedback loop. Figure 1 outlines the mechanisms assumed to be essential for the immune–target interaction. The target may be any biological material such as bacteria, viruses or immunogenic tumor cells susceptible to an immune response. The temporal change of the target population size T is determined by the difference between their reproduction and their elimination. It is assumed that the reproduction rate is proportional to the target size. The elimination of the targets as the result of the interaction with specific immune components (effectors E) is considered to be proportional to the contact rate between the targets and the effectors.

Thus, the temporal change of the target population is described by the differential equation

$$\frac{dT}{dt} = rT - kTE$$

with non-negative rate constants r and k.

We define the immune competence E as the elimination capacity of the immune system with respect to that special target. E may be measured, e.g., by the concentration of certain immune cells, like cytotoxic T-cells, natural killer cells, or by the concentration of certain antibodies.

The immune competence E is supposed to be constituted by three different factors:

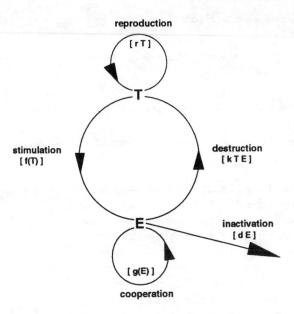

FIG. 1. Scheme of the essential mechanisms of interaction between a target population T and the effectiveness E of the immune system against this target. For details see text.

(1) The targets trigger processes in the immune system leading to competence against them. For example, in the presence of targets nonspecific precursor cells, or not yet activated T-cells are transformed into specific helper cells, cytotoxic T-cells or plasma cells producing specific antibodies. The velocity of this stimulation is described by a function $f(T)$ which for specificity is given by

$$f(T)=p\frac{T^u}{m^v+T^v} \quad (T\geq 0) \tag{1}$$

with positive constants p, m, u and v, $u\leq v$. Depending on the parameters u and v there exist three different shapes of the stimulation function $f(T)$ as illustrated by Figs. 2(a)–2(c). All these functions are bounded accounting for the fact that the precursor population is limited. The sigmoid increase in the case $u>1$ emphasizes that a small amount of targets may be more or less ignored by the immune system. This effect is known as low-zone unresponsiveness. The high-zone unresponsiveness,

$u<v$, is characterized by a decrease of immune response stimulation under high target burden. The parameter p represents the precursor pool size.

(2) The immune reaction is additionally strengthened by autocatalytic and/or cooperative reinforcement of immune activation processes. This means, for example, that competent immune effector cells are able to proliferate and/or to stimulate themselves or precursor cells for increased proliferation or differentiation. The resulting increase rate of immune competence is modeled by the function

$$g(E)=s\frac{E^n}{c^n+E^n} \tag{2}$$

whose graph qualitatively looks like Fig. 2(a) ($n=1$) or Fig. 2(b) ($n>1$). The sigmoid shape takes into account that a critical number of immune cells may be necessary in order to realize the cooperative and autocatalytic effect.

(3) Finally a term $-d\cdot E$ represents the finite lifetime of the immune competent cells or agents, with a positive death rate constant d.

A summary of the mathematical model for the interaction of the immune system and the target is given by the following system of two ordinary differential equations:

$$\frac{dT}{dt}=rT-kTE, \tag{3}$$

$$\frac{dE}{dt}=f(T)+g(E)-dE. \tag{4}$$

The system contains three nonlinear terms, TE, $f(T)$ and $g(T)$. It will be shown in the subsequent discussion that the interaction of these three factors is essential for the large variety of different types of behavior the model is admitting.

There is already a considerable number of low dimensional models (not more than three equations) in the literature. We point to the list[11–21] which is not claimed to be complete. These models are more or less related to the model presented here.

The essential feature of our model is the cooperation of the nonlinearities which has a great number of dramatic effects, in fact, observed in real immune responses. Most of the

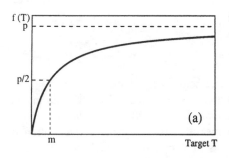
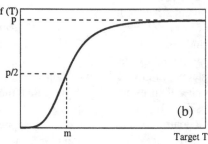
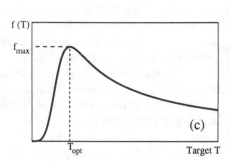

FIG. 2. Graph of the stimulation function $f(T)$ for three different sets of parameters: (a) $u=v=1$; (b) $u=v>1$; (c) $1<u<v$

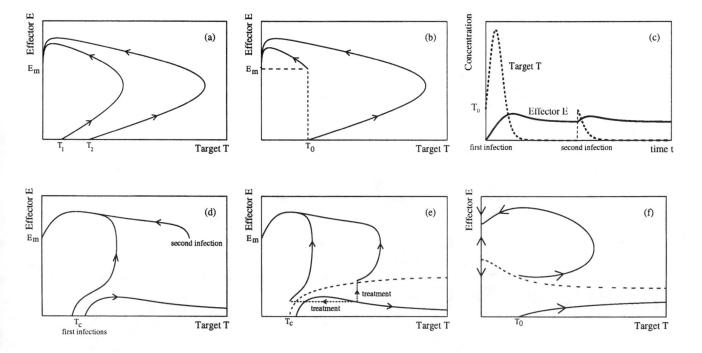

FIG. 3. Figures show numerical solutions of the model equations (3) and (4). (a) Trajectories in the phase plane corresponding to two differently strong infections. (b) Primary and secondary response represented in the phase plane and (c) in the time domain. (d) Essential increase of immune defense efficiency in a secondary response leading to a rejection of a much higher infectious dose than during a primary response. (e) Therapeutic interventions, indicated by dotted lines. (f) Example that any primary infection may be lethal despite the existence of an immune state. Values of parameters for the computation of the trajectories: r, k, p, s = 2.3, 2, 1, 2.5 [(a), (b), (c)]; 0.15, 0.1, 0.7, 2 [(d), (e)]; 1.2, 1, 0.28, 2 (f); u, v, n = 1, 1, 1 [(a), (b), (c)]; 1, 2, 3 [(d), (e)]; 2, 2, 3, (f).

models in the literature are less nonlinear, and thus are not able to produce this richness of behavior. Of course, there is overlap with the model of this paper, and some of them have special properties which ours is missing. It remains a future task to establish a reasonable relationship between the low-dimensional models contained in the literature.

II. RESULTS OF ANALYTICAL INVESTIGATIONS OF THE MODEL

The time courses of the immune competence E and of the targets T are determined as the solutions of the differential equation system (3) and (4). Of course, each of the solutions depends on an initial condition $T(0)$, $E(0)$. Though there is no analytic expression for the solutions $T(t)$, $E(t)$, $t \geq 0$, one of the advantages of the model is that a nearly complete phase plane analysis can be carried out, and thus a nearly complete overview of the qualitative behavior of the model is possible. Without giving details here of this analysis, in the following we shall use mainly phase portraits in the T-E plane to illustrate and to characterize the different types of behavior that may happen depending on the values of the constant parameters.

Note that by linear rescaling of E, T and t, it can be achieved that $m = c = d = 1$, so the model contains just seven independent parameters.

Figure 3(a) shows two trajectories $[T(t), E(t)]_{t \geq 0}$ in the phase plane solving the system of differential equations. They start from initial conditions $(T_1, 0)$ and, respectively, $(T_2, 0)$ corresponding to two infections of different strength, $T_1 < T_2$. No specialized immune effectors are present at the

time of infection, $t = 0$, $E(0) = 0$. In response to the targets the concentration and/or the activity of immune competent cells starts to increase. Moving along the trajectories the system finally converges towards the so-called immune state $(0, E_m)$, where no targets but only "memory cells" exist.

In case of a second infection the initial condition is (T_0, E_m), $T_0 > 0$, and the immune system will respond faster. This is illustrated by Fig. 3(b) showing a primary and a secondary response with the same amount of infectious particles T_0. The temporal relationship between first and second infection is illustrated more pronouncedly in the time domain, see Fig. 3(c). In reality the secondary response can be so strong and fast, that a reinfection is often not recognized as for instance in the case of rubella (German measles). This type of behavior of the model occurs if the parameters satisfy the conditions

$$n = u = v = 1; \quad s > 1 \quad \text{and} \quad r/k < s - 1$$

(note that there may be still other regimes in parameter space where the same type of behavior occurs). This can be proved by discussing the vector field in the T-E plane defined by the right hand side of the differential equations, in particular by discussing the direction of flow in those areas of the phase plane which are separated by the nullclines $dT/dt = 0$ and $dE/dt = 0$. This analysis reveals that under the above conditions on the parameters the system has exactly two steady states (T and E constant), namely $(0,0)$ and $(0, E_m)$, $E_m = s - 1$. The first one turns out to be repelling, the second one is globally attractive in the domain $T \geq 0$, $E > 0$.

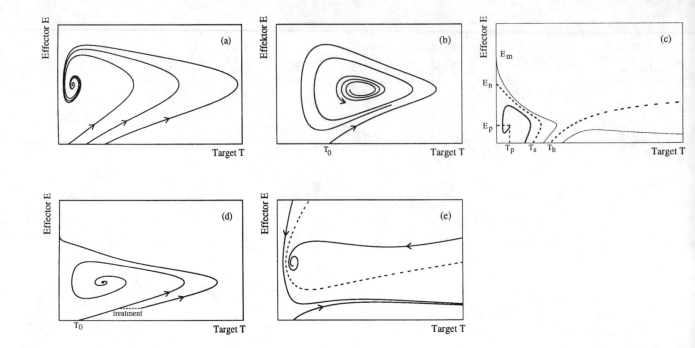

FIG. 4. Chronic coexistence of targets and effectors (a) in a steady state and (b) in a limit cycle. (c) Dose dependent outcome of an infection. (d) Paradox behaviors: a benefit effect from target increase, and (e) a target reduction or immune improvement may be lethal. Parameter values for (a)–(e), respectively: $r=4.5, 0.5, 0.3, 2.7, 0.6$; $k=3, 1, 1, 4.5, 0.5$; $p=3, 0.35, 0.7, 1, 0.7$; $s=0.5, 1.75, 2, 1.5, 1.6$; $u=2, 4, 1, 2, 1$; $v=2, 4, 2, 2, 2$; $n=1, 3, 3, 9, 3$.

Under other conditions on the parameters it may happen that the steady state $(0,E_m)$ is only locally attractive, for instance if

Condition (C):

$$n>1; \quad u<v; \quad s>s_1; \quad \max f(T)>f_1;$$

$$0<E_1<r/k<E_m$$

and r and k are sufficiently small. Here $s_1=n/\sqrt[n]{(n-1)^{n-1}}$, $f_1=z(E_1)$ where E_1 is the local maximum of the function $z(E)=E-g(E)$. The constant E_m is the largest solution of $E^n-sE^{n-1}+1=0$.

In case of condition (C) there exists a threshold $T_c>0$, such that whenever the infection dose $T_0>T_c$ the solution satisfies $T(t)\rightarrow\infty$, $E(t)\rightarrow0$ as $t\rightarrow\infty$, i.e., no immune state will be reached and the disease is lethal, see Fig. 3(d). Closer analysis shows that there is a separatrix [dashed curve in Fig. 3(e)] limiting the domain of attraction ("attraction basin") of the immune state $(0,E_m)$. From the last two figures one can observe that with a second infection a higher infection dose can be tolerated than with the first one, a behavior which is well known for instance from cholera.

Beyond reproducing such facts the discussion of the model gives a deeper look on the prognosis and may lead to the discovery of strategies on how to interfere with the immune system or the pathogen target in order to cure the patient or at least to keep the disease under control.

An example can be concluded from Fig. 3(e). Assume the infection dose satisfies $T_0>T_c$, i.e., without treatment the disease would be lethal. A treatment should aim at bringing the system on the other side of the separatrix into the domain of attraction of the immune state. This can be

achieved either by improving the immune competence (vertical dotted line) or by target reduction (horizontal dotted line), e.g., by antibiotics therapy, or by a combination of these two strategies.

The model also reproduces the behavior found with infections by smallpox. Here a primary infection ($E_0=0$, $T_0>0$) is generally lethal. However, by vaccination or by a previous infection with cowpox (a virus which is much less virulent than smallpox) an immune state $E_m>0$ can be achieved. In fact, competent immune effectors generated against cowpox are also able to recognize and eliminate smallpox infected cells at least up to a certain degree. This situation is represented by our model if condition (C) is satisfied and r and k are sufficiently large. For an illustration see Fig. 3(f) where again the boundary of the attraction basin of the immune state is indicated by a dashed curve.

Such a basin where the immune system can eliminate the targets does not always exist, for example if the "pathogenity constant" r/k exceeds a certain value E^* [denoting the supremum of the E-components of all points on the nullcline $0=f(T)+g(E)-E$]. In this case, the target population always grows to infinity and no immunity is achieved.

Another situation where a complete target elimination cannot be reached arises if

$$n=1, \quad u=v, \quad s<1 \quad \text{and} \quad 0<r/k<E^*.$$

Under this condition a steady state (T_p,E_p), $E_p=r/k$, exists where both components are positive as illustrated in Fig. 4(a). Targets and immune competent cells coexist in an equilibrium, representing a more or less dangerous chronic disease. Hepatitis B and Salmonella are examples of this type.

The coexistence state is globally attractive for all initial conditions different from (0,0). The movement into the positive steady state may be either oscillatory [Fig. 4(a)], e.g., if

$$0 < g'(r/k) < 1 - \sqrt{4kT_p f'(T_p)}$$

or monotone if

$$1 - \sqrt{4kT_p f'(T_p)} < g'(r/k) < 1.$$

A different type of coexistence is represented by a limit cycle [Fig. 4(b)] where target size and immune competence permanently oscillate around an unstable steady state. Such a limit cycle occurs for instance if

$$n > 1; \quad u = v; \quad s_0 < s < s_1; \quad p > f_1; \quad E_1 < r/k < E_2.$$

In addition to the constants defined with (C) the value of s_0 is given by

$$s_0 = 4n/\sqrt[n]{(n-1)^{(n-1)} + (n+1)^{(n+1)}}$$

and E_2 denotes the local minimum of the function $z(E) = E - g(E)$. Herpex simplex and malaria are examples of diseases which may show a periodic or nearly periodic time course.

Oscillatory dynamics of the immune response has not yet found the attention it deserves. There is apparently a variety of autoimmune diseases, like multiple sclerosis and recurrent inflammations in various organs (e.g., gastrointestinal tract), which show more or less regular sequences of outbreaks. The model clearly shows this oscillatory behavior, which would occur even under much more general conditions on the parameter constants, if the model equations (3) and (4) would be modified more realistically by including time delay effects. Such a time delay model could be, e.g.,

$$\frac{dT}{dt} = rT(t-\tau) - kT(t)E(t),$$

$$\frac{dE}{dt} = f(T(t-\delta)) + g(E(t-\Delta)) - dE(t).$$

The positive delay constants τ, δ, Δ take into account times necessary for molecule production, proliferation, differentiation of cells, transport, etc. It is well known from the theory of differential-delay equations that time delays strongly support oscillatory behavior in these systems. However, we do not go into any analysis of this delay model. Instead, we continue with system (3) and (4).

There are even situations with five steady states: (0,0) saddle, $(T_1, r/k)$ asymptotically stable, $(T_2, r/k)$ unstable, $(0, E_n)$ saddle, and $(0, E_m)$ asymptotically stable, see Fig. 4(c), where the unstable state is not specially marked (E_n is the smallest positive solution of $E^n - sE^{n-1} + 1 = 0$, E_m the largest one). Parameters are as in condition (C), however $0 < r/k < E_1$ and r and k sufficiently small. Then the development of a disease strongly depends on the dose of infection. There are two thresholds, T_S and T_h. A small target dose, $T_0 < T_S$, leads to permanent coexistence of targets and immune competent cells. However, a medium infectious dose, $T_S < T_0 < T_h$ generates an optimal immune response with elimination of the infectious germs, while a high infectious dose, $T_0 > T_h$, cannot be controlled by the immune system. When the immune system has achieved a memory state $(0, E_m)$ a secondary infection will generally lead to that state.

The model also predicts the apparently paradox situation that instead of reducing the target burden, the opposite treatment, an increase in the number of targets, can be of benefit for the patient. As illustrated in Fig. 4(d), by this treatment the immune system escapes the state of coexistence leading again to the elimination of the pathogens and to the creation of an immune state. This case of the model, occurring for example if

$$n > 1; \quad u = v; \quad s > s_1; \quad p > f_1; \quad r/k < E_1$$

gives a rationale for active vaccination under certain conditions.

To be more accurate, an active vaccination operates generally with living but inactivated cells which are not able to reproduce themselves, i.e., $r = 0$ for these cells, or $r < 0$ because of degradation. A modification of the model takes this into account by distinguishing between active (T) and inactivated (T_i) targets:

$$\frac{dT}{dt} = rT - kTE, \tag{5}$$

$$\frac{dE}{dt} = f(T + T_i) + g(E) - E, \tag{6}$$

$$\frac{dT_i}{dt} = -d_i T_i - kT_i E. \tag{7}$$

Another paradoxical situation is predicted by the model [Fig. 4(e)] in the case that

$$n = 1; \quad u < v; \quad s - 1 < r/k < E^*.$$

Here an attempt to cure a patient from the chronic disease by immune stimulation or target reduction could lead to death after a short time of benefit. This situation occurs if the separatrix is crossed during the treatment.

III. CHAOTIC BEHAVIOR

Real time series data of the immune state of patients often look rather irregular. Figure 5(a) shows an empirical example of the number of phenotypically identified natural killer cells (CD 16^+, CD 56^+) versus total tumor size during the course of a metastatic disease (Fibrosarcoma). The number of peripheral blood derived NK cells was determined once every four or five weeks over a period of 475 days. The tumor load was evaluated on the basis of the diameters of several individual lesions registered on x-ray pictures. Both, the number of NK cells and tumor volume exhibit during this period a seemingly "chaotic" behavior: they fluctuate irregularly and apparently unpredictably. Sometimes the tumor even reduces its volume.

The model presented here is not able to produce any kind of chaotic behavior, since it is only two-dimensional. However, we can show that chaos can be induced if at least one of the parameters instead of being constant changes periodically. In this way we obtained the data of Fig. 5(b), where the tumor production rate r has been assumed to

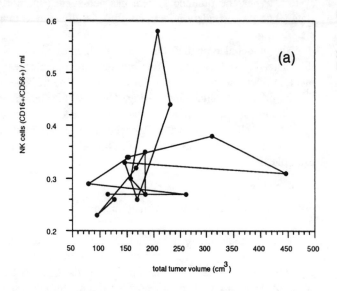

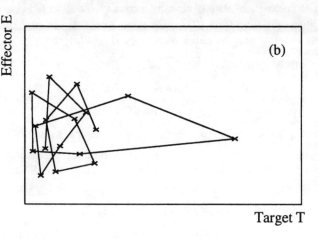

FIG. 5. (a) The NK cell and tumor relationship of a patient suffering from fibrosarcoma. (b) Calculations from the model based on the assumption of sinusoidally changing tumor reproduction rate. Chosen values are $r = 0.7$, $k = 1$, $p = 0.5$, $s = 1.4$, $u = v = 1$, $n = 3$, $\omega = 0.97$, $A = 0.7$; only points of the trajectory separated by 25 time units are plotted.

change sinusoidally and temporally equidistant samples have been taken from the trajectory. Hereby we demonstrate that even a chaotic behavior of the immune system can possibly be generated by a very small number of simple, fully deterministic conditions. Moreover, this model shows that uncorrelated data [like in Fig. 5(a)] do not necessarily exclude a strong connection between the measured quantities.

Of course, by these very few remarks on "chaotic behavior" we neither claim that the empirical data truly exhibit what is called "deterministic chaos" (which probably cannot be shown) nor do we suggest that our low dimensional model explains in any detail those irregular data.

IV. CONCLUSION

Here we stop this introductory discussion of the model. There are still more types of dynamic behavior occurring in other domains of the parameters.

In our opinion, there are at least two advantages of this rather simple and idealistic model which neglects many details. First of all, it shows clearly that the combination of a few mechanisms and interaction rules, as described by the right hand sides of our differential equations (3) and (4), can lead to a large variety of qualitatively different types of immune reactions corresponding to the large variety of phenomena in different diseases or even within a single disease. Second, the well developed techniques of phase plane analysis allow a nearly complete analytical discussion of the two-dimensional model, a goal that generally cannot be reached with high-dimensional systems. Of course, we do not claim, that more complicated models with more variables, for reviews see Refs. 22–27, become superfluous or even lose their significance by this approach. An introductory presentation of our model was given in Ref. 28.

ACKNOWLEDGMENTS

The clinical data were kindly provided by Dr. R. Schietzel, Department of Radiology, Gemeinschaftskrankenhaus Herdecke. This work was supported by Karl Doerken-Stiftung.

[1] K. S. Zaenker (editor), Kommunikationsnetzwerke im Koerper: Psychoneuroimmunologie—Aspekte einer neuen Wissenschaftsdisziplin (Spektrum Akademischer Verlag, Heidelberg, 1991).

[2] I. G. Kevrekidis, A. D. Zecha, and A. S. Perelson, "Modeling dynamical aspects of the immune response: T cell proliferation and the effect of IL–2," in Theoretical Immunology I, edited by A. S. Perelson (Addison–Wesley, New York, 1988), pp. 167–197.

[3] S. Michelson, "Immune surveillance: Towards a tumor-specific model," in Theoretical Immunology II, edited by A. S. Perelson (Addison–Wesley, New York, 1988), pp. 37–55.

[4] B. C. Batt and D. S. Kompala, "Verification of immune response optimality through cybernetic modeling," J. Theor. Biol. 142, 317–340 (1990).

[5] R. Antia, B. Levin, and P. Williamson, "A quantitative model suggests immune memory involves the colocalization of B and Th cells," J. Theor. Biol. 153, 371–384 (1991).

[6] R. J. De Boer, A. S. Perelson, and I. G. Kevrekidis, "Immune network behavior—I. From stationary states to limit cycle oscillations," Bull. Math. Biol. 55, 745–780 (1993).

[7] R. J. De Boer, A. S. Perelson, and I. G. Kevrekidis, "Immune network behavior—II. From oscillations to chaos and stationary states," Bull. Math. Biol. 55, 781–816 (1993).

[8] I. A. Sidorov and A. A. Romanyukha, "Mathematical modeling of T-cell proliferation," Math. Biosci. 115, 187–232 (1993).

[9] B. Sulzer, J. L. Van Hemmen, A. U. Neumann, and U. Behn, "Memory in idiotypic networks due to competition between proliferation and differentiation," Bull. Math. Biol. 55, 1133–1182 (1993).

[10] I. Guckenheimer and P. Holmes (editors), Nonlinear Oscillations, Dynamical Systems, and Bifurcations of Vector Fields (Springer-Verlag, New York, 1983).

[11] A. M. Molchanov, "Biophysics of complex systems. Mathematical models. Multibarrier immunity," Biophysics 16, 500–506 (1971).

[12] A. M. Molchanov, V. G. Nazarenko, and I. G. Shaturnyi, "Biophysics of complex systems. Mathematical models. Analysis of the model of single-barrier immunity," Biophysics 16, 692–697 (1971).

[13] G. I. Bell, "Predator–prey equations simulating an immune response," Math. Biosciences 16, 291–314 (1973).

[14] B. F. Dibrov, M. A. Livshits, and M. V. Volkenstein, "Mathematical models of immune processes," J. Theor. Biol. **65**, 609–631 (1977).

[15] B. F. Dibrov, M. A. Livshits, and M. V. Volkenstein, "Mathematical models of immune processes. II. Kinetic features of antigen–antibody interactions," J. Theoret. Biol. **69**, 23–39 (1977).

[16] P. Waltman and E. Butz, "A threshold model of antigen-antibody dynamics," J. Theor. Biol. **65**, 499–512 (1977).

[17] S. J. Merill, " A model of the stimulation of B-cells by replication antigen —I, II," Math. Biosci. **41**, 125–155 (1978).

[18] A. Albert, M. Freedman, and A. S. Perelson, "Tumors and the immune system: The effects of a tumor growth modulator," Math. Biosci. **50**, 25–58 (1980).

[19] J. R. Hiernaux and R. Lefever, "Population dynamics of tumors attacked by immunocompetent killer cells," in Ref. 3, pp. 19–35.

[20] A. R. McLean and T. B. L. Kirkwood, "A model of human immunodeficiency virus infection in T helper cell clones," J. Theor. Biol. **147**, 177–203 (1990).

[21] V. A. Kuznetsov, I. A. Makalkin, M. A. Taylor, and A. S. Perelson, "Non-linear dynamics of immunogenic tumors: Parameter estimation and global bifurcation analysis," Bull. Math. Biol. **56**, 295–321 (1994).

[22] R. R. Mohler, C. Bruni, and A. Gandolfi, "A systems approach to immunology," Proc. IEEE **68**, 964–990 (1980).

[23] G. I. Marchuk and I. N. Belykh (editors), *Mathematical Modelling in Immunology and Medicine* (North-Holland, Amsterdam, 1982).

[24] G. I. Marchuk (editor), *Mathematical Models in Immunology* (Optimization Software INC, Publication Division, New York, 1983).

[25] S. Levin (editor), *Immunology and Epidemiology* (Springer-Verlag, Berlin, 1985).

[26] A. S. Perelson (editor), *Theoretical Immunology I, II* (Addison–Wesley, Redwood City, CA, 1988).

[27] D. Prikrylova, M. Jilek, and J. Waniewski, *Mathematical Modeling of the Immune Response* (CRC Press, Boca Raton, FL, 1992).

[28] D. P. F. Moeller and O. Richter (editors), *Fortschritte der Simulation in Medizin, Biologie und Oekologie* (Technische Universitaet Clausthal, Clausthal, 1992).

Shift of a limit cycle in biology: From pathological to physiological homeostasia*

Daniel Claude

Laboratoire des Signaux et Systèmes, C.N.R.S.—E.S.E., Plateau de Moulon, 91190 Gif-sur-Yvette, France

(Received 10 May 1994; accepted for publication 21 September 1994)

Biological systems may show homeostatic behaviors that are similar to the ones of forced dynamic systems with a stable limit cycle. For a large class of dynamic systems, it is shown that a shift of a pathological limit cycle over the physiological limit cycle can never be executed by means of a control with a desired periodicity. The above statement shows that the only possibility is to reduce as much as possible the dimensions of a small residual limit cycle. Moreover, it is possible to give some information about the structure of feedback laws that would allow the shift of the limit cycle. The fact that it is generally not possible to recover a physiological limit cycle from a pathological one, results into the fear of never or hardly ever reaching a physiological behavior, and it seems that any hope of therapeutics is given up. This leads to introduce the locking concept, which permits system parameters to change and provides the basis for an adaptive and iterative control, which allows a step by step approach and to finally reach the physiological limit cycle. © *1995 American Institute of Physics.*

I. INTRODUCTION

Biology has essentially a nonlinear character and biological systems may show homeostatic behaviors,[1] which are similar to the ones of dynamic systems with a stable limit cycle.[2] This is the case of the adrenal-postpituitary system (see Refs. 3–7), which shows a limit cycle that can be physiological or pathological, according to the circumstances. Moreover, as many biological systems, the adrenal-postpituitary system is forced by the circadian synchronization "night–day" and the limit cycle has a circadian period.

Homeostasia[1] has an autonomous character, but for hormonal regulations it can be considered to administrate similar but exogenous hormones. The biological system does not make any difference between endogenous and exogenous hormones, thus providing the bases for therapeutics.

Therefore, as in the case of the adrenal-postpituitary system,[4,7] the aim of the control designs for therapeutical actions is to change a pathological limit cycle through a physiological one. From the control viewpoint, this means that physicians should reduce the gap between the behavior of the controlled pathological system and the physiological one. However, it is advisable to keep their natural periodicity for the endogenous hormones to avoid, by concatenation of imbalances, serious biological disorders. Consequently, the control law will have the same periodicity. However, in this case it is proved here, by generalization of demonstrations given in Refs. 7 and 8, that it is not possible to find the physiological rhythm again through a dynamical model of the controlled pathological system. From the control viewpoint, this means that one should not try to obtain an asymptotical convergence of the associated error toward zero.[8] The only possibility consists of reducing as much as possible a small residual limit cycle. Moreover, it is possible to give some information about the structure of feedback laws that would allow the shift of a limit cycle.

The fact that it is generally not possible to recover a physiological limit cycle from a pathological one, results into the fear of never or hardly ever reaching a physiological behavior, and thus it seems that any hope of therapeutics is given up. This leads to introducing the locking concept, which permits system parameters to change and provides the basis for an adaptive and iterative control which allows a step by step approach and to finally reach the physiological limit cycle (cf. Ref. 7 in the case of the adrenal-postpituitary system).

II. MODEL OF A HORMONAL COUPLE WITH A HOMEOSTATIC LIMIT CYCLE AND ITS CONTROL

Let us consider two *endogenous hormonal agents* represented by two variables x and y, with positive constraints as a result of the natural boundaries of hormonal concentrations. The modeling is based on the fact that the evolution of the biological system, represented by the couple (x,y) is simultaneously controlled by the changes of the variable $\mathscr{X}=x+X$ and variable $\mathscr{Y}=y+Y$, where X and Y represent the *exogenous hormonal agents*, which form the bases for therapeutical actions.

Thus, it is permitted to propose the following state-space description of the behavior of a hormonal couple in cases where there are no specific stimuli:

$$\dot{x}=D_1(\kappa_1,p_1,\mathscr{X},\mathscr{Y},S),$$
$$\dot{y}=D_2(\kappa_2,p_2,\mathscr{X},\mathscr{Y},S), \tag{2.1}$$

where κ_1, κ_2, p_1, and p_2 are vectorial constant parameters and $S(t)$ is a synchronizer, common in chronobiology.

When the controls X, Y, and the synchronizer S are zero, $(0,0)$ is a critical point of system (2.1).[2]

Model (2.1) represents the system both in the physiological and in the pathological case. The first one is represented by the parameters $\kappa^{\varphi}=(\kappa_1^{\varphi},\kappa_2^{\varphi})$, which determine the developments of D_1^{φ} and D_2^{φ}. The second one is determined by different parameters $\kappa^{\psi}=(\kappa_1^{\psi},\kappa_2^{\psi})$, characterizing D_1^{ψ} and D_2^{ψ}. Parameters p_1, p_2 are supposed to be common to both

*In homage to François Rabelais and to the "substantificque mouelle."

the pathological and physiological systems. We assume that D_1 and D_2 are linear functions of parameters κ_1 and κ_2, respectively. This fact is natural in modeling.

When $X=0$ and $Y=0$, the physiological system, as well as the pathological system, admit a specific stable limit cycle with a period T, under the influence of the synchronizer, which possesses a period T, which is circadian, for example with a model of the adrenal-postpituitary system (cf. Refs. 6 and 7).

The therapeutical strategy consists in searching the temporal rules to be followed by the exogenous hormones X and Y so that, after a transient period, the state of the controlled system (2.1) get as close as possible to a physiological behavior with the constraints $X \geqslant 0$, $Y \geqslant 0$, $x \geqslant 0$, $y \geqslant 0$. However, in order to preserve biologic rhythms (Ref. 9) for endogenous hormones, as well as other biological systems, which depends directly or indirectly on this particular hormonal production, it is appealing to have a periodic evolution with a period T for pathological endogenous hormones. Thus, in the case that $(\mathscr{X}, \mathscr{Y})$ follows the physiological limit cycle, $\mathscr{X}=x+X$, $\mathscr{Y}=y+Y$, x and y should be functions with a period T, and consequently $X=\mathscr{X}-x$ and $Y=\mathscr{Y}-y$ should all have a period T. Thus, after a transient period, the exogenous hormones should be periodical functions of period T, which produces an attractive pharmacopoeia.

Through the usual control and decoupling techniques, one defines a new state $(x, y, \mathscr{X}, \mathscr{Y})$, and the pathological system (2.1) can be rewritten as a nonlinear system of the following type, where a_1 and a_2 now represent the new control, and s_1, s_2 the measurable outputs:

$$\dot{x}=D_1(\kappa_1^\psi, p_1, \mathscr{X}, \mathscr{Y}, S),$$

$$\dot{y}=D_2(\kappa_2^\psi, p_2, \mathscr{X}, \mathscr{Y}, S),$$

$$\dot{\mathscr{X}}=D_1(\kappa_1^\varphi, p_1, \mathscr{X}, \mathscr{Y}, S)+a_1,$$

$$\dot{\mathscr{Y}}=D_2(\kappa_2^\varphi, p_2, \mathscr{X}, \mathscr{Y}, S)+a_2, \qquad (2.2)$$

$$s_1=\mathscr{X},$$

$$s_2=\mathscr{Y},$$

this system being submitted to the constraints $\mathscr{X} \geqslant x \geqslant 0$, $\mathscr{Y} \geqslant y \geqslant 0$ and $\mathscr{X}$, as well as $\mathscr{Y}$ bounded.

The actual control law is given by

$$(X,Y)=(\mathscr{X}-x, \mathscr{Y}-y), \qquad (2.3)$$

and the aim of control (X,Y) is to give $(\mathscr{X}, \mathscr{Y})$ the same behavior as physiological hormones.

III. SHIFT OF A LIMIT CYCLE

The model (2.1) has, in the physiological case, as well as in the pathological case, the same synchronizer S with T as its period.

Thus, the physiological system,

$$\dot{x}=D_1(\kappa_1^\varphi, p_1, \mathscr{X}, \mathscr{Y}, S),$$

$$\dot{y}=D_2(\kappa_2^\varphi, p_2, \mathscr{X}, \mathscr{Y}, S),$$

$$s_1=\mathscr{X}, \qquad (3.1)$$

$$s_2=\mathscr{Y},$$

with the controls $X=0$ and $Y=0$, is supposed to have a stable limit cycle (x^φ, y^φ), which represents a periodic function of period T and which is called a *physiological limit cycle*.

Thus, we have

$$x^\varphi(T)=x^\varphi(0)+\int_0^T D_1[\kappa_1^\varphi, p_1, x^\varphi(\tau), y^\varphi(\tau), S(\tau)]d\tau,$$

$$y^\varphi(T)=y^\varphi(0)+\int_0^T D_2[\kappa_2^\varphi, p_2, x^\varphi(\tau), y^\varphi(\tau), S(\tau)]d\tau,$$

and consequently, if we note

$$\tilde{D}_1^\varphi(\tau)=D_1[\kappa_1^\varphi, p_1, x^\varphi(\tau), y^\varphi(\tau), S(\tau)]$$

and

$$\tilde{D}_2^\varphi(\tau)=D_2[\kappa_2^\varphi, p_2, x^\varphi(\tau), y^\varphi(\tau), S(\tau)],$$

we find

$$\int_0^T \tilde{D}_1^\varphi(\tau)d\tau=0 \quad \text{and} \quad \int_0^T \tilde{D}_2^\varphi(\tau)d\tau=0. \qquad (3.2)$$

Likewise, the pathological system,

$$\dot{x}=D_1(\kappa_1^\psi, p_1, \mathscr{X}, \mathscr{Y}, S),$$

$$\dot{y}=D_2(\kappa_2^\psi, p_2, \mathscr{X}, \mathscr{Y}, S),$$

$$s_1=\mathscr{X}, \qquad (3.3)$$

$$s_2=\mathscr{Y},$$

with the controls $X=0$ and $Y=0$, is also supposed to have a *pathological limit cycle* (x^ψ, y^ψ), with the same period T.

Then we define the maps Φ_1 and Φ_2 with the parameters κ_1 and κ_2, respectively,

$$\Phi_1(\kappa_1)=\int_0^T D_1[\kappa_1, p_1, x^\varphi(\tau), y^\varphi(\tau), S(\tau)]d\tau,$$

$$\Phi_2(\kappa_2)=\int_0^T D_2[\kappa_2, p_2, x^\varphi(\tau), y^\varphi(\tau), S(\tau)]d\tau. \qquad (3.4)$$

As D_1 and D_2, respectively, are $\mathbb{R}$-linear functions of κ_1 and κ_2, these maps constitute two $\mathbb{R}$-linear forms, and we suppose that they are not identical to zero.

For example, for the adrenal-postpituitary system, we have (cf. Ref. 7)

$$\Phi_1(0,1,0,0,0,0)$$

$$=\Phi_2(0,1,0,0,0,0)=\int_0^T [x^\varphi(\tau)-y^\varphi(\tau)]^2 d\tau \neq 0,$$

because in this case $x^\varphi-y^\varphi \neq 0$.

Moreover, as we have $\Phi_1(\kappa_1^\varphi)=0$ and $\Phi_2(\kappa_2^\varphi)=0$ from (3.2), the kernel of Φ_1 is defined by a hyperplane that contains the physiological parameters κ_1^φ as well as ker Φ_2, which is a hyperplane containing the physiological parameters κ_2^φ.

Proposition 3.1: If $\Phi_1 \neq 0$ and $\Phi_2 \neq 0$, a necessary and sufficient condition for the existence of a continuous control of period T, after a transient period, which allows the output of pathological system (3.3) to follow the limit cycle (x^φ, y^φ) is

$$\kappa_1^\psi \in \ker \Phi_1 \quad \text{and} \quad \kappa_2^\psi \in \ker \Phi_2. \tag{3.5}$$

$\triangle$ If for time $t \geq 0$, there should be a periodic control (X,Y) of period T, which would give the trajectory (x^φ, y^φ) for the outputs of system (3.3), it should be true that $\mathscr{X} = x^\varphi$, $\mathscr{Y} = y^\varphi$, and $\mathscr{X}$ and $\mathscr{Y}$ should be periodic functions of period T. Consequently, the endogenous variables $x = \mathscr{X} - X$ and $y = \mathscr{Y} - Y$ should also have a period T. Thus, the endogenous variables $x(t)$ and $y(t)$ of system (3.3), given by the following equations:

$$x(t) = x(0) + \int_0^t D_1[\kappa_1^\psi, p_1, x^\varphi(\tau), y^\varphi(\tau), S(\tau)] d\tau,$$

$$y(t) = y(0) + \int_0^t D_2[\kappa_2^\psi, p_2, x^\varphi(\tau), y^\varphi(\tau), S(\tau)] d\tau, \tag{3.6}$$

would be periodic of period T.

Therefore, we would have $x(T) = x(0)$ and $y(T) = y(0)$. Hence, if we note

$$\tilde{D}_1^\psi(\tau) = D_1[\kappa_1^\psi, p_1, x^\varphi(\tau), y^\varphi(\tau), S(\tau)]$$

and

$$\tilde{D}_2^\psi(\tau) = D_2[\kappa_2^\psi, p_2, x^\varphi(\tau), y^\varphi(\tau), S(\tau)],$$

we have

$$\int_0^T \tilde{D}_1^\psi(\tau) d\tau = \Phi_1(\kappa_1^\psi) = 0$$

and

$$\int_0^T \tilde{D}_2^\psi(\tau) d\tau = \Phi_2(\kappa_2^\psi) = 0.$$

Thus,

$$\kappa_1^\psi \in \ker \Phi_1 \quad \text{and} \quad \kappa_2^\psi \in \ker \Phi_2.$$

Moreover, one finds

$$X(t) = x^\varphi(t) - x(0) - \int_0^t \tilde{D}_1^\psi(\tau) d\tau,$$

$$Y(t) = y^\varphi(t) - y(0) - \int_0^t \tilde{D}_2^\psi(\tau) d\tau. \tag{3.7}$$

However, it is easy to verify that X and Y are periodic of period T for $t \geq 0$. Indeed, for any t, we have

$$X(t+T) - X(t)$$

$$= x^\varphi(t+T) - x^\varphi(t) - \int_0^{t+T} \tilde{D}_1^\psi d(\tau) + \int_0^t \tilde{D}_1^\psi(\tau) d\tau$$

$$= -\int_0^T \tilde{D}_1^\psi(\tau) d\tau - \int_T^{t+T} \tilde{D}_1^\psi(\tau) d\tau + \int_0^t \tilde{D}_1^\psi(\tau) d\tau.$$

Making use of the T periodicity of $\tilde{D}_1^\psi(\tau)$, we can write

$$\int_T^{t+T} \tilde{D}_1^\psi(\tau) d\tau = \int_0^t \tilde{D}_1^\psi(\tau) d\tau.$$

Therefore, we have

$$X(t+T) - X(t) = -\int_0^T \tilde{D}_1^\psi(\tau) d\tau = -\Phi_1(\kappa_1^\psi) = 0,$$

because $\kappa_1^\psi \in \ker \Phi_1$. The same result can be established for function Y. Thus $[x(t), y(t)]$, given by Eq. (3.6), is the only solution of Eq. (3.3):

$$\dot{x} = D_1[\kappa_1^\psi, p_1, (x+X), (y+Y), S],$$

$$\dot{y} = D_1[\kappa_2^\psi, p_2, (x+X), (y+Y), S], \tag{3.8}$$

with $[x(0), y(0)]$ as the initial conditions, and X, Y given by relations (3.7).

Reciprocally, if $\kappa_1^\psi \in \ker \Phi_1$ and $\kappa_2^\psi \in \ker \Phi_2$, X, Y, given by Eqs. (3.7), are periodic functions of T. Moreover, system (3.3), with $[x(0), y(0)]$ as the initial conditions, and (X,Y) given by (3.7) as control law, has for solutions $x(t)$ and $y(t)$ given by Eqs. (3.6). Therefore, we have

$$\mathscr{X}(t) = x(t) + X(t) = x^\varphi(t),$$

$$\mathscr{Y}(t) = y(t) + Y(t) = y^\varphi(t).$$

So, for $t \geq 0$ we found a periodic continuous control law of period T, which allows the outputs of the pathological system (3.3) to follow the physiological limit cycle. $\triangle$

Remark 3.1: The positivity constraints for X, Y, x, y have not been taken into account.

Remark 3.2: As a hyperplane is a subset of measure zero, the conditions $\kappa_1^\psi \in \ker \Phi_1$ and $\kappa_2^\psi \in \ker \Phi_2$ are not generic.

Corollary 3.1: If $\kappa_1^\psi \notin \ker \Phi_1$ or $\kappa_2^\psi \notin \ker \Phi_2$, the control law $(a_1, a_2) = (0,0)$ applied to the pathological system (2.2) does not permit $(\mathscr{X}, \mathscr{Y})$ to reach the physiological limit cycle with a periodic continuous control (X,Y) of period T.

Corollary 3.2: If $\mathscr{X}$ and $\mathscr{Y}$ are, respectively, equal to x^φ and y^φ, and if $\kappa_1^\psi \notin \ker \Phi_1$ or $\kappa_2^\psi \notin \ker \Phi_2$, the trajectory $[x(t), y(t)]$ of system (3.3) diverges.

$\triangle$ For any t, the solutions of system (3.3) verify

$$x(t+T) - x(t) = \int_t^{t+T} \tilde{D}_1^\psi(\tau) d\tau$$

$$= \int_0^T \tilde{D}_1^\psi(\tau) d\tau + \int_T^{t+T} \tilde{D}_1^\psi(\tau) d\tau$$

$$- \int_0^t \tilde{D}_1^\psi(\tau) d\tau.$$

Making use of the T periodicity of D_1^ψ, we can write

$$\int_T^{t+T} \tilde{D}_1^\psi(\tau) d\tau = \int_0^t \tilde{D}_1^\psi(\tau) d\tau,$$

therefore we have

$$x(t+T) - x(t) = \int_0^T \tilde{D}_1^\psi(\tau) d\tau = \Phi_1(\kappa_1^\psi)$$

and

$$y(t+T)-y(t)=\int_0^T \tilde{D}_2^\psi(\tau)d\tau=\Phi_2(\kappa_2^\psi).$$

These relations show that we obtain:

$$x(T)-x(0)=\Phi_1(\kappa_1^\psi),$$
$$y(T)-y(0)=\Phi_2(\kappa_2^\psi).$$ (3.9)

Therefore, as $\Phi_1(\kappa_1^\psi)\neq 0$ or $\Phi_2(\kappa_2^\psi)\neq 0$, the trajectory during $[kT,(k+1)T]$ is obtained from the trajectory defined during $[(k-1)T,kT]$ by applying a constant affine drift and the trajectory diverges.   △

Theorem 3.1: In general, no control law allows the outputs of pathological system (3.3) to follow the physiological limit cycle.

△ This statement is directly deduced from Remark 3.2 and Proposition 3.1.   △

Now, if we consider that physiological as well as pathological systems are structurally stable,[2] the notion of a limit cycle must be enlarged to the set of the limit cycles of physiological or pathological systems (2.1) with the parameters $\kappa^{\varphi'}$ or $\kappa^{\psi'}$ chosen within a neighborhood of κ^φ or κ^ψ, respectively.

Moreover, all these systems being forced by the same synchronizer S, the fact that they have limit cycles of period T is quite suitable.

Thus, in the case where the parameters $\kappa^{\psi'} = (\kappa_1^{\psi'},\kappa_2^{\psi'})$ of system (3.3) verify

$$\kappa_1^{\psi'} \in \ker \Phi_1' \quad \text{and} \quad \kappa_2^{\psi'} \in \ker \Phi_2',$$

where Φ_1' and Φ_2' indicate the hyperplanes associated with the physiological limit cycle $(x^{\varphi'},y^{\varphi'})$, and Proposition 3.1 shows that the resulting control law (X',Y') of period T, applied to the pathological system with parameters $\kappa^{\psi'}$ allows $\mathscr{X},\mathscr{Y}$ to follow $x^{\varphi'}$ and $y^{\varphi'}$.

However, if we choose $\kappa^{\psi''}=(\kappa_1^{\psi''},\kappa_2^{\psi''})$ within a neighborhood of $\kappa^{\psi'}$, so that $\kappa_1^{\psi''} \notin \ker \Phi_1'$ or $\kappa_2^{\psi''} \notin \ker \Phi_2'$, and if we apply control law (X',Y'), Corollary 3.2 shows that a divergent trajectory is obtained. This fact indicates that the open loop control law (X',Y') is unstable. Thus, it is impossible to recover the physiological behavior given by an equation of the type (3.1), and it is necessary to search a control law that allows the controlled pathological system to follow a limit cycle close to the physiological limit cycle. Moreover, due to the additionally pharmacokinetical constraints on exogenous hormonal variations, generally one ought to envisage to reduce as much as possible the dimensions of a small residual limit cycle obtained by the difference between the output of the controlled pathological system and the physiological limit cycle.

IV. FEEDBACK LAW

In order to reduce, as much as possible, the dimensions of a small residual limit cycle with the controlled pathological system and to avoid the disadvantage of an open loop control law, we may envisage the use of a feedback law. Then we may consider the system (2.2):

$$\dot{x}=D_1(\kappa_1^\psi,p_1,\mathscr{X},\mathscr{Y},S),$$
$$\dot{y}=D_2(\kappa_2^\psi,p_2,\mathscr{X},\mathscr{Y},S),$$
$$\dot{\mathscr{X}}=D_1(\kappa_1^\varphi,p_1,\mathscr{X},\mathscr{Y},S)+a_1,$$
$$\dot{\mathscr{Y}}=D_2(\kappa_2^\varphi,p_2,\mathscr{X},\mathscr{Y},S)+a_2,$$ (4.1)
$$s_1=\mathscr{X},$$
$$s_2=\mathscr{Y},$$

and with the aim of creating a deformation of the physiological vector field, we take for a_1, a_2 a feedback law of the type

$$a_1=F_1(\theta_1,x,\mathscr{X},y,\mathscr{Y},S),$$
$$a_2=F_2(\theta_2,x,\mathscr{X},y,\mathscr{Y},S),$$ (4.2)

with θ_1,θ_2, as vectorial constant parameters, and where F_1, F_2 denote linear functions of parameters θ_1 and θ_2, respectively, so that

$$F_1(0,x,\mathscr{X},y,\mathscr{Y},S)=0 \quad \text{and} \quad F_2(0,x,\mathscr{X},y,\mathscr{Y},S)=0.$$

From a medical point of view, it would be very interesting to take a feedback law of the type

$$a_1=G_1(\theta_1,\mathscr{X},\mathscr{Y},S),$$
$$a_2=G_2(\theta_2,\mathscr{X},\mathscr{Y},S),$$ (4.3)

where G_1, G_2 denotes linear functions of parameters θ_1 and θ_2, respectively. This feedback law only measures the blood concentration of $\mathscr{X}$ and $\mathscr{Y}$ hormones. However, the same demonstrations as in Sec. III can be applied and we find the following.

Proposition 4.1: In general, there is no feedback law (a_1,a_2) of type (4.3) that allows $(\mathscr{X},\mathscr{Y})$ to follow a limit cycle of period T, and that allows (x,y) to follow a limit cycle of period T as well.

△ Let E_1 and E_2 be defined by the equalities

$$E_1(\kappa_1,\theta_1,p_1,\mathscr{X},\mathscr{Y},S)=D_1(\kappa_1,p_1,\mathscr{X},\mathscr{Y},S)$$
$$+G_1(\theta_1,\mathscr{X},\mathscr{Y},S),$$
$$E_2(\kappa_2,\theta_2,p_2,x,\mathscr{X},y,\mathscr{Y},S)=D_2(\kappa_2,p_2,\mathscr{X},\mathscr{Y},S)$$ (4.4)
$$+G_2(\theta_2,\mathscr{X},\mathscr{Y},S).$$

In particular, we have

$$D_1(\kappa_1^\psi,p_1,\mathscr{X},\mathscr{Y},S)=E_1(\kappa_1^\psi,0,p_1,\mathscr{X},\mathscr{Y},S),$$
$$D_2(\kappa_2^\psi,p_2,\mathscr{X},\mathscr{Y},S)=E_2(\kappa_2^\psi,0,p_2,\mathscr{X},\mathscr{Y},S).$$

Thus, as for Theorem 3.1, generally no feedback law, given by G_1 and G_2, allows the parameters $(\kappa_1^\varphi,\theta_1)$ and $(\kappa_1^\psi,0)$ as well as $(\kappa_2^\varphi,\theta_2)$ and $(\kappa_2^\psi,0)$, respectively, to belong to the same vectorial hyperplane.   △

Thus, the only possibility is to search feedback laws that are based both on a global concentration of the hormones $\mathscr{X}$ and $\mathscr{Y}$ and the production of the x and y endogenous pathological hormones, which is predictable by means of Eq. (3.3).

Moreover, with the control laws X and Y, which are periodic functions of period T, it is interesting to force Eqs. (4.1) by expressions of the type

$$a_1 = F_1(\theta_1, x, \mathscr{X}, y, \mathscr{Y}, S) = \tilde{F}_1(\tilde{\theta}_1, \mathscr{X} - x) + \beta_1,$$

$$a_2 = F_2(\theta_2, x, \mathscr{X}, y, \mathscr{Y}, S) = \tilde{F}_2(\tilde{\theta}_2, \mathscr{Y} - y) + \beta_2, \qquad (4.5)$$

with β_1, β_2 as two constant parameters. Then, if the system (4.1), without the synchronizer S, admit a stable limit cycle and is structurally stable, it is reasonable to obtain a robust control law with respect to only small parameter variations or small deformations of the control law, the synchronizer maintaining the periodicity.

This method has been applied to a model of the adrenal-postpituitary system (cf. Ref. 7), and the parameters θ_1, β_1 and θ_2, β_2 have been computed to reduce as much as possible the dimensions of a small residual limit cycle.

V. CONCLUSION

Particular controls in biology, aiming at therapeutical actions, consist of the shift of a limit cycle from a pathological to a physiological homeostasia.

For a large class of nonlinear model of biological systems with homeostasia described by a stable limit cycle, we have shown that, in general, it is not possible to recover a physiological limit cycle from a pathological limit cycle by means of any control law with a desired period. The only possibility is to reduce as much as possible the dimensions of a small residual limit cycle.

From a practical point of view, one might conclude that there are cases where it is impossible to reach a physiological behavior, and thus give up any hope of therapeutics. However, a feasible approach is based on a locking thesis. This thesis presumes in the therapeutical act, that the pathological system parameters may reach the physiological ones, by a reversible movement, which is the only possibility that allows to control the system during a bounded time. This leads us to introduce *the locking concept.*

This notion can be formulated in the following way: *in some pathologies, when the controlled system follows a periodic behavior for a rather long time, it will copy it by adapting its parameters, now behaving as an uncontrolled system.*

Indeed, we suppose that the biological system cannot make the difference between the endogenous and the exogenous hormones, and thus it "ignores" that it is controlled.

We may note that this locking thesis appears, in particular, in psychiatry, and especially in the work of Watzlawick and Weakland,[10] and from our point of view behind the conditional reflex of Pavlov and the impregnation concept of Lorenz. In biology, a reversible example of locking is given by the engram of dental occlusion: the cerebral image of dental interdigitation can, in fact, change,[11] but the evolution toward another position may have a rather long transient period.

Possible locking of nonlinear oscillators suggest a nonlinear adaptive control process of imbalances, since system parameters can change and iterative control allows a step-by-step approach to finally reach the physiological limit cycle (cf. Ref. 7 for the adrenal-postpituitary system).

In order to be complete in this paper, one should note that if the constraint to have hormonal evolutions and control laws with the same period as the one of the synchronizer can be removed, then the search for almost periodic functions (cf. Ref. 12, for example) may lead to other interesting approximations of the physiological behavior.

[1] *International Dictionary of Medicine and Biology* (Wiley, New York, 1986).

[2] L. Perko, *Differential Equations and Dynamical Systems* (Springer-Verlag, New York, 1991).

[3] E.-E. Baulieu and P. A. Kelly, *Hormones: From Molecules to Disease* (Hermann, Paris, 1990).

[4] E. Bernard-Weil, "Lack of response to a drug: A system theory approach," Kybernetes **14**, 25–30 (1985).

[5] E. Bernard-Weil, "Interactions entre les modèles empirique et mathématique dans la vasopressino-corticothérapie de certaines affections cancéreuses," in *Régulations Physiologiques: Modèles Récents,* edited by G. Chauvet and J. A. Jacquez (Masson, Paris, 1986), pp. 133–155.

[6] E. Bernard-Weil, "A general model for the simulation of balance, imbalance and control by agonistic–antagonistic biological couples," Math. Modelling **7**, 1587–1600 (1986).

[7] D. Claude and N. Nadjar, "Nonlinear adaptive control of adrenal-postpituitary imbalances and identifiability analysis," J. Math. Biosci. **121**, 155–192 (1994).

[8] D. Claude, "Shift of a limit cycle in biology and error equation," J. Math. Syst. Estimation Control **4**, 85–97 (1994).

[9] *Biologic Rhythms in Clinical and Laboratory Medicine,* edited by Y. Touitou and E. Haus (Springer-Verlag, New York, 1992).

[10] P. Watzlawick and J. H. Weakland, *The Interactional View, Works of the Mental Research Institute Palo Alto, 1967–1974* (Norton, New York, 1977).

[11] A. G. Petrovic, J. J. Stutzman, and J. M. Lavergne, "Mechanisms of cranio-facial growth and modus operandi of functional appliances: A cell-level and cybernetic approach to orthodontic decision making," *Cranio-facial Growth Theory and Orthodontic Treatment,* edited by D. S. Carlson, Cranio-facial Growth Series 23, Center for Human Growth & Development (The University of Michigan, Ann Arbor, MI, 1990).

[12] J. K. Hale, *Oscillations in Nonlinear Systems* (McGraw-Hill, New York, 1963).

"Dynamical confinement" in neural networks and cell cycle

J. Demongeot, D. Benaouda, and C. Jézéquel
TIMC–IMAG, University J. Fourier of Grenoble, Faculty of Medicine, 38 700 La Tronche, France

(Received 26 May 1994; accepted for publication 21 September 1994)

In this paper randomization of well-known former mathematical models is proposed (i.e., the Hopfield model for neural networks and the Hahn model for the cell cycle) in order to facilitate the study of their asymptotic behavior: in fact, we replace the determination of the stability basins for attractors and boundaries by the study of a unique (or a small number of) invariant measure(s), whose distribution function maxima (or, respectively, percentile contour lines) correspond to the location of the attractors (or, respectively, boundaries of their stability basins). We give the name of "confinement" to this localization of the mass of the invariant measure(s). We intend to show here that the study of the confinement is in certain cases easier than the study of underlying attractors, in particular if these last are numerous and possess small stability basins (for example, for the first time we calculate the invariant measure in the random Hopfield model in a case for which the deterministic version exhibits many attractors, and in a case of phase transition). © *1995 American Institute of Physics.*

I. INTRODUCTION

Neural networks and, more generally, cell populations present complex dynamics explaining their anatomic and functional characteristics (e.g., their 3-D morphology, their endocrine or memory properties, ...). If we suppose that these collective living systems are observable on their asymptotically stable trajectories, other than for certain transient periods after perturbations (sensory stimulation, feeding, heating, pH change,...), the essential part of their dynamical study can be summarized by determining their attractors (or respectively, confiners) in the deterministic (or respectively, stochastic) version of their mathematical models. Each perturbation can cause changes in stability basins (hence a change of the attractor observed after perturbation), loss, or restoration of synchrony. These important features in the behavior of neurons or cells may be responsible for cell populations being placed on a survival attractor in the case of a pathologic perturbation, or in a synchronous mode for secreting a hormone at particular times, or for evoking a same potential activity (recordable for example by EEG or PET scanner), or for causing a same recall memory phenomenon. In this paper, we will study such collective behaviors using the stochastic version of simple models of neural networks or cell populations in order to simplify the study of the attractors and their stability properties by focusing on their invariant measure. Therefore, we will present archetypal mathematical models to illustrate the power of concepts important in biomedical applications, related to the invariant measure such as confiners, stochastic isochrons, phase transition, or Kolmogorov–Sinaï entropy. First we will study the stochastic version of the Hopfield neuronal model, the aim of which is not an exact fit with physiological reality, but to simply introduce the central notion of phase transition, i.e., the multiplicity of invariant measures. Then we will study the stochastic version of the Hahn cell cycle model, in order to introduce the notion of Kolmogorov–Sinaï entropy which can be used to quantify synchrony phenomena.

II. NEURAL NETWORKS

The random version of the Hopfield neural network is defined by the following stochastic evolution equation, available for each neuron i amongst the N neurons of the network R:

$$P[x_i(t+1)=a|x_j(t),j \in V_i]$$
$$=e^{a\Sigma_{j \in V_i} w_{ij}x_j(t)/T}/(1+e^{\Sigma_{j \in V_i} w_{ij}x_j(t)/T}),$$

where $x_i(t+1)$ is the activity of the neuron i at time $(t+1)$, V_i is a neighborhood of i, w_{ij} is the synaptic weight between j and i, and T is the temperature of the network R. If $T=0$, we then recover the deterministic version of the Hopfield model.

A. Block-sequential invariant measure for the random Hopfield model

Let us now consider a modular neural network R made from the union of n subnetworks R_r $(r=1,...,n)$, each having m neurons, with $N=nm$ (see Fig. 1). For the sake of simplicity, we suppose that R_r's are identical, synaptic weights w_{ij} $(i,j=1,...,N;i \neq j)$, are symmetrical, and w_{ii}'s $(i=1,...,N)$ are equal to 0. We then have the following.

Lemma 1: The invariant measure of the neural network is given by:

$$\mu(A)=\sum_{R \supset B} e^{\langle\langle B,A\rangle\rangle+\langle A\rangle},$$

where

$$\langle\langle B,A\rangle\rangle=\sum_{k=1}^{n} \sum_{i \in B_k,j \in A^k} w_{ij},$$

where

$$B_k=B\cap(\underset{r=1}{\overset{k}{\cup}} R_r)$$

and

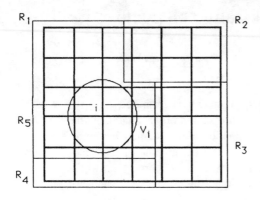

FIG. 1. Network R, union of five subnetworks R_r ($r=1,...,5$).

$$A^k = A \cap (\bigcup_{r=k}^{n} R_r),$$

and where

$$\langle A \rangle = \sum_{i,j \in A; i<j} w_{ij}.$$

Proof: The general coefficient $M_{A,C}$ of the Markovian matrix M giving the probability to move from the configuration A in R to the configuration C in R, after synchronously updating the m neurons of a subnetwork, and successively the subnetworks R_r ($r=1,...,n$), is given by

$$M_{A,C} = e^{\langle\langle C,A\rangle\rangle} \bigg/ \sum_{R \supset B} e^{\langle\langle B,A\rangle\rangle}.$$

It is easy then to check that μ is invariant for M by remarking that:

$$\sum_{R \supset A} e^{\langle\langle C,A\rangle\rangle + \langle A \rangle} = \sum_{R \supset A} e^{\langle\langle A,C\rangle\rangle + \langle C \rangle}. \qquad \blacksquare$$

Using Lemma 1 above we can easily obtain the same formula for the invariant measure μ as those calculated in the massively parallel case ($n=1$) and in the pure sequential case ($m=1$).[1-3] It is convenient to concretely represent the way in which the corresponding distribution functions concentrate their probability mass. We have defined[4-6] the notion of dynamical confinement in order to deal with this concentration by simply generalizing the definition of an attractor. If there is an invariant measure, it is easy to show that the p-confiner is simply the set surrounded by contour lines in the state space of the system containing $100p$ percent of the total probability mass [see Fig. 2(a), with $p=0.6$].

In the present case, if the synaptic weights are symmetrical and the diagonal weights w_{ii} are non-negative, then all attractors of the network R are the same fixed configurations both in the sequential and in the parallel case.[7] The stability basins of these attractors, however, are different. This is revealed by looking at the localization of the two distribution functions. We can study this concentration through the notion of 1-D confinement. Figure 2(b) shows the parallel confiner, which is different from the sequential confiner, proving that

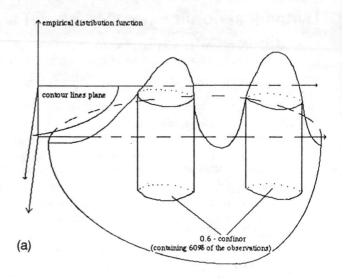

(a)

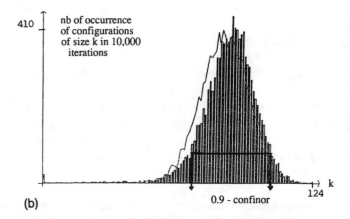

(b)

FIG. 2. (a) 2-D confinement phenomenon. (b) 1-D confinement phenomenon in the case of sequential (continuous distribution function) and parallel (black bars histogram) updating.

the parallel distribution function favors the occurrence of high size configurations (numerical experiments on a SIMD MasPar 8192 machine correspond to a 128×128 neural network, the first size showing a significant difference (level $=0.001$) between the two distributions).

B. Finite range phase transition

The finite range phase transition occurs when the coefficients $M_{A,C}$ of the Markovian matrix M verify the so-called K-cyclic Perron–Fröbenius rule:[8] (1) the eigenvalue 1 of M is multiple of order K; (2) for each eigenvector μ_i ($i=1,...,K$) associated to the eigenvalue 1, we have

$$\|\mu_i M\| \leqslant a \|\mu_i\| + b, \quad \text{where } 0<a<1 \quad \text{and } 0<b,$$

which ensures the existence of an asymptotically stable K-cycle of measures $\mu_1,...,\mu_K$. It is easy to build examples of 2-cycles for the stochastic Hopfield model, as in Refs. 8 and 9. In Fig. 3, we have represented the landscape corre-

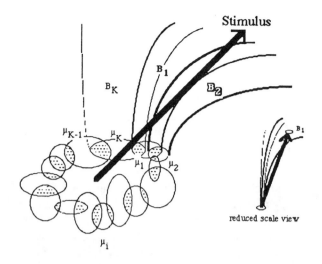

FIG. 3. Confiners and stochastic isochrons landscape.

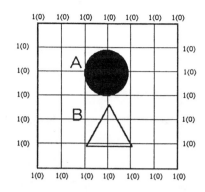

FIG. 4. Definition of a cylinder and choice of boundary conditions 1's (or 0's).

sponding to a K-cycle of empirical asymptotic measures. For example, in the case of the empirical confiner C_1 of μ_1, we have added its p-stability basin B_1 (called stochastic isochron[4-6]), which is simply the region confining $100p$ percent of the empirical mass corresponding to the configurations $C_1 = A(t_1)$, $A(t_1-K),...,A(t_1-iK),...$, observed in the transient phase. Empirical period K is the smallest integer which minimizes $A = \Sigma_{i,j} \text{Area}(C_i \cap C_j)$ and we can define the notion of periodic confinement noise rate by $\rho = 2A/K(K-1)\text{Area}(\cup_i C_i)$. The landscape of confiners and stochastic isochrons is very important to concretize the recall memory capacity of the network. To illustrate, let us suppose that we can move the confiner annulus by an instantaneous stimulus vector to a region where there is no overlapping amongst basins, such as a region which intersects only B_1. Then, after applying this stimulus to a collection of asynchronous networks identical to R after a certain transient phase, we obtain a synchrony of all stimulated networks the behavior of which is then the same as that of a nonstimulated network beginning in the confiner of μ_1 at the time the stimulus is applied. The neurons of the stimulated networks can evoke a similar synchronous potential activity, such as those recordable by EEG or PET scanner, or cause the same recall memory phenomenon, since they are able to pass a certain threshold because of synchrony. Among the possible applications, we can consider that the bulbar respiratory generator[10-12] and an insect locomotion generator[13] both correspond to a finite range transition behavior. Indeed, in each of these examples the real data show a stochastic periodic behavior which leads to an "annulus" confiner and to a sub-confinement phenomenon showing a dispatching of this annulus (Fig. 3) into subsets corresponding to the different observed phases. To follow up on Ref. 4, it is then possible to estimate this dynamical confinement by using estimators made from the empirical density.

C. Thermodynamic phase transition

The thermodynamic phase transition occurs when the size of the network R tends to infinity. In general, the limit invariant measure is unique and particularly it does not depend on the boundary conditions (1 or 0) of the sequence of networks. This explains the fact that numerous numerical experimentalists choose toric (or periodic) boundaries. Unfortunately, as in the case of the Ising model in solid-state physics, there exist certain parametric circumstances for which the thermodynamic limit (obtained with only 1's or only 0's on the boundaries of a sequence of networks tending in size to infinity) exhibits two completely distinct invariant measures μ_1 and μ_0. In the following, we will analyze a simple network in which we can study such a behavior analytically.

An important concept for proving the existence of thermodynamic phase transitions is that of a cylinder. The cylinder $[A,B] = \{x_j = 1, j \in A; x_j = 0, j \in B\}$ is only the event corresponding to the occurrence of 1's on A and of 0's on B (with any state of the neurons outside of $A \cup B$; cf. Fig. 4).

If we systematically seek out the linear equations linking each cylinder's measure, we find two types of such equations: the first type always verified in a product space like $\{0,1\}^R$ (projective equations), and the second available for each conditional rule such as that defining a random neural network (conditional equations). These equations are

(1) projective equations:

$$\forall A \ni i, \mu([A,B]) + \mu([A\setminus\{i\}, B \cup \{i\}]) = \mu([A\setminus\{i\}, B]),$$

(2) conditional equations:

$$\forall R \ni i, \mu([\{i\}, \varnothing])$$

$$= \sum_{i \notin A, B; A \cup B = R\setminus\{i\}; A \cap B = \varnothing} \Phi(A,B)\mu([A,B]),$$

where $\Phi(A,B) = e^{\Sigma j \in V_i \cap A} w_{ij}/T / (1 + e^{\Sigma j \in V_i \cap A} w_{ij}/T)$.

If we note $L = R\setminus\{i\}$ and, for any subset K of L, j_K is the smallest index of the neurons of K, L being ordered from 1 to $|L|$, we can define the matrix M corresponding to the coefficients of the equations above:

$$\mu([L,\phi]),\mu([L\setminus\{1\},\{1\}]),\mu([L\setminus\{2\},\{2\}])..\mu([K,L\setminus K]),\mu([K\setminus\{j_K\},L\setminus K\cup\{j_K\}])..\mu([\phi,L])$$

$$\begin{vmatrix} 1 & 1 & 0 & \cdots & 0 & & 0 & \cdots & 0 \\ 1 & \vdots & 0 & \vdots & 1 & \cdots & 0 & \vdots & 0 & \cdots & 0 \\ 0 & \vdots & 0 & \vdots & 0 & 1 & \vdots & 1 & \cdots & 0 \\ 0 & 0 & 0 & 0 & 0 & \cdots & 1 \end{vmatrix} = \mathbf{M}.$$

$$|\phi([L,\phi]),\ \Phi([L\setminus\{1\},\{1\}]),...,\ \Phi([K,L\setminus K]),\ \Phi([K\setminus\{j_K\},L\setminus K\cup\{j_K\}]),...,\Phi([\phi,L])|$$

Then we can easily prove Lemma 2, and Theorem 1 which holds true in the simple case of the Ising model (with nearest neighbors w_{ij}'s isotropic and translation invariant):

Lemma 2:

$$\text{Det } M=0 \Leftrightarrow \sum_{L\supset K} (-1)^{|L-K|}\Phi(K,L\setminus K)=0.$$

Theorem 1: In the case of the 2-D Ising model, let us define: $w_{ii}=u_0/2, w_{ij}=u_1$ and $a=u_0/2+u_1$. Then we have (a) Det $M=0 \Leftrightarrow u_0/2+2u_1=0$, which is simply the classical Ising phase transition condition, by adding (b) Ker $M \cap \zeta \neq \phi$, where ζ is the simplex generated by the cylindrical probabilities $\mu([K,L\setminus K])$ when K describes the subsets of L.

Simulations show the differences between probabilities for observing 1 in the central neuron of the network R with boundaries of 1 or of 0. Notably 0.014 ($p=0.05$) is the significant threshold frequently passed by the differences observed, after 10 000 iterations in the asymptotic state on a MasPar 8192 for network sizes up to 512×512 (see Table I).

III. CELL POPULATIONS

Recent publications show that we can model the cell cycle in terms of the limit cycle in a phase plane whose variables are enzymatic concentrations[14] or microscopic observables.[15] Figure 5 exhibits an analog of an empirical confiner for such variables.

A. The Hahn model of the cell cycle

The cell cycle describes the different physiological states a cell traverses from the time of its birth to the instant at which it divides. Four successive phases can be distinguished: the presynthetic phase G_1, during which the different components of the cell increase in number, the phase of nucleic acid synthesis S, the premitotic phase G_2, and the mitotic phase M during which the cell undergoes a change in structure with condensation of the chromosomes resulting in a discontinuous process in which two daughter cells are produced. The four phases of the cell cycle can be further decomposed into different states. In mathematical models of the cell cycle, the fundamental variables considered are the rates at which the cells traverse the different physiological states and the state density function. We assume that the systems are described in terms of n states, these states corresponding to well-defined biochemical and metabolic criteria. The state of the cell population at time t is described by $\bar{u}(t)=[u_1(t),...,u_i(t),...,u_n(t)]$, where $u_i(t)$ is the size of the fraction of the cell population in state i at time t. The dynamical system describing the change in state i is given by the equation $\bar{u}(t+1)=A\bar{u}(t)$.

The elements of the matrix A are assumed to be constant. These elements represent the rates at which the cells traverse the cycle. The matrix A is given by

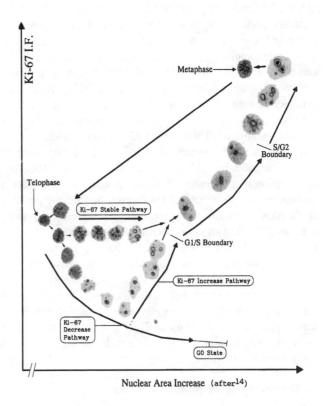

FIG. 5. Empirical confiner in the (Ki-67 fluorescence intensity, nuclear area) plane.[14]

TABLE I. Differences between probabilities to observe 1 in the central neuron of the network R, respectively, with boundaries of 1 or of 0 for different network sizes.

u_0	8192	128×128	32 768	256×256	512×512
1.5	0.001	0.0065	0.005	0.0085	0.0105
1.75	0.003	0.0105	0.009	0.001	0.0005
2	0.02	0.0085	0.004	0.03	0.021
2.25	0.0245	0.028	0.036	0.0165	0.0005
2.5	0.065	0.029	0.164	0.016	0.0605
2.75	0.0505	0.007	0.1455	0.11	0.015
3	0.2565	0.1865	0.367	0.2865	0.052

$$A \equiv \begin{bmatrix} \alpha_1 & 0 & 0,...,Q\gamma_{n-1} & Q\beta_n \\ \beta_1 & \alpha_2 & 0,...,0 & Q\gamma_n \\ \gamma_1 & \beta_2 & \alpha_3 0,...,0 & 0 \\ \vdots & \vdots & \vdots & \vdots \\ 0 & 0 & 0,...,\beta_n & \alpha_n \end{bmatrix}.$$

Here Q represents the mean number of daughter cells at mitosis ($1 < Q \leq 2$), α_i represents the probability that the cell remains in state (i) between observation times t and $t+1$, and β_i (or, respectively, γ_1) is the probability that the cell passes to the next state of the cycle (or, respectively, to the state which follows that) at time $t+1$: the matrix A is then simply that of a Lotka–Leslie matrix. We assume that $\alpha_i + \beta_i + \gamma_i \leq 1$ and $(1 - \alpha_i - \beta_i - \gamma_i)$ is the death rate in the population at state (i). The case $\alpha_i = \alpha$, $\beta_i = \beta$, $\gamma_i = \gamma$ for any i, corresponds to the case where the cells traverse the different phases of the cycle with the same dynamics. This condition corresponds to the model introduced by Hahn.[16] Its continuous analog[17] can be written as follows:

(a) $\dfrac{\partial u}{\partial t} + \beta(i)\dfrac{\partial u}{\partial i} = -\mu(i)u,$

where $\mu(i) = 1 - \alpha(i) - \beta(i)$, if $\gamma(i) = 0$, for any i;

(b) $\dfrac{\partial u}{\partial t} + (\beta + 2\gamma)\dfrac{\partial u}{\partial i} - \gamma\dfrac{\partial^2 u}{\partial i^2} = -\mu u,$

where $\mu = 1 - \alpha - \beta - \gamma$. The partial differential equation (a) is quasilinear, strictly hyperbolic,[18,19] and the equation (b) is linear with a solution $u(t,i) = Ke^{rt+li}$, with $u(0,i) = f(i)$ and $u(t,0) = \int_0^n Qm(i)u(i,t)di$, where $m(i) = \beta$, for $n-1 < i \leq n$, $m(i) = \gamma$, for $n-2 < i \leq n-1$, and $m(i) = 0$, elsewhere.

The asymptotic growth rate r of the model is given by: $r = \text{Log } \lambda$, where λ is the dominant eigenvalue of the matrix A. As is well known, if $N(t)$ denotes the population size at time t, we have: $N(t) = \Sigma_{i=1}^n u_i(t)$, then $\lim_{t\to\infty} \text{Log}[N(t)/N(t-1)] = r$. Hence the parameter r represents the rate of increase of total cell population size when the stable cell cycle distribution is attained.

B. Dynamical entropy

The relationship between the different states in the cell cycle can be characterized by Fig. 6. This figure is the same graph associated with matrix A and characterizes the different states the cell traverses.

The dynamical behavior of the cell population can be considered in terms of the temporal sequence of states. A cell in the mitotic state has the following possible offspring, each index k representing a state: $...(k-2)(k-2)k(k+1) \times (k+3)(k+3)...$

Genealogy is the term used to describe one such temporal sequence of states. We can distinguish between both backward and forward genealogies. A backward genealogy represents the sequence of states that a cell traversed before it reached its present state. A forward genealogy describes the sequence of states its descendants will enter as the population evolves. Formally, a genealogy is a sequence

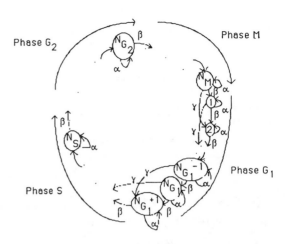

FIG. 6. Relationship between different states in the cell cycle.

$x = (...x_{-1}, x_0, x_1 ...)$, where the elements x_i correspond to different physiological states, and the index i corresponds to time. Let Ω denote the set of all genealogies, and let μ denote a probability measure on Ω which is invariant under the time translation operator $T: (Tx)_i = x_{i-1}$. Let $H_\mu(T)$ denote the Kolmogorov–Sinaï entropy of the dynamical system (Ω, μ, T). Then $r = \text{Log } \lambda$ satisfies a variational principle described on the space of genealogies. We have, in the hyperbolic[18,19] case:

$$\text{Log } \lambda = \sup_\mu \left(H_\mu(T) + \int \Phi \, d\mu \right),$$

where $\Phi(x) = \text{Log } a_{x_0 x_1}$ is a potential function defined on the set of genealogies Ω. The potential function Φ associates with each genealogy $x = (...x_{-1}, x_0, x_1 ...)$ a real number $\text{Log } a_{x_0 x_1}$, which depends only on the two indices x_0, x_1. We recall that a_{ij} is the (i,j)th entry of the matrix A. There is a unique measure $\mu = \bar{w}$, for which the above maximum is attained. From A, we define a probability matrix P as follows: $p_{ij} = a_{ij}v_j/\lambda v_i$, where $\bar{v} = (v_i)$ is the normalized eigenvector associated to the dominant eigenvalue λ of A; P is simply the transition matrix of the Markov process which relates x_i to $(Tx)_i = x_{i-1}$. We have: $\Sigma_{j=1}^n p_{ij} = 1$, for $i = 1,...,n$, and $\bar{w} = (w_i)$ is the stationary distribution of P: $\bar{w}P = \bar{w}$.

The dominant eigenvalue λ admits the decomposition:[20]

$$\text{Log } \lambda = r = H + \int \Phi \, d\mu,$$

where

$$H = -\sum_{i,j} w_i p_{ij} \text{ Log } p_{ij}$$

and

$$\int \Phi \, d\mu = \sum_{i,j} w_i p_{ij} \text{ Log } a_{ij}.$$

We call H population entropy, and $\int \Phi \, d\mu$ the reproductive potential. The macroscopic parameters r, H, and $\int \Phi \, d\mu$ can be explicitly calculated in terms of the model where α_i, β_i, γ_i satisfy the condition $\alpha_i = \alpha$, $\beta_i = \beta$, $\gamma_i = \gamma$. In this case, the matrix A is quasicirculant, and its eigenvalues are given by $\lambda_j = \alpha + \beta(Qj)^{1/n} + \gamma(Qj)^{2/n}$, where j is the jth root of 1; hence the dominant eigenvalue of A is equal to $\lambda = \alpha + \beta Q^{(1/n)} + \gamma Q^{(2/n)}$. The stable age distribution is then given by $\bar{v} = [\bar{Q}, \bar{Q}Q^{1/n}, \ldots, \bar{Q}Q^{(n-1)/n}]$, where $\bar{Q} = (1 - Q^{-(1/n)})/(1 - Q^{-1})$.

The transition matrix $P = (p_{ij})$ verifies

$$
P = \begin{bmatrix}
\alpha & 0 & \cdots & & 0 & \gamma Q^{2/n} & \beta Q^{1/n} \\
\beta Q^{1/n} & \alpha & & & & & \gamma Q^{2/n} \\
\gamma Q^{2/n} & \beta Q^{1/n} & \alpha & & & & 0 \\
0 & \gamma Q^{2/n} & \beta Q^{1/n} & & & & \vdots \\
\vdots & & & \gamma Q^{2/n} & & & \\
& & & & & \alpha & 0 \\
0 & 0 & 0 & \cdots & 0 & \beta Q^{1/n} & \alpha
\end{bmatrix}
$$

and $\bar{w}$ is uniform. Then the population entropy H and the reproductive potential $\int \Phi \, d\mu$ are equal to

$$
H = \frac{-\alpha}{\lambda} \text{Log}\left(\frac{\alpha}{\lambda}\right) - \frac{\beta Q^{1/n}}{\lambda} \text{Log}\left(\frac{\beta Q^{1/n}}{\lambda}\right)
$$
$$
- \frac{\gamma Q^{2/n}}{\lambda} \text{Log}\left(\frac{\gamma Q^{2/n}}{\lambda}\right),
$$

and

$$
\int \Phi \, d\mu = \frac{\alpha}{\lambda} \text{Log} \, \alpha + \frac{\beta Q^{1/n}}{\lambda} \text{Log}(\beta Q) + \frac{\gamma Q^{2/n}}{\lambda} \text{Log}(\gamma Q).
$$

The parameter H describes the variations in the rates at which the cell traverses the different cycle states. A sensitivity study of H can be done in the spirit of Ref. 21, when β is changed to $\beta^* = \beta/\eta$ and α to $\alpha^* = (\eta - \beta)/\eta$, for k control states. H is then changed to: $H_\eta = [(n-k)H^* + k\eta H^{**}]/(n-k+k\eta)$, where $H^* = -\alpha/\lambda^* \, \text{Log}(\alpha/\lambda^*) - \beta/\lambda^* \, \text{Log}(\beta/\lambda^*)$ and $H^{**} = -\alpha^*/\lambda^* \, \text{Log}(\alpha^*/\lambda^*) - \beta^*/\lambda^* \, \text{Log}(\beta^*/\lambda^*)$, and λ^* is the perturbed dominant eigenvalue as studied in Ref. 21.

C. Entropy as a measure of synchrony

The analytical properties of H, namely description in terms of the complexity of the cell cycle and characterization as a measure of the rate of decay of synchrony, can be made explicit by considering a description of the model in terms of the genealogies it induces. The study of the case of finite range phase transition for P (e.g., when $\alpha = \gamma = 0$, $\beta = Q = 1$) permits exhibition of a cycle of $\bar{w}$ measures (an n cycle in the given example), and hence to draw the landscape of confiners and stochastic isochrons of the successive measures of the cycle in order to find the stimuli capable of causing a lasting synchrony if H (calculated for the barycenter of the measures of the cycle) is small. In practice, data obtained from microscopy (see Fig. 5) can be used in order to estimate

these confiners and stochastic isochrons, by replacing the natural measure by the empirical density corresponding to the observations.

IV. CONCLUSION

We have shown the interest of the notion of dynamical confinement for studying phase transition and synchrony problems both for neural networks and cell populations. This notion is directly related to the concept of dynamical attraction in the case of deterministic dynamical systems,[4–6] but permits study of the landscape of empirical confiners and stochastic isochrons from data (cf. Fig. 3) in order to prepare new experiments by seeking the noise level (calculating the confinement noise rate ρ above and the approximate entropy[22]) and the best synchronizing stimuli. To end, let us note that this entire article has dwelt on the existence of an invariant measure or of an asymptotic cycle of measures for the stochastic models presented above. In general, this is true unless there are asymptotic phase transitions which can occur in an open set of parameter values.[23]

[1] T. Hervé, J. M. Dolmazon, and J. Demongeot, "Random field and neural information: A new representation for multi-neuronal activity," Proc. Natl. Acad. Sci. USA **87**, 806–810 (1990).

[2] O. Francois, "Ergodicité des processus neuronaux," C. R. Acad. Sci. **310**, 435–440 (1990).

[3] O. Francois, J. Demongeot, and T. Hervé, "Convergence of self-organizing stochastic neural network processes," Neural Networks **5**, 277–282 (1992).

[4] J. Demongeot, C. Jacob, and P. Cinquin, "Periodicity and chaos in biological systems: New tools for the study of attractors," *Life Science Series* (Plenum, New York, 1987), Vol. 138, pp. 255–266.

[5] J. Demongeot and C. Jacob, "Confineurs: Une approche stochastique," C. R. Acad. Sci. **56**, 206–210 (1989).

[6] J. Demongeot and C. Jacob, "Confiners, stochastic equivalents of attractors," in *Stochastic Modeling in Biology: Relevant Mathematic Concepts and Recent Applications*, edited by P. Tautu (World Scientific, Singapore, 1990), pp. 309–327.

[7] F. Fogelman, E. Goles, and G. Weisbuch, "Transient length in sequential iteration of threshold functions," Discrete Appl. Math. **6**, 95–98 (1983).

[8] J. Losson and M. C. Mackey, "Statistical cycling in coupled map lattices," Phys. Rev. E **50**, 843–856 (1994).

[9] J. Komornik, "Asymptotic periodicity of the iterates of weakly constrictive Markov operators," Tohoku Math. J. **38**, 15–27 (1986).

[10] T. Pham Dinh, J. Demongeot, P. Baconnier, and G. Benchetrit, "Simulation of a biological oscillator: The respiratory rhythm," J. Theor. Biol. **103**, 113–132 (1983).

[11] J. Demongeot, P. Pachot, P. Baconnier, G. Benchetrit, S. Muzzin, and T. Pham Dinh, "Entrainment of the respiratory rhythm: Concepts and technics of analysis," in *Concept and Formalizations in the Control of Breathing*, edited by G. Benchetrit *et al.* (Manchester University Press, Manchester, 1987), pp. 217–232.

[12] P. Baconnier, G. Benchetrit, P. Pachot, and J. Demongeot, "Entrainment of the respiratory rhythm: A new approach," J. Theor. Biol. **164**, 149–162 (1993).

[13] F. Gruau, "Efficient computer morphogenesis: A pictorial demonstration," Santa Fe Institute Research Report No. 94-04-027, 1-25, 1994.

[14] A. Goldbeter, "A minimal cascade model for the mitotic oscillator involving cycling and cdc2 kinase," Proc. Natl. Acad. Soc. USA **88**, 9107–9112 (1991).

[15] S. du Manoir, P. Guillaud, E. Camus, D. Seigneurin, and G. Brugal, "Ki-67 labeling in post-mitotic cells defines different Ki-67 pathways within the $2c$ compartment," Cytometry **12**, 455–463 (1991).

[16] G. M. Hahn, "Mammalian cell populations," Math. Biosci. **6**, 295–304 (1970).

[17] J. Demongeot and L. Demetrius, "Relation between discrete and continuous models of the cell cycle: macroscopic properties," to appear in Math. Pop. Studies.

[18] L. Ta-tsien, *Global Classical Solutions for Quasilinear Hyperbolic Systems* (Wiley–Masson, Paris, 1993).

[19] C. Chiu and F. C. Hoppenstaedt, "Mathematical models and computer simulation for synchronization of bacterial culture growth," to appear in J. Math. Biol.

[20] J. Demongeot and L. Demetrius, "Entropie et valeur adaptative. Une étude empirique: la France de 1985 à 1980," Population **1**, 109–134 (1989).

[21] H. Caswell, "A general formula for the sensitivity of population growth rate to changes in life history parameters," Theoret. Pop. Biol. **14**, 215–230 (1978).

[22] S. M. Pincus, "Approximate entropy as a measure of system complexity," Proc. Natl. Acad. Sci. USA **88**, 2297–2301 (1991).

[23] R. L. Dobrushin, "Applications of the animal model to the Ising contour model," *Ecole d'Eté de Probabilités de St. Flour XIV*, Lecture Notes in Mathematics (Springer-Verlag, Heidelberg, 1994).

A minimal single-channel model for the regularity of beating in the sinoatrial node

Michael R. Guevara and Timothy J. Lewis[a]
Department of Physiology and Centre for Nonlinear Dynamics in Physiology and Medicine, McGill University, Montreal H3G 1Y6, Canada

(Received 30 June 1994; accepted for publication 7 December 1994)

It has been suggested that the normal irregular beating of the heart is a manifestation of deterministically chaotic dynamics. Evidence proffered in support of this hypothesis includes a $1/f$-like power spectrum, a small noninteger correlation dimension, and self-similarity of the time series. The major cause of the normal fluctuations in heart rate is the impingement of several neural and hormonal control systems upon the sinoatrial node, the natural pacemaker of the heart. However, intrinsic fluctuations of beat rate can be seen in the isolated node, devoid of all neural and hormonal inputs, and even in a single cell isolated from the node. The electrical activity in such a single cell is generated by ions flowing through discrete channels in the cell membrane. We decided to test the hypothesis that the fluctuations in beat rate in a single cell might be due to the fluctuations in the activity of this population of single channels. We thus assemble a model consisting of 6000 channels and probe its dynamics. Each channel has one or more gates, all of which must be open to allow current to flow through the channel. Since these gates are thought to open and close in a random manner, we model each gate by a Markov process, assigning a pseudorandom number to each gate every time that it changes state from open to closed or vice versa. This number, in conjunction with the classical voltage-dependent Hodgkin–Huxley-like rate constants that control the speed with which a gate will open or close, then determines when that gate will next change state. We also employ a second method that is much more efficient computationally, in which one computes the lifetime of the ensemble of 6000 channels. We show that the Monte Carlo model has behavior consistent with the hypothesis that the irregular beating seen experimentally in single nodal cells is due to the (pseudo)random opening and closing of single channels. However, since the pseudorandom number generator used in the simulations is deterministic, one cannot state that the activity in the model is random (or stochastic). Thus, it would be premature to claim that the irregularity of beating in a single nodal cell is accounted for by the *stochastic* behavior of a population of a few thousand single channels lying in the membrane of the cell. Finally, we consider some implications of our work for the naturally occurring *in situ* fluctuations in heart rate ("heart rate variability"). © *1995 American Institute of Physics.*

I. INTRODUCTION

We are all well aware of the fact that our own hearts do not beat with a perfectly regular rhythm. Three lines of evidence exist that might lead one to speculate that this irregular beating is a manifestation of chaotic dynamics: (i) the correlation dimension of the electrocardiogram is not an integer,[1–3] suggesting the existence of a strange attractor; (ii) there is self-similarity,[4–6] reminiscent of many chaotic systems; and (iii) there is a $1/f$-like power spectrum,[4,7] which it is known can occur in intermittency.[8,9] Kobayashi and Musha[7] raised two possibilities for the origin of the $1/f$ spectrum: it is either intrinsic to electrical activity in the membrane of the sinoatrial node (SAN), the natural pacemaker of the heart, or it is generated by the neural feedback systems that control heart rate. It is at present difficult to realistically model the entire cardiovascular system with its myriad of feedback control loops. It is even difficult to model the isolated SAN, since it is an extended, inhomogeneous structure,[10–12] the details of which are still under investigation. We therefore decided to formulate a model of a single SAN cell, in which fluctuations in beat rate are produced by the opening and closing of single channels in the cell membrane, in order to ascertain the extent to which these processes, which are presently thought to be random, might account for the irregular beating seen experimentally in single SAN cells.[13–15] We then go on to discuss the relevance of our work for the regularity of beating in the intact heart ("heart rate variability").

II. METHODS

There are several ionic models of spontaneous activity in the SAN.[16] We have chosen to use the model of Irisawa and Noma,[17] simplifying it by removing the fast inward sodium current I_{Na} and the pacemaker current I_h (more commonly termed I_f). This reduced "minimal" model thus has only three currents: I_s (the slow inward calcium current), I_K (the delayed rectifier potassium current), and I_l (the time-independent background or "leak" current). We did not take the further simplifying step of making activation of I_s time independent.[18]

We use two methods to simulate single-channel dynam-

[a]Present address: Department of Mathematics, University of Utah, Salt Lake City, Utah 84112.

ics. In both methods, one assumes that gates behave independently of one another, i.e., there is no "cooperativity." In the first method,[19–21] each gate of each channel is treated individually: one can thus refer to it as the "simple" method.[20] We illustrate this approach using the I_K current, which in the Irisawa–Noma description has but one activation variable (raised to the first power), and no inactivation variable. There is thus only one gate controlling each I_K channel: when that gate is open, the channel conducts; when it is closed, the channel does not conduct. The activation gate of each I_K channel has a pseudorandom number (drawn from a uniform distribution on (0,1]) assigned to it when it changes state from open to closed or vice versa. The Hodgkin–Huxley-like rate constants α_p and β_p for the macroscopic I_K current, which are nonlinear functions of the transmembrane voltage, control the duration that that particular gate will remain in its present configuration (i.e., open or closed). The Hodgkin–Huxley-like equation governing the activation variable p is

$$\frac{dp}{dt} = \alpha_p(1-p) - \beta_p p. \tag{1}$$

In the traditional interpretation, p gives the fraction of I_K activation or "p" gates open at any given time t. In the simple method, when one is following an individual I_K channel that opens at time t_{open}, one assigns a pseudorandom number r to the gate at that time. One then numerically integrates until the time t_{close} such that

$$-(\ln r) = \int_{t_{open}}^{t_{close}} \beta_p[V(t)]dt. \tag{2}$$

At time t_{close} the channel flips from the open state to the closed state. A new pseudorandom number is then assigned to the gate, and Eq. (2) is then used once again to compute the time to the next opening of the gate, but with β_p being replaced by α_p and t_{open} and t_{close} switched in the limits of the integral. The transmembrane potential V is computed using forward Euler integration of the equation

$$\frac{dV}{dt} = -(I_s + I_K + I_l)/C, \tag{3}$$

where C is the cell capacitance, i.e., $V(t + \delta t) = V(t) + (dV/dt)\delta t$, where δt is the integration step size, which is fixed at 0.1 ms in the computations presented below involving the simple method. The smallest activation or inactivation time constant in the range of potentials considered here is the activation time constant of I_s, which approaches 1 ms at depolarized potentials, and so is an order of magnitude larger than δt.

In the second method (adopted with modification from method 2a of Ref. 19), which we term the "complex" method, one keeps track of the ensemble of channels.[14,15,19,22] We illustrate this method for the case where one has both I_s and I_K channels present, and no others. At each step of the numerical procedure, one keeps track of the number of I_K gates (or equivalently, channels) in each of the two possible states: open (N_{Ko}) and closed (N_{Kc}). Since it follows from the Irisawa–Noma description of I_s that there is one activation and one inactivation gate for each

channel, there are four possible states for each I_s channel. One therefore notes at each step of the procedure the number of I_s channels in each of these four states: N_{scc} (activation and inactivation gate both closed), N_{sco} (activation gate closed, inactivation gate open), N_{soc} (activation gate open, inactivation gate closed), and N_{soo} (both activation and inactivation gates open). At time t, one then calculates a realization of the lifetime Δt of that state of the ensemble from

$$\Delta t = -(\ln r)/[\alpha_p N_{Kc} + \beta_p N_{Ko} + \alpha_d(N_{scc} + N_{sco})$$
$$+ \beta_d(N_{soc} + N_{soo}) + \alpha_f(N_{scc} + N_{soc})$$
$$+ \beta_f(N_{sco} + N_{soo})], \tag{4}$$

where r is a pseudorandom number drawn from a uniform distribution on (0,1] at time t, α_d and β_d are the rate constants for the activation variable (d) of I_s, and α_f and β_f are the rate constants for the inactivation variable (f) of I_s. Once Δt is known, one must then decide which of the six possible transitions actually occurs at time $t + \Delta t$. This is obtained by calculating the probability of occurrence of each of these transitions [e.g., the probability of the transition being the one in which a closed p gate opens is given by $\alpha_p N_{Kc}$ divided by the overall rate constant appearing in the denominator of Eq. (4)]. One then places six intervals next to one another, with lengths corresponding to each of the six probabilities calculated above. By construction, the sum of the lengths of these intervals is one, since one of the six transitions must occur. To decide which transition occurs, one then determines into which of these six intervals a second pseudorandom number drawn from a uniform distribution on [0,1] falls. Simple forward Euler integration of Eq. (3) is then used to determine $V(t + \Delta t)$: i.e., $V(t + \Delta t) = V(t) - (I_s + I_K + I_l)\Delta t/C$.

The error in the complex method is associated with the fact that the voltage is actually changing during the time Δt, and so the rate constants and the assorted probabilities are also changing. One can keep this error within bounds by not allowing the change in voltage during Δt to exceed a certain maximum limit.[19] In our algorithm, when $V(t + \Delta t)$ exceeds $V(t)$ by more than 0.4 mV in absolute value, Δt is halved (successively if need be) and the calculations of the currents and $V(t + \Delta t)$ redone until the desired accuracy is achieved. For continuous Hodgkin–Huxley-like equations (i.e., not for the single-channel model), it can be proven that this time-step-halving algorithm converges.[23] Since the probability of an event occurring in a time Δt is independent of the prior history of the system, one can simply carry out the drawing procedure described above at time $t + \Delta t$ to continue the simulation, without affecting the validity of the process.[19]

Computations were run in single precision (approximately seven significant decimal digits) on a DECsystem 2100. Programs were written in FORTRAN77 and the system-supplied double precision library subroutine RAND was used to produce pseudorandom numbers to determine open- and closed-times of gates as outlined above.

III. RESULTS

The Irisawa–Noma model follows the Hodgkin–Huxley formalism, and is thus formally a deterministic system of continuous nonlinear ordinary differential equations. We shall refer to this model as the "continuous" model. From the physiological viewpoint, this type of model corresponds to a situation in which each ionic current flows through an infinite number of channels, each of infinitely small conductance. However, it is now established that there are a finite number of individual channels in the cell membrane, each with a discrete conductance. In what follows, the model constructed as a population of finite-conductance single channels, each opening and closing as time progresses, will be referred to as the "single-channel" model.

The first step in producing the single-channel model from the continuous model is to estimate the number of channels in a single SAN cell. Since I_K has a linear open-channel current–voltage relationship,[24] one has

$$I_K = P_o N_K \gamma_K (V - E_K), \tag{5}$$

where V is the transmembrane voltage, P_o is the probability that the activation gate (and therefore the channel itself) will be open at that voltage, N_K is the number of I_K channels, γ_K is the single-channel conductance, and E_K is the reversal potential for I_K. An estimate of γ_K of 1.6 pS at physiological external $[K^+]$ has been made from extrapolation of the results of single-channel voltage-clamp experiments carried out at unphysiologically high values of external $[K^+]$.[24] Using Eq. (5)—suitably modified to include a fast inactivation process not included in the Irisawa–Noma model—an estimate of N_K of 1054 ± 254 $(n=13)$ has been made from experiments carried out in cells with an average capacitance of about 35 pF.[24] We use $N_K = 1000$ and $C = 35$ pF in the model below.

The value of γ_s has been estimated to be about 4 pS from noise analysis carried out in small strips cut out of the SAN.[25] We are not aware of any experimentally derived estimates of the number of I_s channels (N_s) in isolated SAN cells. We therefore calculated a value of N_s that would be appropriate for the Irisawa–Noma model. Since I_s rectifies in this model, we computed the slope conductance of the fully activated, noninactivated current at its reversal potential of 40 mV, which is positive to where rectification sets in. This leads to a value of 0.6 mS cm^{-2}. For a single cell capacitance of 35 pF, this results in a single-cell conductance of 21 nS. Given the single-channel conductance of 4 pS, one arrives at $N_s = 5250$. This results in a channel density of 1.5 μm^{-2} (assuming the usual specific capacitance of 1 μF cm^{-2}), which is within the range of 0.1–5.0 μm^{-2} reported for neonatal and adult ventricular cells (see Refs. 26 and 27 and references therein). In the model below we use $N_s = 5000$.

Figure 1(a) shows a voltage-clamp simulation, in which the activation variable p of I_K in the continuous model is plotted as a function of time. At $t=0$ ms, p is set to zero, corresponding to clamping the transmembrane potential to a very negative value. The voltage is then stepped up to a potential of +50 mV at $t=0$ ms, producing almost complete activation (i.e., $p=1.0$) of the current, and then down to -50

mV at $t=2000$ ms. The variable in the single-channel model corresponding to p is the fraction of I_K channels open. Figure 1(b) shows this fraction for the case when the cell has 1000 I_K channels, which is the number used in our single-cell model. Figures 1(c) and 1(d) show the results when the number of I_K channels (N_K) is reduced to 100 and then further to 10. Note the increase in the "noise," especially visible upon clamping down to $V = -50$ mV.

Figure 2 shows a voltage-clamp protocol carried out in the single-channel model $(N_K = 1000)$ in which the voltage is first stepped to a clamp potential of 0, -20, or -40 mV at $t=0$ ms to activate I_K, followed by a step down to -50 mV at $t=2500$ ms to deactivate the current. As expected, one sees effects due to the voltage dependence of steady-state activation and the time constant of activation. The trace at the bottom of the figure shows a record of the activity in one of the thousand I_K channels upon clamping to 0 mV. It is clear that the mean open time is larger at the more depolarized clamp potential than at the more hyperpolarized holding potential.

Figure 3(a) shows the transmembrane potential as a function of time in the deterministic three-current minimal Irisawa–Noma model. The trace is smooth, since, as already mentioned, it is produced by a continuous system of differential equations. Figure 3(f) shows the corresponding trace produced by the single-channel model, with channel numbers as estimated above (5000 for I_s, 1000 for I_K). Note the more irregular look of the trace, especially during the pacemaker potential. Figures 3(b) and 3(g) show the total current (I_{tot}) in the two models, while Figs. 3(c) and 3(h) give the individual currents. In the single-channel model, the background current (I_l) is left in its continuous Hodgkin–Huxley form (see Sec. IV). Note that the fluctuations visible in I_K in Fig. 3(h) are considerably smaller in amplitude than those in I_s. Figure 3(i) shows the fraction of I_K and I_s channels open in the single-channel model, while Fig. 3(d) gives the analogous traces (p and df, respectively) in the deterministic model. Figure 3(j) shows the fraction of the d (I_s activation) and f (I_s inactivation) gates open. (The fraction of I_K channels open [Fig. 3(i)] also gives the fraction of p gates open.) These three traces of the fractions of d, f, and p gates open [Figs. 3(i) and 3(j)] show time courses similar to those of the activation and inactivation variables (d, f, p) in the deterministic model [Figs. 3(d) and 3(e)]. While the amplitudes of the fluctuations in the numbers of I_s and I_K channels open [Fig. 3(i)] are roughly comparable, there seem to be larger fluctuations in the number of d gates open than in the number of f gates open [Fig. 3(j)]. In this 750 ms run, the d, f, and p gates open and close about 10^5, 2×10^4, and 10^3 times, respectively. Thus the mean value of the lifetime Δt of the ensemble of channels [Eq. (4)] is about 6 μs.

Figure 4(a) shows 10 s of spontaneous activity in the single-channel model. The first cycle of this activity was shown earlier in Fig. 3(f) on an expanded time scale. Figure 4(b) is a tachogram, giving the ith interbeat interval (IBI$_i$) as a function of interval number (i), calculated from a 50 s long simulation. A joint interval distribution[28] or scattergram of this data, in which each IBI—apart from the first—is plotted versus the preceding IBI is presented in Fig. 4(c). The inter-

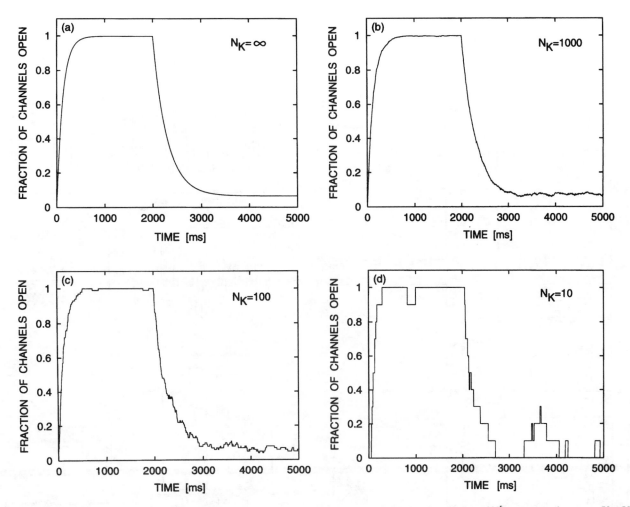

FIG. 1. Simulation of voltage-clamp step. All I_K channels closed at $t=0$, at which time V is stepped to 50 mV. At $t=2000$ ms, a step down to -50 mV is made. (a) Continuous Hodgkin–Huxley-like model. (b)–(d) Single-channel model with 1000 (b), 100 (c), and 10 (d) I_K channels. In (a)–(c), integration step size is 0.1 ms, and data points are plotted every 1 ms. In (b)–(d), "simple" simulation method is used.

val histogram[29] is shown in Fig. 4(d), while the serial correlation coefficients (R_j) are shown in Fig. 4(e).[15,30,31] Note the rapid decline in the R_j. The persistence of positive small nonzero values for $j \geq 1$ is due to the slow drifts in IBI evident in Fig. 4(b).[30] Scrambling the IBIs with a pseudorandom number generator results in the R_j oscillating equally positive and negative about the zero baseline (see also Fig. 2-2 of Ref. 31). This rapid decline to zero for $j > 1$ shows the lack of dependence of any given IBI on the preceding IBIs.

Figure 4 showed results for one simulation run, starting out with a particular seed value for the pseudorandom number generator. Figure 5 shows IBIs for four other runs, each starting out with a different seed value. While it is apparent that the details of each run are quite different, the mean IBI of the five-run ensemble is 398 ms and the mean coefficient of variation (standard deviation divided by mean) of IBI for the ensemble is 3.8%. This ensemble mean IBI is extremely close to the value of 395 ms obtained in the continuous model [Fig. 3(a)], using a variable time-step algorithm with an identical upper limit (0.4 mV) on the change in voltage allowed during one integration time step.[32]

When N_s and N_K are decreased by a factor of 10 (to 500

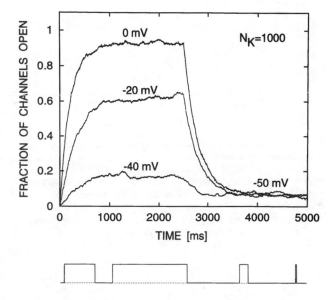

FIG. 2. Top: Simulation of voltage clamp step in single-channel model of 1000 I_K channels. All I_K channels are closed at $t=0$, at which time V is stepped to 0, -20, or -40 mV, and then down to -50 mV at $t=2500$ ms. Bottom: Time series from one of the 1000 channels during the simulation involving the step to 0 mV. The "simple" simulation method was used, with 0.1 ms integration step size, and data points plotted every 1 ms.

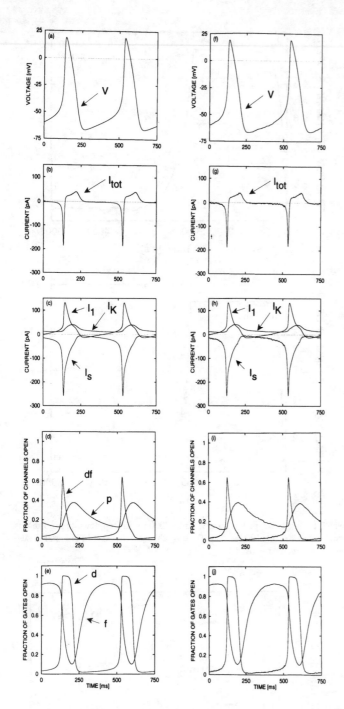

FIG. 3. 750 ms run of spontaneous activity in continuous (left panel) and single-channel (right panel) models. (a),(f) V; (b),(g) I_{tot}; (c),(h) I_s, I_K, I_l; (d) df,p; (i) fractions of I_s, I_K channels open; (e) d,f; (j) fractions of d,f gates open. Initial conditions (left panel): $V=-60$ mV, $d=0.003\,115\,67$, $f=0.910\,749$, $p=0.171\,578$. Initial conditions (right panel): $V=-60$ mV, fractions of gates open correspond to initial conditions on d,f,p as stated for the left panel. Not all data points computed are plotted. The "complex" simulation method was used in the right panel.

and 100, respectively), with tenfold increase in single-channel conductance so as to leave the total conductance unchanged, there is a marked increase in the irregularity of beating, with the coefficient of variation of the IBI increasing to about 12%.

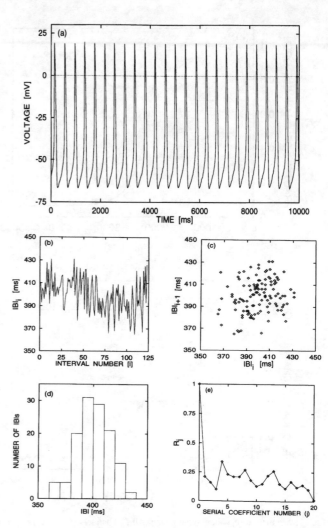

FIG. 4. 50 s run of spontaneous activity in the single-channel model. (a) First 10 s of transmembrane potential. (b) Tachogram. (c) IBI scattergram. (d) IBI histogram. (e) IBI serial correlation coefficients. Mean IBI=400 ms, coefficient of variation of IBI=3.7%. Same initial conditions as in Fig. 3. In (a), not all computed data points are plotted. Computation time for 50 s run is about 20 min. "Complex" simulation method is used.

IV. DISCUSSION

A. Comparison with experimental data

In healthy human subjects the coefficient of variation for a run of between 25 and a few hundred heart beats is on the order of 10%–15%.[33,34] In 36 h recordings from isolated rat hearts, the coefficient of variation also seems to be of about the same magnitude.[35] In the isolated rabbit SAN, the coefficient of variation for one 300-beat run was much smaller, being about 0.4%.[36] Since the isolated SAN is a population oscillator consisting of many coupled cells, one would expect it to be considerably more regular than a single SAN cell.[36,37] This is indeed the case: in runs ranging from 34 to 136 beats in 14 single SAN cells, the coefficient of variation ranged between 1.4% and 2.8%, averaging 2.0%.[15] The value obtained in our model of 3.8% [Figs. 4(b) and 5] is thus about double this experimental value. The most obvious candidate to account for this discrepancy is an underestimation of one or more of the numbers of single channels and/or overestimation of the single-channel conductance(s). A

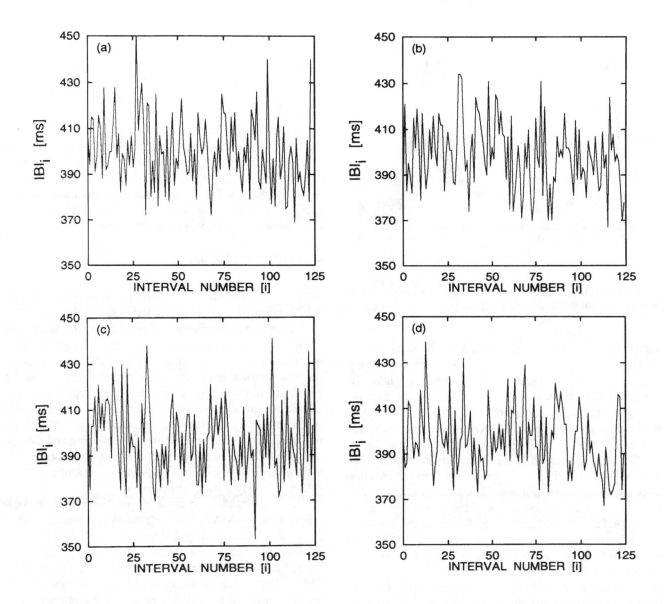

FIG. 5. Tachograms resulting from four simulation runs in the single-channel model, starting with different seeds for the pseudorandom number generator. Mean IBI and coefficient of variation of IBI: (a) 400 ms, 3.9%; (b) 399 ms, 3.8%; (c) 397 ms, 4.1%; (d) 396 ms, 3.6%. "Complex" simulation method is used.

simple random-walk-to-threshold model of the pacemaker potential predicts that the coefficient of variation of IBI should be inversely proportional to the square-root of the number of channels present in the membrane.[37] Coupling together several "stochastic" SAN cells produces a result consistent with this estimate.[14] Thus one would expect that increasing the number of I_s channels from our standard value of 5000 to 10 000 should lead to a coefficient of variation of about 2.7%. While this is indeed exactly what one finds in the model, this value lies at the upper end of the range of reported experimental values. In a recent report involving a more detailed SAN model,[16] in which the estimated number of I_s channels is 10 000, the mean coefficient of variation for three 100-beat runs was found to be 2.2%.[15] Our conclusion from the above results is that the single-channel fluctuations in the two currents I_s and I_K suffice to account for the major part of the fluctuations in IBI experimentally observed in single SAN cells.

B. Problems with the single-channel model

In the Irisawa–Noma model, both I_K and I_s rectify. In the simulations presented above, we have treated the rectification as residing in the single-channel conductance: i.e., we have made the conductance of the open channel (i.e., the single-channel conductance) a function of voltage. However, the I_K channel is linear in nodal cells,[24] and it is a relatively fast voltage-dependent inactivation process that lies at the root of the rectification.[24] Since this inactivation process is not included in the Irisawa–Noma description of I_K, we did not include it in our model. In addition, the Irisawa–Noma equations for I_K were derived from voltage-clamp experiments carried out on the rabbit SAN. In the guinea-pig SAN, the major component of I_K present is not $I_{K,r}$, but rather $I_{K,s}$.[38]

While I_s rectifies in the SAN,[39] I_s channels have a linear current–voltage relationship in ventricular cells.[27] To make

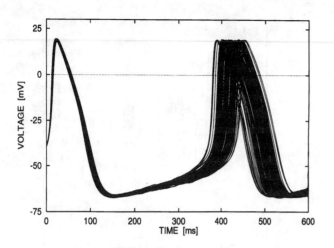

FIG. 6. Superimposed cycles from 50 s run, the first 10 s of which was shown in Fig. 4(a). Cycles all start off at $t=0$ when V crosses -40 mV on the action potential upstroke.

matters far worse, the simple four-state kinetic scheme for I_s used here is probably an oversimplification in the SAN, since I_s channels have much more esoteric kinetics in ventricular cells, including bursting due to the presence of multiple closed states.[26] Thus, future work will be needed to explore how the rectification, multiple closed-state properties, and species differences change the results presented above.

We have not formulated the background current I_l of the Irisawa–Noma model as a population of single channels since we do not feel that it is realistic to do so at the present time. First of all, the ionic nature of the background current in the SAN is still undetermined. A chloride-sensitive current has been described,[40] and more recent work describes a current carried by both Na^+ and K^+ ions.[41] In neither case has the single-channel conductance been reported. Second, the I_l current in the Irisawa–Noma model is presumably a sum of these (and perhaps other yet to be determined) background currents, as well as other currents, such as the Na^+–K^+ pump current. Thus we feel that it is premature to include these currents in a single-channel model.

C. Implications for the intact SAN

There are two major problems in extrapolating the above results to the intact SAN. First, SAN cells form an inhomogeneous population (see Ref. 42 for a recent review of the ionic currents in SAN cells), with, for example, some cells possessing much more I_{Na},[11,43] I_h,[44] or $I_{Ca,T}$ (Ref. 45) than others. This inhomogeneity is reflected in the fact that even simple visual inspection of the records of spontaneous activity in single cells shows differences in the origin of the IBI fluctuations: e.g., fluctuation in action potential duration can account for anywhere between 20% and 50% of the IBI fluctuation in different cells (see Fig. 1 of Ref. 13, Figs. 4.1 and 4.5 of Ref. 14). In our model, only a small part (roughly 20%) of the IBI fluctuation is traceable to fluctuations in action potential duration (Fig. 6). While our minimal model might be a reasonably good caricature of cells from the central part of the SAN, cells from the more peripheral parts of the node can possess significant amounts of I_{Na} and I_f. It

remains to be seen what happens to the regularity of beating in single-channel models of cells that depend on I_{Na} and/or I_f for generation of spontaneous activity. The unusually small single-channel conductance of I_f (Ref. 46) might result in more regular beating in cells that depend upon I_f for pacemaking.

A second problem is that the coupling between cells in the SAN is anisotropic and highly inhomogeneous,[47] with much better coupling in the periphery than in the center.[10] The implications for this in terms of the regularity of beating in a population oscillator remain unexplored. In addition, the gap-junctional channels that provide this cell-to-cell coupling themselves gate in a stochastic manner.[14]

D. Random or chaotic?

"Anyone who considers arithmetical methods of producing random digits is, of course, in a state of sin" [J. von Neumann (1951), quoted in Ref. 48].

The above computations show that the fluctuations in IBI in a model formulated as a population of single channels is consistent with the experimental data. Thus, it is unlikely that chaos would have any role in generating the irregular beating of isolated cells, unless one could replace the stochastic interpretation of the kinetics of single channels with a chaotic one.[49,50] Unfortunately, there is at the present time no foolproof way of deciding whether the opening and closing of a single channel (i.e., an experimental record corresponding to the simulation shown in the lower part of Fig. 2) is deterministically chaotic or stochastic.

In addition, there is another consideration. A system-supplied pseudorandom number generator subroutine is used in the simulations presented above. This algorithm is deterministic, *not* random or stochastic, since one always obtains the same sequence if one starts with the same seed value. This routine belongs to the class of linear congruential generators which have at their heart a piecewise-linear one-dimensional finite-difference equation of the form

$$I_{i+1}=MI_i+N \text{ (mod } m\text{)}, \qquad (6)$$

where I_i is the ith random integer generated, and M, N, and m are well-chosen integer constants, with $M,N \geqslant 1$, $m \geqslant 0$.[48,51,52] For $N=0$, one speaks of a (pure) multiplicative congruential generator. For judicious choices of the constants in Eq. (6), the deterministic sequence of integers produced has a very long repetition period, low serial correlation, and passes many of the statistical tests of randomness.[48,51,52] However, for $M>1$, the real (in contrast to integer) counterpart of Eq. (6) generates chaotic behavior.[53] Thus one can make the argument—even in the case of exact integer arithmetic implementation on a computer, with no roundoff or truncation errors—that the output of Eq. (6) has more in common with a chaotic process than with a stochastic one.

A single-channel model of squid axon membrane replicates much of the irregular appearance of experimental traces that are claimed to be chaotic.[54] However, since that single-channel model presumably used a deterministic pseudorandom number generator, the conclusion that a *stochastic* single-channel population mechanism can account for the irregularity seen in the experimental traces is premature. Similar remarks hold for single-channel models of bursting pancreatic β cells (see Sec. IV F). Nevertheless, it is unlikely that the interpretation of the results of these simulations would be changed, in terms of their characterization using simple phenomenological measures, should the pseudorandom sequence be replaced with a sequence of numbers that would be universally accepted as being truly random (e.g., one obtained from radioactive decay or a noise diode[48]). Indeed, it is unlikely that any presently available technique would be able to discriminate between the two sets of simulations, given the output voltage tracing from the model as input data.

The opening or closing of a channel, which is a protein, is usually taken as being caused by a conformational change in that molecule, which is governed by the laws of quantum mechanics. Thus, as previously stated,[31] deterministically nonperiodic dynamics can only occur in single channels should the Copenhagen (statistical) interpretation of quantum mechanics be replaced by a deterministic mechanism. While Einstein's opposition to the Copenhagen interpretation is oft cited ("God does not play dice with the universe"),[55] one can also adopt the view—formulated in a recent study of whether the toss of a die is chaotic—that "even if a process in principle is deterministic, we may consider it as random if the complexity involved is so high that we cannot relate cause and effect in detail."[56] Or perhaps, more poetically stated: "In a sense, randomness, like beauty, is in the eye of the beholder."[52]

E. Heart rate variability: Chaos in the intact heart?

Our study does not rule out the possibility that chaotic activity might occur in the beating of an isolated SAN cell over the long term (e.g., due to the presence of intracellular biochemical feedback mechanisms with time delays). Chaos might equally well occur, even in the short term, when many individually oscillating pacemaker cells are coupled together to form an intact isolated SAN. There are many intracardiac feedback mechanisms (e.g., stretch of the SAN caused by pulsation of the sinoatrial nodal artery) that operate to control nodal rate,[57] as well as numerous neural and hormonal regulatory systems. These systems all depend on ion-channel gating and neurotransmitter release for their action, and hence have stochastic components. Their characteristic response times range from less than a second (e.g., the baroreceptors) to days (e.g., control of blood volume by the kidney), and their feedback gains span many orders of magnitude.[58] It is thus not surprising that IBI[4,7] and blood pressure[59] have broadband power spectra. In addition, ultradian frequency components have been described in heart rate and blood pressure of intact animals,[60] and in the beat rate of isolated hearts.[35] In respiration, where self-similar phenomenology has also been described,[61] there are several discrete components in the power spectrum with frequencies ranging over more than two orders of magnitude.[62]

A decrease in heart rate variability (HRV) has been reported in several disease states, including diabetes,[63] injury to the central nervous system,[64] and congestive heart failure.[65] Decreased HRV predicts a greater mortality after myocardial infarction[66] as well as an increased chance of

sudden cardiac death in patients with coronary heart disease.[34] In obstetrics, loss of HRV in the fetal tachogram is a dire prognostic sign,[67] and, at the other end of life, HRV decreases with age.[63,68,69] In essential hypertension, several studies report a decrease in HRV (see Ref. 33 and references given in Ref. 70), while at least one study reports unchanged HRV.[71] Assuming that fluctuations in heart rate are due to some underlying chaotic mechanism, it is thus tempting to raise the question: "Is it healthy to be chaotic?"[72] However, while HRV might be reduced in hypertension, blood pressure (BP) variability is increased (see references in Ref. 70). Thus, while one could take the decreased HRV variability as a sign of disease in the hypertensive individual, one could equally well conclude from the increased BP variability that the hypertensive individual is in fact "healthier" than the normotensive individual. A similar remark holds for the concomitant decrease in HRV and increase in BP variability with age.[63,68,69,71]

When studying any control system, one should always keep in the back of one's mind consideration of which variable is the controlled variable. The major system for short term regulation of the arterial BP is the carotid baroreceptor reflex. Removal of this "buffer" reflex leads to a great increase in BP variability, but a fall in HRV.[58,73] Individuals (normal or hypertensive) who have a higher baroreceptor reflex gain (slope of line relating IBI to systolic BP) have a lower BP variability, but a higher HRV.[70,74] The conclusion must be that one is observing the response of a controller that is attempting to *reduce* variability in blood pressure (the controlled variable), at the unavoidable expense of increasing variability in heart rate (an effector branch of the feedback loop). In fact, reverting to a perhaps old-fashioned interpretation of the concept of homeostasis, one could make the case that the body is in fact trying to produce a steady state in the blood pressure.

The baroreceptor feedback loop could conceivably be the origin of the $1/f$ spectrum in IBI,[4,7] since there is a $1/f$ falloff in the spectrum of the blood pressure waveform.[59] Indeed, in an isolated heart preparation—in which there are perforce no extra-cardiac regulating systems present—the IBI spectrum could not be "reasonably" fit to a power law during normal conditions.[75]

F. Other applications of the single-channel model

There are several other situations in cardiac electrophysiology in which the single-channel form of the model might be useful in investigating effects to which membrane noise might contribute:[49] e.g., the beat-to-beat fluctuations in action potential duration during 1:1 rhythm in paced isolated ventricular cells, irregular Wenckebach rhythms in isolated ventricular cells,[49] irregular "chaotic" dynamics in periodically stimulated cells,[76,77] Shil'nikov chaos occurring in the Irisawa–Noma model,[32] and annihilation of activity in spontaneously beating preparations.[78] Finally, there are many other noncardiac situations in which chaotic activity has been claimed to exist and in which we believe approaches similar to single-channel modeling will be useful: e.g., bursting activity in pancreatic β-cells,[79,80] rhythmic activity in smooth muscle (e.g., in gut, arterioles, and uterus), intracellular calcium oscillations, neurotransmitter release at nerve terminals (e.g., resulting in the EEG), and pulsatile release of hormones by neurons.

ACKNOWLEDGMENTS

We thank D. Kaplan for helpful discussions on pseudo-random number generators, J. Outerbridge and A. Yehia for help with computers, and C. Pamplin for help in typing the manuscript. This work was supported by an operating grant from the Medical Research Council (MRC) of Canada. The initial part of this work was carried out by T. Lewis as his senior-year undergraduate research project (1986–87).

[1] A. Babloyantz and A. Destexhe, "Is the normal heart a periodic oscillator?," Biol. Cybern. 58, 203–211 (1988).

[2] J. P. Zbilut, G. Mayer-Kress, and K. Geist, "Dimensional analysis of heart rate in heart transplant recipients," Math. Biosci. 90, 49–70 (1988).

[3] G. Mayer-Kress, F. E. Yates, L. Benton, M. Keidel, W. Tirsch, S. J. Poppl, and K. Geist, "Dimensional analysis of nonlinear oscillations in brain, heart and muscle," Math. Biosci. 90, 155–182 (1988).

[4] J. P. Saul, P. Albrecht, R. D. Berger, and R. J. Cohen, "Analysis of long term heart rate variability: Methods, $1/f$ scaling and implications," in IEEE Computers in Cardiology (IEEE Computer Society, Silver Spring, 1987), pp. 419–422.

[5] A. L. Goldberger, D. R. Rigney, and B. J. West, "Chaos and fractals in human physiology," Sci. Am. 262(2), 42–49 (1990).

[6] N. A. J. Gough, "Fractals, chaos, and fetal heart rate," Lancet 339, 182–183 (1992).

[7] M. Kobayashi and T. Musha, "$1/f$ fluctuation of heartbeat period," IEEE Trans. Biomed. Eng. BE-29, 456–457 (1982).

[8] P. Manneville, "Intermittency, self-similarity and $1/f$ spectrum in dissipative dynamical systems," J. Phys. 41, 1235–1243 (1980).

[9] I. Procaccia and H. Schuster, "Functional renormalization-group theory of universal $1/f$ noise in dynamical systems," Phys. Rev. A 28, 1210–1212 (1983).

[10] W. K. Bleeker, A. J. C. Mackaay, M. Masson-Pévet, L. N. Bouman, and A. E. Becker, "Functional and morphological organization of the rabbit sinus node," Circ. Res. 46, 11–22 (1980).

[11] D. Kreitner, "Electrophysiological study of the two main pacemaker mechanisms in the rabbit sinus node," Cardiovasc. Res. 19, 304–318 (1985).

[12] I. Kodama and M. R. Boyett, "Regional differences in the electrical activity of the rabbit sinus node," Pflügers Arch. 404, 214–226 (1985).

[13] T. Opthof, A. C. G. van Ginneken, L. N. Bouman, and H. J. Jongsma, "The intrinsic cycle length in small pieces isolated from the rabbit sinoatrial node," J. Mol. Cell. Cardiol. 19, 923–934 (1987).

[14] R. Wilders, "From single channel kinetics to regular beating," Doctoral thesis, University of Amsterdam, Amsterdam, 1993.

[15] R. Wilders and H. J. Jongsma, "Beating irregularity of single pacemaker cells isolated from the rabbit sinoatrial node," Biophys. J. 65, 2601–2613 (1993).

[16] R. Wilders, H. J. Jongsma, and A. C. G. van Ginneken, "Pacemaker activity of the rabbit sinoatrial node. A comparison of mathematical models," Biophys. J. 60, 1202–1216 (1991).

[17] H. Irisawa and A. Noma, "Pacemaker mechanisms of rabbit sinoatrial node cells," in Cardiac Rate and Rhythm, edited by L. N. Bouman and H. J. Jongsma (Martinus Nijhoff, The Hague, The Netherlands, 1982), pp. 35–51.

[18] M. R. Guevara, A. C. G. van Ginneken, and H. J. Jongsma, "Patterns of activity in a reduced ionic model of a cell from the rabbit sinoatrial node," in Chaos in Biological Systems, edited by H. Degn, A. V. Holden, and L. F. Olsen (Plenum, London, 1987), pp. 5–12.

[19] E. Skaugen and L. Walløe, "Firing behavior in a stochastic nerve membrane model based upon the Hodgkin–Huxley equations," Acta Physiol. Scand. 107, 343–363 (1979).

[20] J. R. Clay and L. J. DeFelice, "Relationship between membrane excitability and single channel open–close kinetics," Biophys. J. 42, 151–157 (1983).

[21] L. J. DeFelice and J. R. Clay, "Membrane current and membrane potential from single-channel kinetics," in Single-Channel Recording, edited by B. Sakmann and E. Neher (Plenum, New York, 1983), pp. 323–342.

[22] W. van Meerwijk, "Qualitative models for cardiac pacemakers and their interaction," Doctoral thesis, Leiden University, Leiden, 1988.

[23] B. Victorri, A. Vinet, F. A. Roberge, and J.-P. Drouhard, "Numerical integration in the reconstruction of cardiac action potentials using Hodgkin–Huxley-type models," Comput. Biomed. Res. 18, 10–23 (1985).

[24] T. Shibasaki, "Conductance and kinetics of delayed rectifier potassium channels in nodal cells of the rabbit heart," J. Physiol. (London) 387, 227–250 (1987).

[25] W. Osterrieder, Q.-F. Yang, and W. Trautwein, "Conductance of the slow inward channel in the rabbit sinoatrial node," Pflügers Arch. 394, 85–89 (1982).

[26] A. Cavalié, D. Pelzer, and W. Trautwein, "Fast and slow gating behavior of single calcium channels in cardiac cells. Relation to activation and inactivation of calcium-channel current," Pflügers Arch. 406, 241–258 (1986).

[27] T. F. McDonald, A. Cavalié, W. Trautwein, and D. Pelzer, "Voltage-dependent properties of macroscopic and elementary calcium channel currents in guinea pig ventricular myocytes," Pflügers Arch. 406, 437–448 (1986).

[28] M. ten Hoopen and J. P. M. Bongaarts, "Probabilistic characterization of R-R intervals," Cardiovasc. Res. 3, 218–226 (1969).

[29] D. W. Simborg, R. S. Ross, K. B. Lewis, and R. H. Shepard, "The R-R interval histogram," J. Am. Med. Assoc. 197, 145–148 (1966).

[30] D. H. Perkel, G. L. Gerstein, and G. P. Moore, "Neuronal spike trains and stochastic point processes. I. The single spike train," Biophys. J. 7, 391–418 (1967).

[31] M. R. Guevara, "Chaotic cardiac dynamics," Doctoral thesis, McGill University, Montreal, 1984.

[32] M. R. Guevara and H. J. Jongsma, "Three ways of abolishing automatically in sinoatrial node: ionic modeling and nonlinear dynamics," Am. J. Physiol. 262. H1268–H1286 (1992).

[33] R. J. Bagshaw, A. Fronek, L. H. Peterson, and H. F. Zinsser, "Dispersion of blood pressure and heart rate in essential hypertension," IEEE Trans. Biomed. Eng. BE-22, 508–512 (1975).

[34] G. J. Martin, N. M. Magid, G. Myers, P. S. Barnett, J. W. Schaad, J. S. Weiss, M. Lesch, and D. H. Singer, "Heart rate variability and sudden death secondary to coronary artery disease during ambulatory electrocardiographic monitoring," Am. J. Cardiol. 60, 86–89 (1987).

[35] G. D. Tharp and G. E. Folk, Jr., "Rhythmic changes in rate of the mammalian heart and heart cells during prolonged isolation," Comp. Biochem. Physiol. 14, 255–273 (1965).

[36] H. J. Jongsma and L. Tsjernina, "Factors influencing regularity and synchronization of beating of tissue cultured heart cells," in Cardiac Rate and Rhythm, edited by L. N. Bouman and H. J. Jongsma (Martinus Nijhoff, The Hague, The Netherlands, 1982), pp. 397–414.

[37] J. R. Clay and R. L. DeHaan, "Fluctuations in interbeat interval in rhythmic heart-cell clusters. Role of membrane voltage noise," Biophys. J. 28, 377–389 (1979).

[38] J. M. B. Anumonwo, L. C. Freeman, W. M. Kwok, and R. S. Kass, "Delayed rectification in single cells isolated from guinea pig sinoatrial node," Am. J. Physiol. 262, H921–H925 (1992).

[39] A. Noma, H. Kotake, S. Kokubun, and H. Irisawa, "Kinetics and rectification of the slow inward current in the rabbit sinoatrial node cell," Jpn. J. Physiol. 31, 491–500 (1981).

[40] I. Seyama, "Characteristics of the anion channel in the sino-atrial node cell of the rabbit," J. Physiol. (London) 294, 447–460 (1979).

[41] N. Hagiwara, H. Irisawa, H, Kasanuki, and S. Hosoda, "Background current in sino-atrial node cells of the rabbit heart," J. Physiol. (London) 448, 53–72 (1992).

[42] H. Irisawa, H. F. Brown, and W. Giles, "Cardiac pacemaking in the sinoatrial node," Physiol. Rev. 73, 197–227 (1993).

[43] H. I. Oei, A. C. G. van Ginneken, H. J. Jongsma, and L. N. Bouman, "Mechanisms of impulse generation in isolated cells from the rabbit sinoatrial node," J. Mol. Cell. Cardiol. 21, 1137–1149 (1989).

[44] J. C. Denyer and H. F. Brown, "Rabbit sino-atrial node cells: isolation and electrophysiological properties," J. Physiol. (London) 428, 405–424 (1990).

[45] N. Hagiwara, H. Irisawa, and M. Kameyama, "Contribution of two types of calcium currents to the pacemaker potentials of rabbit sino-atrial node cells," J. Physiol. (London) 395, 233–253 (1988).

[46] D. DiFrancesco, "Characterization of single pacemaker channels in cardiac sino-atrial node cells," Nature (London) 324, 470–473 (1986).

[47] J. J. Duivenvoorden, "Electrotonic current spread in the rabbit sinoatrial node," Doctoral thesis, University of Amsterdam, Amsterdam, 1989.

[48] J. Moshman, "Random number generation," in *Mathematical Methods for Digital Computers*, edited by A. Ralston and H. S. Wilf (Wiley, New York, 1967), Vol. II, pp. 249–263.

[49] M. R. Guevara, "Mathematical modeling of the electrical activity of cardiac cells," in *Theory of Heart*, edited by L. Glass, P. Hunter, and A. McCulloch (Springer-Verlag, New York, 1991), pp. 239–253.

[50] L. S. Liebovitch and T. I. Toth, "A model of ion channel kinetics using deterministic chaotic rather than stochastic processes," J. Theor. Biol. **148**, 243–267 (1991).

[51] D. E. Knuth, *The Art of Computer Programming* (Addison–Wesley, Reading, MA, 1969), Vol. 2.

[52] S. K. Park and K. W. Miller, "Random number generators: a good one is hard to find," Commun. ACM **31**, 1192–1201 (1988).

[53] S. Oishi and H. Inoue, "Pseudo-random number generators and chaos," Trans. IECE Jpn. **65**, 534–541 (1982).

[54] L. J. DeFelice and A. Isaac, "Chaotic states in a random world: Relationship between the nonlinear differential equations of excitability and the stochastic properties of ion channels," J. Stat. Phys. **70**, 339–354 (1992).

[55] A. Pais, '*Subtle is the Lord...': The Science and Life of Albert Einstein* (Oxford University Press, Oxford, 1982), pp. 443.

[56] R. Feldberg, M. Szymkat, C. Knudsen, and E. Mosekilde, "Iterated-map approach to die tossing," Phys. Rev. A **42**, 4493–4502 (1990).

[57] D. Jensen, *Instrinsic Cardiac Rate Regulation* (Appleton–Century–Crofts, New York, 1971).

[58] A. C. Guyton, *Textbook of Medical Physiology*, 8th ed. (Saunders, Philadelphia, 1991), pp. 218–219.

[59] G. Parati, M. di Rienzo, S. Omboni, P. Castiglioni, A. Frattola, and G. Mancia, "Spectral analysis of 24 h blood pressure recordings," Am. J. Hyptertens. **6**, 188S–193S (1993).

[60] A. Livnat, J. E. Zehr, and T. P. Broten, "Ultradian oscillations in blood pressure and heart rate in free-running dogs," Am. J. Physiol. **246**, R817–R824 (1984).

[61] B. Hoop, H. Kazemi, and L. Liebovitch, "Rescaled range analysis of resting respiration," Chaos **3**, 27–29 (1993).

[62] L. Goodman, "Oscillatory behavior of ventilation in resting man," IEEE Trans. Biomed. Eng. **BE-11**, 82–93 (1964).

[63] T. Wheeler and P. J. Watkins, "Cardiac denervation in diabetes," Br. Med. J. **4**, 584–586 (1973).

[64] C. Vallbona, D. Cardus, W. A. Spencer, and H. E. Hoff, "Patterns of sinus arrhythmia in patients with lesions of the central nervous system," Am. J. Cardiol. **16**, 379–389 (1965).

[65] A. L. Goldberger, D. R. Rigney, J. Mietus, E. M. Antman, and S. Greenwald, "Nonlinear dynamics in sudden cardiac death syndrome: Heartrate oscillations and bifurcations," Experientia **44**, 983–987 (1988).

[66] R. E. Kleiger, J. P. Miller, J. T. Bigger, Jr., A. J. Moss, and the Multicenter Post-Infarction Research Group, "Decreased heart rate variability and its association with increased mortality after acute myocardial infarction," Am. J. Cardiol. **59**, 256–262 (1987).

[67] E. H. Hon and S. T. Lee, "Electronic evaluation of the fetal heart rate," Am. J. Obstet. Gynecol. **87**, 814–828 (1963).

[68] M. Pagani, F. Lombardi, S. Guzetti, O. Rimoldi, R. Furlan, P. Pizzinelli, G. Sandrone, G. Malfatto, S. Dell'Orto, E. Piccaluga, M. Turiel, G. Baselli, S. Cerutti, and A. Malliani, "Power spectral analysis of heart rate and arterial pressure variabilities as a marker of sympatho-vagal interaction in man and conscious dog," Circ. Res. **59**, 178–193 (1986).

[69] D. T. Kaplan, M. I. Furman, S. M. Pincus, S. M. Ryan, L. A. Lipsitz, and A. L. Goldberger, "Aging and the complexity of cardiovascular dynamics," Biophys. J. **59**, 945–949 (1991).

[70] A. J. S. Coates, J. Conway, P. Sleight, T. E. Meyer, V. K. Somers, J. S. Floras, and J. V. Jones, "Interdependence of blood pressure and heart period regulation in mild hypertension," Am. J. Hyptertens. **4**, 234–238 (1991).

[71] G. Mancia, A. Ferrari, L. Gregorini, G. Parati, G. Pomidossi, G. Bertinieri, G. Grassi, M. di Rienzo, A. Perdotti, and A. Zanchetti, "Blood pressure and heart rate variabilities in normotensive and hypertensive human beings," Circ. Res. **53**, 96–104 (1983).

[72] R. Pool, "Is it healthy to be chaotic?," Science **243**, 604–607 (1989).

[73] C. S. Ito and A. M. Scher, "Hypertension following arterial baroreceptor denervation in the unanesthetized dog," Circ. Res. **48**, 576–586 (1981).

[74] G. Mancia, G. Parati, G. Pomidossi, R. Casadei, M. di Rienzo, and A. Zanchetti, "Arterial baroreflexes and blood pressure and heart rate variabilities in humans," Hypertension **8**, 147–153 (1986).

[75] J. P. Zbilut, G. Mayer-Kress, P. A. Sobotka, M. O'Toole, and J. X. Thomas, Jr., "Bifurcations and intrinsic chaotic and $1/f$ dynamics in an isolated perfused rat heart," Biol. Cybern. **61**, 371–378 (1989).

[76] M. R. Guevara, L. Glass, and A. Shrier, "Phase locking, period-doubling bifurcations, and irregular dynamics in periodically stimulated cardiac cells," Science **214**, 1350–1353 (1981).

[77] J. Hescheler and R. Speicher, "Regular and chaotic behavior of cardiac cells stimulated at frequencies between 2 and 20 Hz," Eur. Biophys. J. **17**, 273–280 (1989).

[78] R. Kapral, "Stochastic dynamics of limit-cycle oscillators with vulnerable phases," J. Chim. Phys. **84**, 1295–1303 (1987).

[79] T. R. Chay and H. S. Kang, "Role of single-channel stochastic noise on bursting clusters of pancreatic β-cells," Biophys. J. **54**, 427–435 (1988).

[80] A. Sherman, J. Rinzel, and J. Keizer, "Emergence of organized bursting in clusters of pancreatic β-cells by channel sharing," Biophys. J. **54**, 411–425 (1988).

Phase resetting and dynamics in isolated atrioventricular nodal cell clusters

Arkady M. Kunysz
Department of Physics and Center for Nonlinear Dynamics—Department of Physiology, McGill University, Montreal, Quebec H3G 1Y6, Canada

Andrew A. Munk and Alvin Shrier
Department of Physiology, McGill University, Montreal, Quebec H3G 1Y6, Canada

(Received 2 June 1994; accepted for publication 7 December 1994)

In the heart, the AV node is the primary conduction pathway between the atria and ventricles and subserves an important function by virtue of its rate-dependent properties. Cell clusters isolated from the rabbit atrioventricular (AV) node beat with a stable rhythm (cycle length: 300–520 ms) and are characterized by slow action potential upstroke velocities (7 to 30 V/s). The goal of this study is to better characterize the phase resetting and the rhythms during periodic stimulation of this slow inward current system. Single or periodic depolarizing pulses (20 ms in duration) were injected into AV nodal cell clusters using glass microelectrodes. Phase resetting curves of both strong, weak as well as discontinuous types were obtained by applying single current pulses of different intensities and latencies following every ten action potentials. Graded responses were elicited in a wide range of stimulus phases and amplitudes. A single premature stimulus caused a transient prolongation of the cycle length. Sustained periodic stimulation, at rates faster than the intrinsic beat rate, resulted in various $N:M$ (stimulus frequency: action potential frequency) entrainment rhythms as well as periodic or irregular changes in action potential morphology. The changes in action potential characteristics were evaluated by computing the area under the action potential trace and above a fixed threshold (-45 mV). We show that the variations in action potential morphology play a major role in the onset of complicated dynamics observed in this experimental preparation. In this context, the prediction of entrainment rhythms using techniques based on the iteration of phase resetting curves (PRCs) is inadequate since the PRC does not carry information directly related to the changes in action potential morphology. This study demonstrates the need to consider graded events which, though not propagated, have important implications in the understanding of dynamical diseases of the heart. © *1995 American Institute of Physics.*

I. INTRODUCTION

In the intact heart, the atrioventricular (AV) node is a small complex structure which plays a crucial role in regulating impulse conduction between the atria and the ventricles. AV nodal cells are in general characterized by slow action potential upstroke velocities (7 to 30 V/s, compared with 100 to 200 V/s for neighboring atrial or ventricular cells) which reflect the relatively slow kinetics of the ionic mechanism underlying electrical activity.[1–3] Under normal conditions, an electrical impulse generated by the primary pacemaker of the heart, the sinoatrial (SA) node, propagates across the atria and reaches the AV node which forms the only normal link between the atria and the ventricles. The functional aspects of the AV node may be summarized as follows: (1) conduction through the AV node is slow (and rate dependent) therefore causing a delay in activation between the atria and the ventricles (coordination of activation); (2) the AV node is able to block impulses propagating from the atria to the ventricles hence protecting the latter from too rapid or complex atrial rhythms (filtering); and (3) under circumstances where the SA node fails in generating the heart rhythm, or when conduction is blocked between the atria and the ventricles, the AV node is capable of serving as a subsidiary pacemaker to the ventricles (pacemaking). In the clinical context, the AV node is therefore often the target of therapeutic or surgical interventions.

Since the pioneering work of Tawara,[4] there has been substantial progress in our understanding of the excitability and conduction properties of the intact AV node. For example, periodic premature stimulation protocols are often used to evaluate nodal excitability and its rate-dependent properties.[5–9] In this procedure, a premature stimulus is introduced at various coupling intervals after sustained periodic pacing at a fixed frequency. The resulting recovery curve (conduction time SH versus recovery time HS) is a representation of the excitability of the AV node. These recovery curves have been incorporated in an iterative mathematical procedure to predict the various rhythms of AV block in patients during atrial stimulation.[5,7]

In the last decade it has been shown that patterns similar to the rhythms of atrioventricular block can be seen *in vitro* in a virtually isopotential preparation of cardiac cells.[10,11] These rhythms could largely be accounted for by analyzing the response of the preparation to single premature stimuli.[10,12] Time-dependent effects (overdrive suppression) analogous to "fatigue" (rate-dependent prolongation in AV nodal conduction time) during periodic stimulation of the AV node[6,8] were observed that could lead to an evolution of the entrainment pattern during the drive.[13] Such *in vitro* experiments may therefore provide a basis for evaluating and modeling the dynamical response of AV nodal tissue to single or premature stimulation. In combination with electrophysiological studies carried out on single cellular preparations using the patch clamp technique, they can provide a better understanding of the spatial organization of the AV nodal tissue and of the ionic mechanisms underlying its functional properties.

In this study we characterize the response of AV nodal clusters to single and periodic stimulation. We investigate the consequences of changes in action potential morphology during periodic stimulation on the complexity of the experimentally observed rhythms. We also observe time-dependent effects which may be analogous to "fatigue" in the intact node.

II. MATERIALS AND METHODS

A. Dissociation procedure

Clusters of AV nodal cells were obtained from New Zealand White rabbits using methods described elsewhere.[14] In the experimental dish, typical cluster size was between 100 and 200 μm. Embryonic chick heart cell aggregates were prepared using the methods developed by DeHaan et al.[15] The aggregates were typically 120 to 180 μm in size and contained approximately 1000 cells. In a maintenance medium containing 1.3 mM of KCl, 85% of the AV nodal cell clusters and 95% of the aggregates showed regular spontaneous activity. At 37 °C, the spontaneous cycle length was, respectively, 300 to 560 ms for AV nodal cell clusters and 470 to 650 ms for atrial cell aggregates.

B. Electrophysiology

Electrical activity was recorded using borosilicate glass microelectrodes filled with 3 M KCl (typical electrode resistance: 40 to 60 MΩ). The transmembrane potential was recorded using an amplifier with negative resistance compensation. The bathing medium was kept at virtual ground by coupling to a current voltage converter (10–100 mV/nA) through an agar salt bridge and a chlorided silver wire. Current pulses were generated by a computer-based stimulation program (Alembic Software, Montreal, Quebec) and injected into the preparation via the same microelectrode used to record the transmembrane potential. Currents were measured to the nearest nA. Voltage and injected current waveforms were monitored on a digital oscilloscope (Textronix 5110) and recorded on a FM instrumentation recorder (HP 3964A, 3 dB frequency response at 3 ips for DC to 1250 Hz) at a tape speed of 3.75 ips for subsequent off-line analysis.

C. Experimental protocols

Phase resetting. Single depolarizing current pulses of fixed amplitude were delivered every tenth spontaneous action potential at an increasing coupling interval through the entire spontaneous cycle. The duration of the pulse was typically 20 ms. This protocol was repeated at several intensities of stimulation.

Overdrive suppression. The preparation was stimulated with increasing numbers of stimuli. Successive trains of 1, 2, 4, 8, 15, 25, 50, 100, and 250 stimuli were delivered, separated by rest periods of approximately 30 s. All measured

interbeat intervals were normalized to the control cycle length defined as the average of the five cycle lengths preceding the drive. The post-drive cycle length was evaluated as a function of stimulation duration.

Periodic stimulation. The preparation was stimulated with trains of 100 stimuli at different pacing frequencies and stimulus amplitudes. Successive episodes of pacing were separated by a 30 s rest period to allow for recovery from stimulation. The period of stimulation was automatically decremented. The entrainment rhythm during periodic simulation was determined by visual inspection of the recorded voltage traces.

D. Data analysis

Off-line analysis was carried out on the digital oscilloscope and by an automated computer system. Magnetic tapes were played back at 15 ips and the voltage waveform was sampled at 1 kHz by an IBM compatible 386 computer through an A/D interface (Omega). Interbeat intervals were calculated from the digitized waveform by a pattern recognition program (Alembic Software). Figures of experimental traces were printed on a laser printer (HP Laserjet III) through a graphing package (SigmaPlot, CorelDraw).

E. Iteration of phase resetting curves (PRCs)

The theory underlying the computation of phase locking based on the iteration of phase resetting curves is discussed at length elsewhere.[10,12,16] Briefly, the response of the preparation to periodic stimulation can be predicted from the corresponding PRC provided that the stimulation does not alter the intrinsic properties of the oscillator. The main idea is that a single stimulus instantaneously resets the phase of the oscillation from one point of the cardiac cycle to another point on the cycle. For a given amplitude of stimulation, the phase resetting curve (PRC) $T(\phi)/T_0$ [where T_0 is the control cycle length and $T(\phi)$ is the perturbed cycle length caused by a stimulus delivered at phase ϕ] describes the perturbation in the cycle length induced by a single stimulus delivered at phase ϕ. Let ϕ_i be the phase of the ith current pulse. We have,

$$\phi_i = f(\phi_{i-1}, \tau) = 1 + \phi_{i-1} - \frac{T(\phi_{i-1})}{T_0} + \tau \quad (\text{mod } 1), \quad (1)$$

where $\tau = T_s/T_0$ with T_s being the cycle length of the stimulus train, and $T(\phi_{i-1})/T_0$ is obtained from the experimentally determined phase response curve (PRC). Under the assumption that ϕ_0 is the phase of the unperturbed spontaneous cycle at which the first stimulus of a train of periodic pulses is delivered, Eq. (1) can be numerically iterated to determine the dynamics.

During periodic stimulation, three types of behavior are observed in Eq. (1): quasiperiodicity, periodic orbits, and chaotic dynamics. The Lyapunov number defined as:

$$\lambda = \lim_{N \to \infty} \frac{1}{N} \sum_{i=1}^{N} \ln|f'(\phi_i, \tau)|, \quad (2)$$

where N is the total number of iterations and $f'(\phi_i, \tau)$ is the first derivative of the function f evaluated at successive phases ϕ_i, can be used to discriminate between these three types of behavior.[17] The Lyapunov number is zero for quasi-periodicity, negative for periodic cycles, and positive for chaos.[18,19]

Before carrying out the iteration procedures, the experimentally obtained phase resetting curves were fitted to analytical functions in order to reduce experimental noise (high local derivatives) due to fluctuations in cycle length. Based on our present understanding of the ionic mechanisms underlying electrical activity in cardiac preparations there is no *a priori* reason to choose a particular function to fit the PRCs. For the two highest amplitudes of stimulation, we used the functions:

$$\frac{T(\phi)}{T_0} = 1 + \frac{b}{\phi - \phi_0} + \frac{b}{\phi_0}, \tag{3}$$

when $\phi \leq \phi_{\text{crit}}$, and

$$\frac{T(\phi)}{T_0} = \phi, \tag{4}$$

otherwise (stimulation induces immediate action potential). Since we assume that there is a rapid return to the limit cycle after the stimulus, the discontinuity in the PRC at ϕ_{crit} (the phase of discontinuity) must be equal to 1,[20] and we have $\phi_{\text{crit}} = (\phi_0^2 + b)/\phi_0$. Because the lowest amplitude stimulus induced almost no change in the cycle length of the preparation, we did not apply the iterative method for this stimulus intensity. The remaining PRC seems to violate the continuity assumption outlined above. This case is analogous to previous experimental observations reported in other cardiac preparations (see, for example, Ref. 17, pp. 113–116), or to phase resetting of integrate-and-fire models.[20] Although the presence of this apparent discontinuity may be attributable to insufficient experimental precision,[17] we nonetheless used a simple piecewise linear function to fit the PRC. The theoretical implications of discontinuous phase resetting are further discussed elsewhere.[17,20] The PRCs were fit using a graphics package (SigmaPlot) on an IBM compatible computer. The exact functions used to fit the experimental curves and the corresponding parameters are presented in the legend of Fig. 4.

III. RESULTS

A. Phase resetting

The response of biological oscillators to a single stimulus depends on the amplitude of the stimulus and the phase of the oscillation where the stimulus is delivered.[10,12,16] Figure 1(A) describes the phase-resetting protocol and defines the measurable quantities used throughout this part of the study. The control cycle length is denoted by T_0. The upstroke of the action potential is defined to have zero phase. A 20 ms depolarizing stimulus introduced every tenth action potential at increasing delay T_s (or phase $\phi = T_s/T_0$) after the upstroke of the action potential induces a perturbed cycle length T_1. The time intervals from the last spontaneous AP to the jth AP following the premature stimulus are denoted

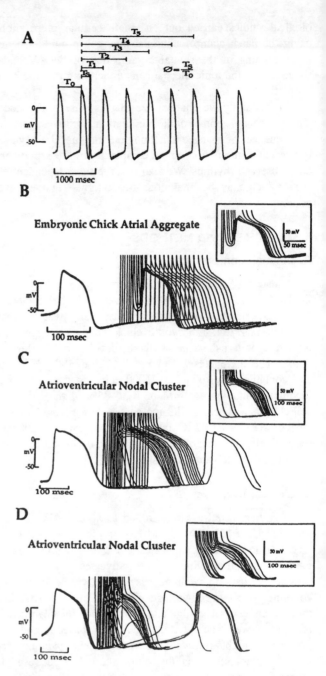

FIG. 1. Description of the phase-resetting protocol [panel (A)] and traces showing response to premature stimulation for two different types of preparations [panels (B)–(D)]. Panel (A): A 20 ms depolarizing stimulus of fixed amplitude is applied every 10 APs at increasing phase $\phi = T_s/T_0$. Panels (B)–(D): Superimposition of traces showing response to premature stimulation for three different preparations as the phase of the stimulus increases. The inserts show the premature APs on a magnified scale. In panel (B) (atrial embryonic chick heart cell aggregate), $T_0 = 500$ ms, amplitude $= 30$ nA. In panels (C) and (D) (AV nodal cell clusters), respectively, $T_0 = 320$ ms, amplitude $= 75$ nA and $T_0 = 550$ ms, amplitude $= 120$ nA. All the data presented in the remaining figures of this study were obtained for preparation (C).

by T_j, $j = 1$ to 5, as described in Fig. 1(A). In Figs. 1(B)–1(D) we present superimposed voltage traces showing the response to stimulation in three different preparations. In all panels, the stimuli appear as off-scale deflections and all the voltage traces are aligned on the upstroke of the last spontaneous action potential before stimulation. For short coupling

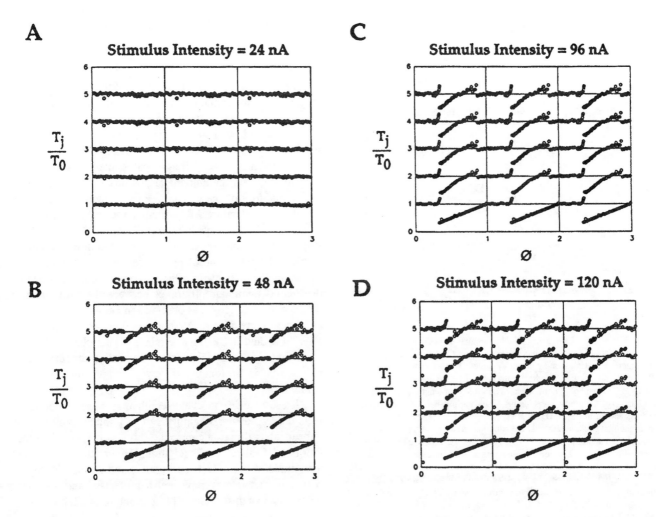

FIG. 2. Phase resetting curves using the protocol described in Fig. 1(A). Current pulses of four different intensities: 24 nA [panel (A)], 48 nA [panel (B)], 96 nA [panel (C)], 120 nA [panel (D)] were introduced every tenth spontaneous action potential. The normalized quantities T_j/T_0, $i=1$ to 5 are plotted as a function of the phase of the stimulus $\phi = T_s/T_0$. T_0 is the average of five control cycle lengths before the stimulus. Panel (A) shows "weak" and panels (C) and (D) show "strong" resetting. In panel (B), "discontinuous" resetting is observed. The lack of vertical translational symmetry may indicate the presence of a time-dependent process.

intervals, the stimulus fails to elicit a premature AP and the onset of the next spontaneous AP is generally delayed. For larger coupling intervals the stimulus evokes a premature action potential. In the atrial embryonic chick heart cell aggregate [Fig. 1(B)], the phase of the stimulus does not significantly affect the size and shape of the premature AP. The traces presented in Figs. 1(C) and 1(D) were obtained from two different AV nodal clusters. The differences in spontaneous action potential morphologies may simply reflect the histological heterogeneity of the AV node.[1,3] In both cases however, the premature action potential amplitudes, upstroke velocities, and durations are strongly affected by the prematurity of the stimulus. This is in agreement with previous observations from the intact AV node[3] and may have important consequences on impulse conduction through the AV node. For example, during sustained periodic stimulation, the presence of graded responses may increase the complexity of the rhythms observed. Also, in the intact heart, a graded response to atrial stimulation may be insufficient to excite neighboring cells therefore resulting in failed conduction.

The experimental protocol explained in Fig. 1(A) can be used to construct the phase resetting curve (PRC) for a given

amplitude of the stimulus. The PRC describes the perturbation in the cycle length induced by a stimulus delivered at various phases of the cycle. The perturbed cycle length T_1/T_0 is plotted as a function of the phase ϕ of the premature stimulus. Under the assumption that the cardiac rhythm is a strongly attracting oscillation with rapid relaxation back to the cycle following the stimulation, the PRC can be used to predict the response of the preparation to sustained periodic stimulation.[10,12,16] In Fig. 2 we present PRCs obtained from an AV nodal cell cluster for four different amplitudes of stimulation. In order to emphasize the general shapes of the curves and the presence of time-dependent effects, we chose to represent T_j, $j=1$ to 5 [as defined in Fig. 1(A)], normalized to control cycle length T_0, versus the phase ϕ. For the same reason, the original data obtained for ϕ between 0 and 1 is also repeated three times on the phase axis. For the lowest intensity of stimulation [24 nA, Fig. 2(A)] a premature stimulus does not perturb the cycle length significantly. The predominance of horizontal lines in this panel is a hallmark of "weak" or "type 1" phase resetting. In Fig. 2(B) (48 nA, moderate intensity), as the phase of the stimulus increases, there is a sudden induction of premature APs pro-

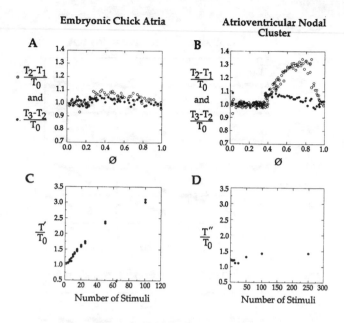

FIG. 3. The effects of single or periodic stimulation on the interbeat interval (IBI) immediately following the pulse. Left-hand panels: atrial embryonic chick aggregate. Right-hand panels: AV node cell cluster. In panels (A) and (B): First and second interbeat intervals (T_2-T_1, open symbols and T_3-T_2, filled symbols), normalized to control cycle length, as a function of the phase ϕ of the premature stimulus. The data in panel (B) corresponds to the PRC shown in Fig. 2(D). In atrial chick heart aggregates, the perturbation in the first cycle length after the stimulus increases with the prematurity of the evoked action potential. In AV nodal clusters, a reverse relationship is observed for a wide range of stimulus phases. However, the perturbation in the second IBI following the stimulus is again an increasing function of the action potential prematurity. In panels (C) and (D): first IBI (T') after cessation of stimulation, normalized to control cycle length T_0, as a function of the number of stimuli applied. In both cases, the period of stimulation was $0.6T_0$ (1:1 entrainment). Note the striking differences in the magnitude of overdrive effects between the two preparations.

ducing large gaps between the segments of the curves: we have an interesting example of an apparently discontinuous phase-resetting curve. In Figs. 2(C) and 2(D) (96 and 120 nA, respectively), as the phase of the stimulus increases, there is first a delay in the onset of the next spontaneous AP. For larger stimulus phases, a premature AP is evoked. The predominance of diagonal lines in these panels indicates "strong" or "type 0" phase resetting. The relationship between "weak," "strong," or discontinuous phase resetting and the dynamics observed during periodic stimulation is discussed thoroughly in the literature.[12,16,20]

Phase resetting normally implies that only the phase of the oscillation is affected by the premature stimulus. However, single stimuli may produce long lasting effects. For instance, in Fig. 2(C), a stimulus at phase $\phi=0.85$ first advances the phase of the oscillation ($T_1\approx0.85$) but after 1 to 5 beats there is a net delay in the phase of the oscillation (for instance: $T_5\approx5.2$). This effect is primarily due to a prolongation of the first interbeat interval following the premature AP (T_2-T_1) and is analogous to phenomena observed in the intact heart. In Fig. 3 we summarize the relationship between the magnitude of this time-dependent effect and the phase of the stimulus as well as the number of stimuli applied. We also draw a comparison between our observations from AV

nodal clusters (right-hand panels) and atrial embryonic chick heart cell aggregates (left-hand panels). In the top panels we show the two first normalized interbeat intervals [$(T_2-T_1)/T_0$ and $(T_3-T_2)/T_0$, respectively] after the premature AP, as a function of the phase of the stimulus. In both preparations, the initiation of a single premature AP is associated with a transient lengthening (up to 10% in atrial embryonic chick heart cell aggregates, up to 40% in clusters of AV nodal cells) of subsequent interbeat intervals. In atrial embryonic chick heart cell aggregates, there is a direct relationship between the amount of post-drive prolongation and the prematurity of the evoked AP (open symbols, first cycle length after premature AP, normalized to control). This time-dependent effect decays in time (filled symbols, second cycle length after premature AP, normalized to control). In clusters of AV nodal cells, there is reverse relationship for the perturbation in the first cycle after the premature AP. However, there is no significant difference between the perturbation in the second cycle length as observed in embryonic chick heart atrial cell aggregates or AV nodal cell clusters [respectively, Figs. 3(A) and 3(B), filled symbols]. This observation suggests that, in AV nodal clusters, two different mechanisms play a role in prolonging the cycle length after premature stimulation.

These changes in cycle length may have important effects on AV nodal excitability. For example, a prolonged interbeat interval may increase the refractoriness of the preparation to forthcoming excitation. Given the considerable magnitude of this effect (up to 40%) and its rapid decay, we speculate that it may represent a protective and stabilizing mechanism against undesirable premature excitation.

B. Overdrive suppression

Overdrive suppression can be defined as a transient suppression of automaticity following sustained periodic stimulation at a frequency faster than the intrinsic rate of the preparation and is the mechanism which ensures, in the intact heart, the domination of the SA node over subsidiary pacemakers[21] (including the AV node). Overdrive suppression has been studied extensively in a variety of preparations, including embryonic chick heart cell aggregates.[13,22] There have been several theoretical attempts to model overdrive suppression in order to account for rate-dependent effects in the heart and for the evolution of rhythms during periodic stimulation.[13,22] In some of these models, the change in the cycle length following a single stimulus was attributed to overdrive suppression. Following periodic stimulation in atrial embryonic chick heart cell aggregates the length of the post-drive pause increases with the number of stimuli and is directly proportional to the action potential frequency during the drive.[22] In Figs. 3(C) and 3(D) we show the length of the first interbeat interval after the drive normalized to control cycle length, T'/T_0, as a function of the number of stimuli applied. In all cases 1:1 entrainment was maintained between the stimulator and the preparation. In atrial aggregates, after 100 stimuli (pacing cycle length=0.6 control cycle length), the spontaneous interbeat interval is three times control. Under similar conditions, in AV nodal cell clusters, we observe only a 50% prolongation of the

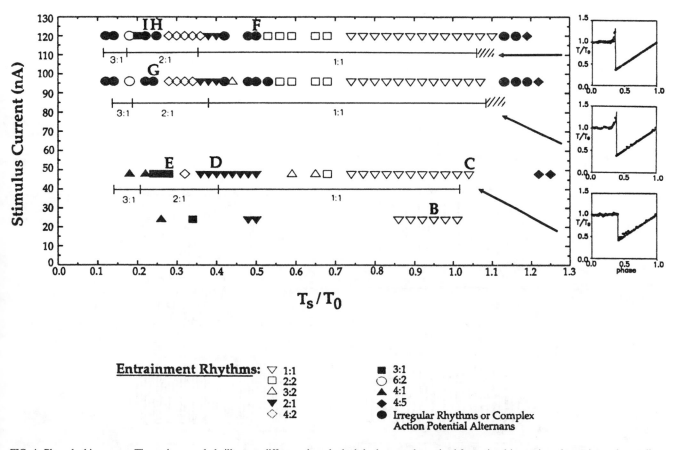

FIG. 4. Phase-locking zones. The various symbols illustrate different phase-locked rhythms, as determined from visual inspection of experimental recordings obtained for four different amplitudes of stimulation, during sustained periodic stimulation for 100 stimuli at different frequencies. The horizontal bars indicate regions where 1:1, 2:1, and 3:1 entrainment was predicted based on the iteration of the PRCs (inserts). In the stippled regions, period doubling bifurcations and irregular dynamics were found. The abscissa is the period of stimulation normalized to control. The amplitude of the stimulus (in nA) is plotted on the vertical axis. The symbols represent 4:1 (▲), 6:2 (○), 3:1 (■), 4:2 (◇), 2:1 (▼), 3:2 (△), 2:2 (□), 1:1 (▽), 4:5 (◆), and irregular rhythms or long period action potential alternans (●). Note the prominence of the 2:2 zone and the large number of irregular looking rhythms. The letters B to I refer to the panels in Fig. 5 where a few experimental traces during sustained periodic stimulation are shown together with information describing the evolution of action potential morphology during the drive. The experimentally measured phase-resetting curves (points) superimposed on the fitted analytical functions (solid curves) used in iterative procedure are shown in the inserts. At the two highest amplitudes of stimulation (discontinuity=1): $T(\phi)/T_0 = 1 + [b/(\phi - \phi_0)] + (b/\phi_0)$ when $\phi \leq \phi_{crit}$ and $T(\phi)/T_0 = \phi$ otherwise. For 120 nA: $b = -0.001\,79$, $\phi_0 = 0.3705$, $\phi_{crit} = 0.3656$. For 96 nA: $b = -0.005\,31$, $\phi_0 = 0.3974$, $\phi_{crit} = 0.3841$. The PRC obtained with 48 nA stimuli was fitted using a piecewise linear function: $T(\phi)/T_0 = a\phi + b$ where $a = 1.06$, $b = 1$ when $\phi \leq 0.408$ and $a = 1$, $b = 0$ otherwise.

spontaneous cycle length (roughly equal to the amount of single stimulus overdrive). Since various cell parameters such as cell input impedance and the ionic basis of activity are different for AV nodal cells than for cells from the surrounding myocardium,[1,2] these results are not surprising. This finding may be consistent with the distinct and specialized functional properties of AV nodal tissue.

C. Periodic stimulation

In the healthy heart, the SA node normally entrains the AV node rhythm in a 1:1 fashion. However, in the clinical context, examples abound of other entrainment rhythms which often correspond to distinct pathological situations. Different mechanisms are generally believed to underly these various rhythms including Wenckebach, reverse or alternating Wenckebach, and Mobitz type II atrioventricular block. Analogous rhythms can also be found in *in vitro* preparations.[10,11] These rhythms can often be predicted using simple theoretical paradigms which suggests that they can be

described in terms of dynamical properties of excitable cardiac tissue.[10,12] In Fig. 4 we identify some of the rhythms observed during periodic stimulation of AV nodal cell clusters with different stimulation frequencies for the four intensities corresponding to the PRCs in Fig. 3. For the three highest amplitudes of stimulation, we draw a comparison between the experimentally observed rhythms (various symbols) and some of the entrainment patterns obtained by iterating the corresponding PRCs (horizontal bars: 1:1, 2:1, 3:1 phase locking; stippled: period doubling bifurcations and irregular dynamics). The experimentally observed patterns of entrainment were determined by visual inspection of the voltage traces. Since there was often an evolution of the rhythms during the drive, only stable rhythms were represented. For reasons of clarity only the most important patterns of entrainment are indicated. For example, at the lowest stimulus intensity, a plethora of quasiperiodic and Wenckebach rhythms can be found between 1:1 and 2:1 entrainment. In general the structure of the phase-locking zones

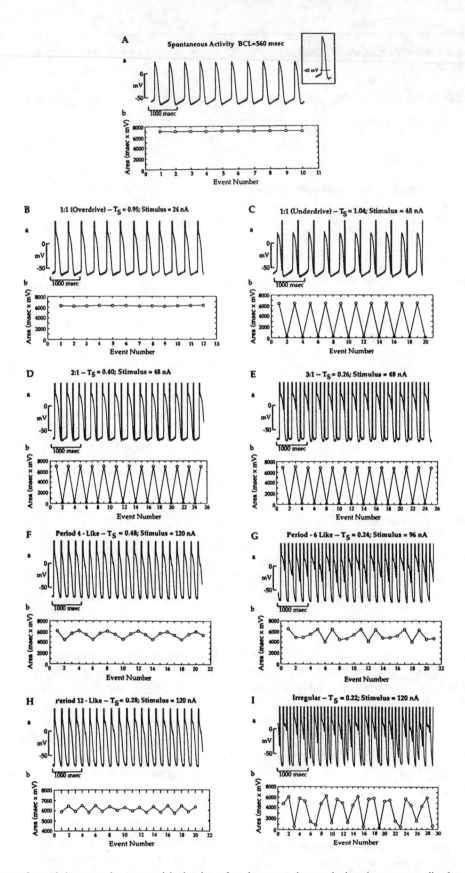

FIG. 5. Experimental traces of recorded transmembrane potentials showing a few chosen entrainment rhythms (see corresponding letters in Fig. 5) observed during sustained periodic stimulation (100 stimuli) at different frequencies and intensities of stimulation. For clarity, only 5 s traces are presented in each panel [Part (a)]. The stimulus artifacts appear as the off-scale vertical deflections. In panel (A), a sample of spontaneous activity is shown. The insert (right corner) describes the procedure for calculating the area under the action potential which corresponds to the area comprised between the experimental AP trace and the threshold fixed at −45 mV. In each panel, the evolution of the area under the AP is shown in Part (b) of the panel. In each panel, the strength, the period of stimulation (normalized to control) and the visually determined entrainment rhythm are indicated. Under certain circumstances, a failed action potential may result in a small but nonzero measured area. In some cases, very complex behavior is observed, associated with marked changes in AP characteristics.

(where the same type of N:M entrainment is found for different frequencies and amplitudes of stimulation) is similar to that observed in other *in vitro* preparations and to the theoretical predictions based on simple models of biological oscillators.[10–12] As the frequency of the stimulation increases, higher degrees of block are observed. The fact that we observe a 2:2 rhythm and 3:2 rhythm for the same amplitude of stimulation (96 nA) deserves special mention. A 2:2 rhythm corresponds to a period-2 oscillation in the phase of the stimulus. As the frequency of stimulation is increased, loss of entrainment will occur for one of the APs in the period-2 cycle: we expect to have 2:1 entrainment (although a narrow band of 3:2 entrainment can sometimes be found). In view of this, our observation is interesting since it may suggest that a slow regenerative process is present that modulates AP duration. This is reminiscent of the rate-dependent modulation of the action potential duration by the transient outward current in ventricular myocytes.[23] In some cases it is possible to drive the preparation in 1:1 fashion at a rate slower than control. Interestingly, there are very large zones where 2:2 and 4:2 entrainment is found. These entrainment patterns as well as the irregular rhythms correspond to situations where the action potential morphology is strongly modulated by stimulation (e.g., AP alternans). Because the PRC does not carry information related to changes in AP morphology induced by premature stimulation, the iteration of the PRC does not predict the existence of the wide regions where this type of complex action potential alternans and irregular dynamics are experimentally observed.

A simple description of the changes in action potential morphology during periodic stimulation can be obtained by calculating the area under the action potential with respect to some arbitrary threshold. In order to illustrate some of the observed rhythms, we show, in Fig. 5, nine voltage traces recorded during periodic stimulation. The rhythms that we chose are indicated in Fig. 4 by capital letters referring to the panels of Fig. 5. Under each trace, we show the corresponding AP area as computed using a trapezoidal integration rule of the voltage traces with respect to the -45 mV threshold [as shown in the insert of Fig. 5(A)]. For presentation reasons, only 5 s traces are shown. Since a large stimulation artifact is present in our recordings, it may sometimes give rise to a small area. A sample of spontaneous activity is shown in Fig. 5(A). Under control conditions, there is no beat-to-beat changes in AP area. The same result holds for 1:1 stimulation as shown in Fig. 5(B). In Fig. 5(C), the preparation is underdriven (stimulus frequency lower than intrinsic rate) in a 1:1 fashion. In this case (and in subsequent panels too), the small area values are due to the stimulus artifact and ought to be ignored. Therefore, as in the previous case [Fig. 5(B)], the area under the AP is constant during the drive. In Figs. 5(D) and 5(E), respectively, examples of 2:1 and 3:1 entrainment are shown. There are again no changes in AP area during the drive. The situation is more complicated in the remaining four panels [(F)–(I)]. In Fig. 5(F), each stimulus evokes an AP but the shape of the AP changes, repeating itself every four stimuli (4:4 entrainment). This alternation in AP parameters is nicely described by the plot of the AP area as a function of time. In a number of similar

cases, visual inspection of rhythms can result in misleading interpretations. The measurement of the area under the AP therefore represents a useful complementary tool in characterizing the observed dynamics. Other complicated rhythms can also be found. For example, in Fig. 5(G), there is a great deal of variability in the shapes of the action potentials, superimposed on a 2:1 rhythm. However, from the evolution of AP area as a function of time, a period-6 oscillation becomes apparent indicating that we have found 12:6 entrainment. Although the periodicity is not as clear in Fig. 5(H), this trace seems to correspond to 12:12 locking between the stimulator and the preparation. In Fig. 5(I), there are erratic changes in action potential morphology during stimulation. This recording is an example of an irregular rhythm. In all cases it is the changes in action potential morphology that account for the complexity of the dynamics. Although our measure of the area does not have a transparent physiological meaning, it is efficient at detecting general changes in AP morphology. In the clinical context, such changes may be important since they may influence impulse propagation through the AV node.

IV. CONCLUSIONS

In this study, we showed that the action potential characteristics of AV nodal cell clusters are modulated by the prematurity of the stimulus. These results are consistent with previous observations from the intact AV node[3] and single cellular preparations.[2] Moreover, single or sustained stimulation induces time-dependent effects that alter the spontaneous activity of the preparation and its excitation properties. During periodic stimulation, we find a variety of entrainment patterns which are analogous to the ventricular rhythms observed during atrial stimulation in the clinical setting. In many of these rhythms, there are large beat-to-beat changes in action potential morphology that increase the complexity of the observed dynamics and are not accounted for by the iteration of the phase resetting curves.

In electrocardiography, the term "concealed conduction" describes a situation where an atrial excitation fails to transverse the entire AV node.[24–26] Although active propagation is interrupted in this situation, remnant electrotonic currents will continue to propagate away from the site of block. The resulting subthreshold activity at sites distal to the site of action potential failure is related to several phenomena that can affect the response of the AV node to subsequent activations (for review, see Pick *et al.*[26]). In view of this, concealed conduction is sometimes related to "electronic inhibition" as described by Antzelevitch and Moe.[25] The possible relationship between these two phenomena is further discussed by Liu *et al.*[24] Our data collected during the phase-resetting protocol clearly shows that a single stimulus can modulate action potential morphology and produce phase-dependent effects on intrinsic cell excitability. During periodic stimulation, we also observe great variability in action potential characteristics. Under *in vivo* conditions, graded responses may be insufficient to propagate through the entire AV node, and contribute to concealed conduction.

"Fatigue" is a rate-dependent prolongation in AV nodal conduction time that may be responsible for the evolution of rhythms often observed experimentally during sustained atrial pacing.[6,8] For example, in healthy patients, atrial stimulation at rates faster than the sinus rate disturbs AV nodal conduction and causes an evolution of rhythms from 1:1 AH conduction toward Wenckebach periods and higher degrees of AH block.[27] In our experimental study, we observed analogous effects. We have shown that a single premature AP can induce a significant change in the following interbeat interval (up to 40%). Periodic stimulation at a rate faster than control is followed by post-drive pause (up to 50%) that, for long episodes of pacing, is virtually independent of the duration of the drive, which is an agreement with previous studies carried out in nodal tissue.[28] This is in contrast with overdrive suppression in atrial embryonic chick heart cell aggregates where the magnitude and the buildup of this effect are much more pronounced.[13,22] This likely reflects the different nature of the underlying ionic mechanisms. Previous studies suggest that, although the sodium pump plays a major role in overdrive suppression in embryonic chick heart atrial cell aggregates,[29] other factors, including increased internal calcium concentration and acetylcholine are determinants of overdrive suppression in nodal (SA) tissue.[28] Since there is a great deal of similarity between SA nodal and AV nodal cells, the same mechanisms may be involved in our experimental observations.

Under normal circumstances, there is 1:1 entrainment between the SA nodal and the AV nodal rhythms. By changing the frequency and the amplitude of the stimulation imposed on the AV nodal cell clusters, we investigated the response of AV nodal tissue to stimulation protocols which may simulate real pathological situations. The resulting rhythms, including Wenckebach and 2:1 block are analogous to experimental or clinical observations. Recently, a number of simple iterative mathematical models were developed to account for the dynamics during periodic stimulation. For example, the structure of the phase-locking zones (different types of $N:M$ entrainment) in an amplitude versus period of stimulation diagram (such as in Fig. 4) can be predicted based on the topology of the experimentally determined PRC[12,16,20] (e.g., "type 1" or "type 0"). To date, most of the studies aimed at studying the dynamics during periodic stimulation were carried out in *in vitro* preparations which consisted of cells characterized by high AP upstroke velocities and hence almost ideal "all or none" responses to stimulation. However, in our preparation, the presence of graded responses plays an important role in increasing the complexity of the dynamics. As a consequence, mathematical models that incorporate both time-dependent effects in the cycle length and changes in action potential morphology must be developed. For example, two pulse protocols could be designed to study the relationship between the areas of successive premature action potentials, as well as the influence of single stimulus overdrive on the phase-resetting properties of the preparation. Subsequently, a theoretical model, in the form of a pluri-dimensional difference equation, could be designed to encompass phase resetting, action potential area, and overdrive, in an attempt to simulate the complex rhythms observed in the experimental context.

There is still a poor understanding of the ionic mechanisms that underly the electrical activity of AV nodal cells.[2] This task is made even more difficult by the diversity of cell profiles found in the AV node.[2,3,14] In the intact heart, a large number of hormonal, neural, and mechanical inputs influence the properties of the AV node. All of these factors can influence the results of *in vivo* studies of the intact AV node, but can be more easily controlled by using our *in vitro* preparation. We hope that a combination of these different complementary approaches will give us a better understanding of how the AV node responds to sustained atrial pacing.

ACKNOWLEDGMENTS

We thank Adam Sherman (Alembic Software, Montreal, Quebec) for computer software used in the experimental protocols and analysis parts of this study, and Cedric Gordon for excellent technical support. We are also indebted to Dr. Leon Glass for making valuable suggestions during the preparation of this manuscript. Financial support was provided the Heart and Stroke Foundation of Canada and the Medical Research Council of Canada (MRC).

[1] F. L. Meijler and M. J. Janse, Physiol. Rev. **68**, 608 (1988).
[2] A. Shrier, R. A. Adjemian, and A. A. Munk, in *Cardiac Electrophysiology: From Cell to Bedside*, edited by D. Zipes and J. Jalife, 2nd ed. (Saunders, Philadelphia, 1995).
[3] J. Billette, Am. J. Physiol. **252**, H163 (1987).
[4] S. Tawara, *Das Reizleitungssystem Des Herzens* (Fisher, Jena, Germany, 1906), pp. 563–584.
[5] A. Shrier, H. Dubarsky, M. Rosengarten, M. R. Guevara, S. Nattel, and L. Glass, Circulation **76**, 1196 (1987).
[6] J. Billette, R. Métayer, and M. St-Vincent, Circ. Res. **62**, 790 (1988).
[7] M. Talajic, D. Papadatos, C. Villemaire, L. Glass, and S. Nattel, Circ. Res. **68**, 1280 (1991).
[8] J. Billette and S. Nattel, J. Cardiovasc. Electrophysiol. **5**, 90 (1994).
[9] M. Delmar and J. Jalife, Ann. NY Acad. Sci. **591**, 23 (1990).
[10] M. R. Guevara, A. Shrier, and L. Glass, Am. J. Physiol. **254**, H1 (1988).
[11] M. R. Guevara, Ph.D. dissertation, McGill University, Montreal, Canada, 1984.
[12] L. Glass, M. R. Guevara, J. Bélair, and A. Shrier, Phys. Rev. A **29**, 1348 (1984).
[13] Z. Wanzhen, L. Glass, and A. Shrier, Circ. Res. **69**, 1022 (1991).
[14] A. A. Munk, R. A. Adjemian, J. Zhao, A. Ogbaghebriel, and A. Shrier, submitted to J. Physiol.
[15] R. L. DeHaan, Dev. Bio. **16**, 216 (1967).
[16] *The Geometry of Biological Time*, edited by A. T. Winfree (Springer-Verlag, New York, 1980).
[17] L. Glass and M. C. Mackey, *From Clocks to Chaos* (Princeton University Press, Princeton, NJ, 1988).
[18] B. L. Hao, *Elementary Symbolic Dynamics and Chaos in Dissipative Systems* (World Scientific, Singapore, 1989).
[19] T. S. Parker and L. O. Chua, *Practical Numerical Algorithms for Chaotic Systems* (Springer-Verlag, New York, 1989).
[20] L. Glass and A. T. Winfree, Am. J. Physiol. **246**, R251 (1984).
[21] M. Vassalle, Circ. Res. **41**, 269 (1977).
[22] A. M. Kunysz, L. Glass, and A. Shrier, submitted to Am. J. Physiol.
[23] S. Kawano and H. Hiraoka, J. Mol. Cell. Cardiol. **23**, 681 (1991).
[24] Y. Liu, W. Zeng, M. Delmar, and J. Jalife, Circulation **88**, 1634 (1993).
[25] C. Antzelevitch and G. K. Moe, Am. J. Physiol. **245**, H42 (1983).
[26] A. Pick and R. Langendorf, in *Interpretation of Complex Arrhythmias* (Lee & Febiger, Philadelphia, 1979), pp. 471–541.
[27] A. Castellanos, A. Interian Jr., M. M. Cox, and R. J. Myerburg, Pace **16**, 2285 (1993).
[28] Y. J. Greenberg and M. Vassalle, J. Electrocardiol. **23**, 53 (1990).
[29] A. Pelleg, S. Vogel, L. Belardinelli, and N. Sperelakis, Am. J. Physiol. **238**, H24 (1980).

Phase-locking regions in a forced model of slow insulin and glucose oscillations

Jeppe Sturis
*Department of Medicine, The University of Chicago, Chicago, Illinois 60637 and Physics Department,
The Technical University of Denmark, DK-2800 Lyngby, Denmark*

Carsten Knudsen
Physics Department, The Technical University of Denmark, DK-2800 Lyngby, Denmark

Niall M. O'Meara
Department of Medicine, The University of Chicago, Chicago, Illinois 60637

Jesper S. Thomsen and Erik Mosekilde
Physics Department, The Technical University of Denmark, DK-2800 Lyngby, Denmark

Eve Van Cauter and Kenneth S. Polonsky
Department of Medicine, The University of Chicago, Chicago, Illinois 60637

(Received 8 December 1992; accepted for publication 8 August 1994)

We present a detailed numerical investigation of the phase-locking regions in a forced model of slow oscillations in human insulin secretion and blood glucose concentration. The bifurcation structures of period 2π and 4π tongues are mapped out and found to be qualitatively identical to those of several other periodically forced self-oscillating systems operating across a Hopf-bifurcation point. The numerical analyses are supplemented by clinical experiments. © *1995 American Institute of Physics.*

I. INTRODUCTION

Phase-locking and other nonlinear dynamic phenomena have been observed in virtually all areas of science and engineering. Human physiology is an example of a field in which an abundance of self-oscillatory subsystems exist, allowing for a variety of nonlinear dynamic phenomena to arise. The present paper deals with an example of such a system, namely the insulin/glucose feedback mechanism in the human body.

The main function of the hormone insulin is to regulate the uptake of glucose by muscle and other cells, thereby controlling the blood glucose concentration. The most important regulator of pancreatic insulin secretion is glucose, and thus insulin and glucose are the two main components of a negative feedback system. In normal humans, ultradian oscillations with an approximate 2-hour period can be observed in pancreatic insulin secretion and blood glucose concentration.[1-3] In addition, more rapid 8–15 min pulses of secretion have also been identified.[4] The two modes of oscillations are clearly distinct phenomena,[1] and it appears that they have different origins. The persistence of rapid pulses in the perfused pancreas[5] and in isolated islets[6] suggests that they are controlled by an intrapancreatic pacemaker mechanism. Because of their relatively high frequency, they are of fairly low amplitude in the systemic circulation of humans. In contrast, the ultradian oscillations are of large amplitude in peripheral blood, especially when insulin secretion is stimulated by glucose administration, and their origin may well be the insulin/glucose feedback system, i.e., the whole-body feedback regulation of glucose and insulin is unstable. We have previously proposed a nonlinear dynamic model of the insulin/glucose feedback system,[7] The model exhibits

self-sustained ultradian oscillations when a constant glucose infusion experiment is simulated.

Additionally, we have shown[8] how the ultradian oscillations in insulin secretion, which persist during constant intravenous glucose infusion, can be entrained to the pattern of an oscillatory glucose infusion. When glucose is infused as a sine wave with a relative amplitude of 33% and a period either 20% below or 20% above the period occurring during constant glucose infusion, the oscillations in glucose concentration and insulin secretion entrain to the pattern of glucose infusion. There are limits to the range within which entrainment can be obtained. Thus, if the period of the oscillatory glucose infusion is outside a certain range, simple 1:1 entrainment can no longer be obtained. In Fig. 1, the result of an experiment first reported in Ref. 8 is shown. Here, the period of infusion was approximately twice as long as the period observed when a constant infusion of glucose was administered, and as a result, two large amplitude oscillations appear for every swing of the glucose infusion. These modes of entrainment can also be accounted for by the model if the simulated pattern of glucose infusion is oscillatory[9] as exemplified in Fig. 1. Other experimental evidence of nonlinear dynamic phenomena in periodically forced physiological systems include phase-locking and global bifurcations in periodically forced chick heart cells,[10] phase-locking in mechanically ventilated cat respiratory systems,[11] and chaos and phase-locking in periodically stimulated squid axons.[12]

In this paper, we extend the experimental evidence of the insulin and glucose oscillations and the entrainment phenomenon by reporting the results of six additional experiments and comparing them to simulations with the model. Subsequently, we move on to a numerical investigation, mapping

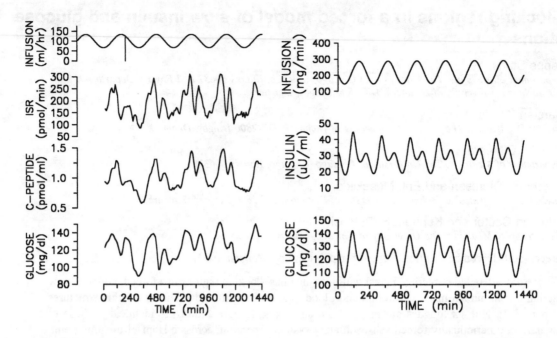

FIG. 1. Left: Glucose infusion study performed in subject A. On this occasion, the period of the glucose infusion was 320 min, and consequently, there were two large amplitude oscillations in glucose, insulin, and insulin secretion rate (ISR) for each oscillation of the infusion. The vertical line in the infusion curve represents a short, accidental interruption in the glucose infusion which was monitored. Redrawn from Ref. 8. Right: Model simulation in which the period of infusion was approximately twice the endogenous period, and a 2:1 type entrainment is produced.

out some of the largest phase-locking regions of the forced model.

II. DESIGN OF CLINICAL EXPERIMENTS

Experimental protocol. Two studies were performed on separate occasions in each of three non-diabetic men (subjects A, B and C; ages 27, 21, and 30 yr; weights 54, 96, and 67 kg; heights 169, 175, and 171 cm). Subject A had been previously studied.[8] After an overnight fast, each subject was admitted to the Clinical Research Center at the University of Chicago. An intravenous catheter was inserted into each arm, one for blood sampling, and one for glucose infusion. Beginning at 0800 hours, glucose (20% dextrose) was administered for 28 hours via a computer-controlled pump (Flo-gard 8000 volumetric infusion pump; Travenol Laboratories, Deerfield, IL). Sampling for glucose, insulin, and C-peptide was performed at 10-min intervals for the final 24 hours of the study. The mean rate of glucose infusion was 6 mg/(kg body weight)/min. For subject A, the pattern of infusion was a sine wave with amplitude and period of 40% and 300 min, and 33% and 78 min in the two studies, respectively. The hypothesis of the first experiment was that another example of 2:1 entrainment would emerge, [i.e., two oscillations in glucose, insulin, and insulin secretion rate (ISR) for every infusion period] while the second study was performed in an attempt to produce a case 1:2 entrainment (i.e., one full oscillation in glucose, insulin, and ISR for every two oscillations in the infusion). Subjects B and C both first received constant glucose infusion, and subsequently an oscillatory glucose infusion with a 33% amplitude and periods of 60 min (subject B) and 480 min (subject C), respectively.

Glucose, insulin, and C-peptide assays. Glucose concentrations were measured with the glucose oxidase technique using a YSI analyzer (Yellow Springs Instrument Co., Yellow Springs, OH). Serum insulin and plasma C-peptide were measured by radioimmunoassay.[13,14]

Data analysis. The raw data were smoothed with a three-point moving average. ISRs were calculated by deconvolution of the smoothed C-peptide data using a two-compartmental model of C-peptide kinetics.[15,16] The kinetic parameters of subject A were calculated in connection with the prior set of experiments[8] while standard parameters were used for subjects B and C.[17]

III. THE MODEL OF THE INSULIN/GLUCOSE FEEDBACK MECHANISM

A detailed description of the model has previously been published.[7] The model was constructed by extracting parameters and qualitative and quantitative features of functional relationships from the results of independent clinical experiments. The model equations are:

$$\frac{dI_p}{dt} = f_1(G) - E\left(\frac{I_p}{V_p} - \frac{I_i}{V_i}\right) - \frac{I_p}{\tau_p}, \quad \frac{dI_i}{dt} = E\left(\frac{I_p}{V_p} - \frac{I_i}{V_i}\right) - \frac{I_i}{\tau_i},$$

$$\frac{dG}{dt} = GI\left(1 + A\,\sin\left(\frac{2\pi t}{P}\right)\right) - f_2(G) - f_3(G)f_4(I_i) + f_5(x_3),$$

$$\frac{dx_1}{dt} = \frac{I_p - x_1}{\tau_d/3}, \quad \frac{dx_2}{dt} = \frac{x_1 - x_2}{\tau_d/3}, \quad \frac{dx_3}{dt} = \frac{x_2 - x_3}{\tau_d/3},$$

where the functional relationships and base case parameters are:

$$f_1 = \frac{209}{1 + \exp(-G/(300V_g) + 6.6)},$$

$$f_2 = 72[1 - \exp(-G/(144V_g))],$$

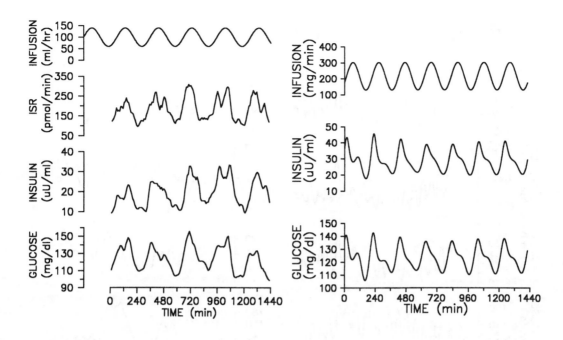

FIG. 2. Left: Clinical experiment in subject A with a period of 300 min and an amplitude of ±40% for the glucose infusion. In this case, the 2:1 entrainment observed in Fig. 1 appears to be lost, in that the second peak is replaced by a "shoulder" in the profiles in some cases and absent in other cases. Right: Corresponding simulation in which the period of infusion was reduced by 8% and the amplitude was increased to 40%.

$$f_3 = 0.01 G/V_g,$$

$$f_4 = \frac{90}{1 + \exp(-1.772 \log(I_i[1/V_i + 1/(E\,\tau_i)]) + 7.76)} + 4,$$

$$f_5 = \frac{180}{(1 + \exp(0.29 x_3/V_p - 7.5))} ;$$

$V_p = 3$ L, $V_i = 11$ L, $V_g = 10$ L, $\tau_p = 6$ min, $\tau_i = 100$ min, $\tau_d = 36$ min, $E = 0.2$ L/min, and $GI = 216$ mg/min.

Insulin secretion is stimulated by glucose (f_1). After its secretion by the pancreas, insulin distributes in the plasma space with a volume of V_p and subsequently it is either degraded according to time constant τ_p or it enters the interstitial fluid with a volume of V_i by diffusion with an effective diffusion constant E. Interstitial insulin, which is degraded slowly (τ_i), enhances glucose utilization (f_4). Additionally, glucose—which is assumed to distribute in one compartment with volume V_g—also enhances its own utilization (f_2, insulin independent uptake, and f_3, insulin dependent uptake). Insulin also inhibits hepatic glucose production (f_5), but there is a time delay between the appearance of insulin in the plasma and its resulting suppressive effect. The pathway of this time delay is presently unknown and therefore it is modeled as a third-order delay with a lag time τ_d. Glucose is infused as a sine wave, mean rate GI, amplitude A, and period P. These three parameters can be varied in the experimental setting. In the following section, we will present numerical simulations as well as perform a two-parameter bifurcation analysis of the forced insulin/glucose model by varying the amplitude and period of the oscillatory glucose infusion while other model parameters are fixed.

IV. SIMULATION AND EXPERIMENTAL RESULTS

In accordance with typical experimental results, simulation of a constant glucose infusion yields self-sustained oscillations of insulin and glucose.[7] The period of the oscillation is approximately 110 min, very close to the experimentally observed period. By simulating oscillatory glucose infusions, entrainment of the insulin and glucose oscillations occurs, providing the forcing period is within a certain range of the natural period.[9] These observations are in complete agreement with our previous experimental results.[8] If the period of infusion is approximately twice that of the endogenous period, a mode of entrainment will be obtained in which the system exhibits two large amplitude oscillations for each period of the forcing. This is also in harmony with our experimental results. The region in which this particular type of entrainment is possible is, however, narrow. When the period of infusion was set at 300 min instead of 320 min and the forcing amplitude increased from 33% to 40%, the result was qualitatively different in that only one large amplitude peak of plasma glucose and insulin secretion could be observed. This experimental result is shown in the left panel of Fig. 2. For comparison, a simulation was performed with a 40% forcing amplitude and a forcing period 8% shorter than the period used for the simulation shown in the right panel of Fig. 1. The result displayed in the right panel of Fig. 2 is similar to the experimental result.

If the infusion period is approximately half that of the natural period of the system, one would expect a 1:2 type of entrainment, i.e., the periodic forcing goes through two oscillations before the system has completed one full cycle. The result of the experiment in which the period of infusion was 78 min is shown in the left part of Fig. 3. During the first

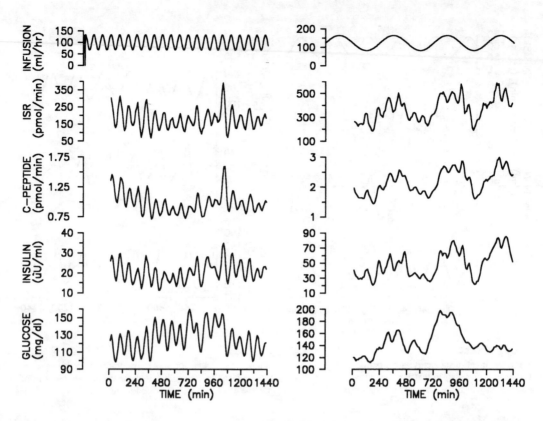

FIG. 3. Left: Clinical experiment in subject A with a period of 78 min and an amplitude of ±33% for the glucose infusion. During the first 16 hours of the study, the mode of oscillation resembles entrainment in a 1:2 fashion in that the troughs in the glucose profile alternate between higher and lower values. After 16 hours, this mode is lost, but it reappears towards the end of the study. Right: Clinical experiment in subject C with a period of 480 min and an amplitude of ±33% for the glucose infusion.

16 hours of the study, the system shows some signs of being entrained in the expected fashion: the troughs of glucose alternate for each infusion cycle. A similar pattern is difficult to discern for the ISR and insulin profiles. After approximately 16 hours, the system loses any sign of 1:2 entrainment, but towards the end of the experiment, the mode reappears. An analogous simulation result (not shown) shows clear 1:2 entrainment. During constant glucose infusion, ultradian oscillations in glucose and insulin secretion occurred in both subjects B and C with an approximate period of 120 min (data not shown). In subject B, during oscillatory glucose infusion with a period of 60 min, the expected 1:2 entrainment pattern did not clearly emerge. Instead, one oscillation in glucose and insulin secretion was evident for each oscillation of the infusion (data not shown), a result very similar to the one obtained in subject A (Fig. 3, left). In subject C, during oscillatory glucose infusion with a period of 480 min, the resulting glucose and insulin secretory profiles revealed 3–5 oscillations for every one oscillation of the infusion (Fig. 3, right). Although one might have expected to observe 4:1 entrainment, the experimental result more closely resembles nonperiodic behavior, e.g., quasiperiodic oscillations.

V. BIFURCATION ANALYSIS OF ENTRAINMENT REGIONS IN THE MODEL

A. Numerical methods

We have used the software package PATH[18] which can locate stable as well as unstable solutions by use of a Newton iteration scheme. The stability of a periodic orbit is determined by calculating the eigenvalues of the derivative of the Poincaré map. A bifurcation point can be located by varying one or two parameters slowly. Once a bifurcation point is found, simultaneous and slow variation of two parameters can automatically be performed by PATH, allowing the curve of bifurcation points which generically exists in a two-parameter case to be traced.

B. Bifurcation analysis of the unforced system

Before analyzing the forced system, it is appropriate to perform some investigation of the autonomous insulin/glucose model. A two-parameter bifurcation diagram is shown in the inset of Fig. 4. Here the rate of glucose infusion GI and the volume V_p of plasma which insulin first enters are the bifurcation parameters. The system is stable for both low and high values of GI and V_p. In the region of intermediate values for these parameters, a stable limit cycle solution exists along with the unstable equilibrium. The boundary between these two regions is a curve of supercritical Hopf-bifurcation points. In the analysis of the forced system, GI is fixed at 216 mg/min and V_p at 3 L. Since the periodic forcing influences the size of GI, a sufficiently large amplitude of the periodic variation will cause GI to take on values for which the autonomous system is stable.

C. Structure of dominant Arnol'd tongues

Figure 4 also presents a phase diagram illustrating all the bifurcation curves which were found in the present numeri-

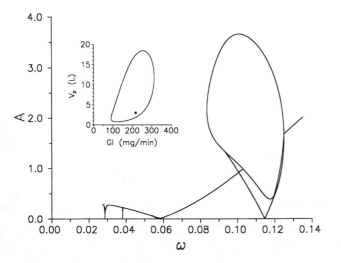

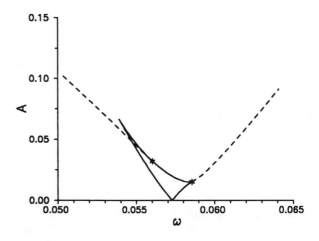

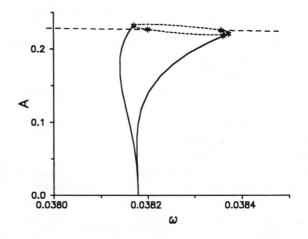

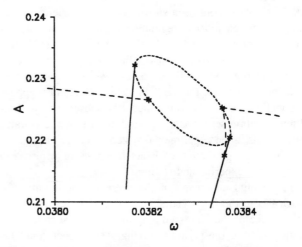

FIG. 4. The inset shows a bifurcation diagram in the V_p-GI plane of the autonomous model; the closed curve represents supercritical Hopf-bifurcations and the asterisk illustrates the parameter combination for the base case simulation. The rest of the figure shows a phase diagram presenting an overview of all the bifurcation curves found in the analysis of the forced model.

cal analysis. Our analysis was confined to regions for which the period of the phase-locked solution was either equal to or twice that of the periodic forcing. In addition to the local bifurcation curves shown in the figure, we have also found evidence of global bifurcations involving chaotic transitions and associated with the codimension 2 bifurcation points, some of which are shown in Fig. 5.

Period 2π regions. The top panel of Fig. 5 shows a magnified region of the tongue for which the forcing period is close to that of the autonomous system. For the lowest amplitudes, both tongue edges are saddle-node bifurcations. As the amplitude increases, both sides of the tongue become torus bifurcation (also denoted Neimark-Sacker bifurcation) curves. The left hand side of the saddle-node edge begins to overlap with the torus edge, turns sharply in a cusp-point, and subsequently connects to the torus part of the edge. At this connection point, the saddle-(stable)node bifurcation becomes a saddle-(unstable)node bifurcation, and the curve continues until it joins the right hand torus edge, at which point the bifurcation again is a saddle-(stable)node bifurcation, and the curve almost simultaneously turns and constitutes the lower right hand side of the tongue. The tongue for which the forcing period is approximately twice that of the period of the autonomous system has the identical qualitative structure as the tongue shown in the top of Fig. 5. Because the period of the steady state solutions in these tongues is equal to the period of the forcing, they are both denoted 2π regions. For low forcing amplitudes, however, in the latter tongue there are almost two full swings in the state variables for each swing of the forcing, but the system only performs a complete cycle with two swings of the forcing. As the amplitude is increased and the period of the forcing differs significantly from twice the period of the autonomous system, the shape of the limit cycle changes so that only one peak in the state variables can be observed. This transition between a solution in which two peaks can be seen in each period to a

FIG. 5. Top panel: Local bifurcation curves in period 2π region for which the period of the forcing is close to the period of the autonomous system. Middle panel: Local bifurcation curves in period 4π regions for which the forcing period is approximately 1.5 times the endogenous period. Bottom panel: Magnification of the region shown in the middle panel. Saddle-node bifurcations are full curves, period-doubling bifurcations are short-dashed curves and torus bifurcations are long-dashed curves. The asterisks denote connections of bifurcation curves—codimension-2 bifurcation points.

solution in which only one peak can be seen (see also Figs. 1 and 2) does not involve a bifurcation, but merely a continuous change in the shape of the limit cycle.

Period 4π tongues. The middle and bottom panels of Fig. 5 illustrate the 4π tongue emerging from the ω-axis at two swings of the periodic forcing for every three oscillations of the autonomous system. Although this region is much smaller than the 4π tongue emerging from the ω-axis at a forcing period equal to half the period of the autonomous system (see full phase diagram in Fig. 4), both regions involve period-doubling, saddle-node and torus bifurcation curves. In particular, the way the curves join appears to be qualitatively identical in the two regions.

VI. DISCUSSION

The present analysis represents an effort to bridge a gap between the field of clinical experimental research and nonlinear dynamics. Our research design was specifically aimed at explaining each individual experimental temporal profile. From the outset, it was assumed that the insulin/glucose feedback regulation is of importance for the genesis and control of the slow, self-sustained oscillations which can be observed in normal man. Administration of oscillatory glucose infusions enabled various modes of entrainment and quasiperiodic behavior to be observed, complementing our previous experimental results.[8]

The agreement between the experimental and simulation results is by no means complete. It was particularly difficult to produce an experimental example of 1:2 entrainment, i.e., one full cycle of the system behavior for every two oscillations in the infusion. One of the most likely explanations for this is the fact that many other self-oscillatory processes exist within the body which influence the insulin-glucose feedback mechanism. For example, the circadian clock and the sleep-wake cycle have both been shown to have independent and strong effects on glucose regulation,[19] and the pulsatile secretion of hormones such as luteinizing hormone (LH) and growth hormone (GH) may also influence the temporal profiles of glucose and insulin secretion. We have shown that this is indeed the case for GH.[20] Since certain features appear to be well-represented by the model, the subsequent numerical investigation serves as an illustration of how the entrainment regions in the experimental system could be structured, but it is not a prediction of exact locations of bifurcation curves in the experimental setting.

A potential advantage of the present experimental approach lies in the improved signal to noise ratio which is a consequence of the increased amplitude of the secretory oscillations due to the periodic forcing. This aspect could facilitate a closer investigation of how other hormones might phase-lock or interact with the insulin/glucose oscillations.

We have recently shown that the pattern of 1:1 entrainment observed during oscillatory glucose infusion in nondiabetic subjects is absent in patients with Type 2 (non-insulin-dependent) diabetes mellitus and even in subjects with only a mild impairment of glucose tolerance.[21] In its present form, those experimental results cannot be reproduced by the mathematical model of the insulin–glucose feedback mechanism. One of the obvious shortcomings of the model is the simple relationship that has been assumed to exist between glucose and insulin secretion. This relationship does not accurately represent the *in vivo* insulin secretory response in a diabetic person. Further development of the model would be useful in elucidating the experimental results observed in diabetes.

A large part of Fig. 4 deals with a region of parameter space which is physiologically unrealistic. Values of A larger than 1 are equivalent to pumping glucose out of instead of into a vein. While such a situation would be impossible to realize experimentally, it is of theoretical interest, and the numerical analyses show that bifurcation phenomena may occur in the unrealistic region of parameter space that are important for the dynamics in the realistic region. For instance, the codimension-2 bifurcation point joining the torus and period-doubling curves in Fig. 4 for (A,ω) $\approx(0.987, 0.103)$ lies very close to the unrealistic region of parameter space. Small variations in one or more of the other model parameters could move this point out of the realistic region. This, however, would not remove the global bifurcations associated with the codimension-2 bifurcation point, but in the experimental situation (assuming that the model accurately describes the experimental system), the global bifurcations would seem to arise out of nowhere because only the region $A \leqslant 1$ could be investigated. We do not have experimental evidence for global bifurcations, but the numerical investigations illustrate the important point that bifurcations may be important even if they occur in an unrealizable part of the parameter region.

Many features of the bifurcation scenario illustrated in the present analysis are qualitatively identical to those observed in the forced Brusselator[22] and in the forced continuous stirred tank reactor model.[23,24] Gambaudo[25] has used a combination of mathematical and numerical analyses and found the same structures in models forced near Hopf-bifurcation points. We refer to those papers for more detailed descriptions of the global bifurcations as well as of the solutions in the different regions.

In conclusion, we have presented clinical experimental and numerical evidence of phase-locking and other modes in human insulin secretion stimulated with oscillatory glucose infusion. Further clinical studies performed in conjunction with appropriate modifications and extensions of the model could improve our insight into some aspects of *in vivo* regulation of insulin secretion.

ACKNOWLEDGMENTS

Supported in part by National Institutes of Health Grant Nos. DK-41814, DK-31842, DK-13941, DK-20595 (Diabetes Research and Training Center) and RR-00055 (Clinical Research Center) and by a NATO Scientific Exchange Programme—Collaborative Research Grant. Dr. Sturis is the recipient of a Research Career Development Award from the Juvenile Diabetes Foundation International.

[1] C. Simon, G. Brandenberger, and M. Follenius, "Ultradian oscillations of plasma glucose, insulin, and C-peptide in man during continuous enteral nutrition," J. Clin. Endocrinol. Metab. **64**, 669–674 (1987).

[2] K. S. Polonsky, B. D. Given, and E. Van Cauter, "Twenty-four-hour profiles and pulsatile patterns of insulin secretion in normal and obese subjects," J. Clin. Invest. **81**, 442–448 (1988).

[3] E. T. Shapiro, H. Tillil, K. S. Polonsky, V. S. Fang, A. H. Rubenstein, and E. Van Cauter, "Oscillations in insulin secretion during constant glucose

infusion in normal man: relationship to changes in plasma glucose," J. Clin. Endocrinol. Metab. **67**, 307–314 (1988).

[4] D. A. Lang, D. R. Matthews, M. Burnett, and R. C. Turner, "Cyclic oscillations of basal plasma glucose and insulin concentrations in human beings," N. Engl. J. Med. **301**, 1023–1027 (1979).

[5] J. I. Stagner, E. Samols, and G. C. Weir, "Sustained oscillations of insulin, glucagon, and somatostatin from the isolated canine pancreas during exposure to a constant glucose concentration," J. Clin. Invest. **65**, 939–942 (1980).

[6] H. F. Chou and E. Ipp, "Pulsatile insulin secretion in isolated rat islets," Diabetes **39**, 112–117 (1990).

[7] J. Sturis, K. S. Polonsky, E. Mosekilde, and E. Van Cauter, "Computer model for mechanisms underlying ultradian oscillations of insulin and glucose," Am. J. Physiol. **260** (Endocrinol. Metab. **23**), E801–E809 (1991).

[8] J. Sturis, E. Van Cauter, J. D. Blackman, and K. S. Polonsky, "Entrainment of pulsatile insulin secretion by oscillatory glucose infusion," J. Clin. Invest. **87**, 439–445 (1991).

[9] J. Sturis, K. S. Polonsky, J. D. Blackman, C. Knudsen, E. Mosekilde, and E. Van Cauter, "Aspects of oscillatory insulin secretion," in *Complexity, Chaos, and Biological Evolution*, edited by E. Mosekilde and Li. Mosekilde (Plenum, New York, 1991), pp. 75–94.

[10] L. Glass, M. R. Guevara, J. Belair, and A. Shrier, "Global bifurcations of a periodically forced biological oscillator," Phys. Rev. A **29**, 1348–1357 (1984).

[11] G. A. Petrillo and L. Glass, "A theory for phase locking of respiration in cats to a mechanical ventilator," Am. J. Physiol. **246** (Regulatory Integrative Comp. Physiol. **15**), R311–R320 (1984).

[12] G. Matsumoto, K. Aihara, Y. Hanyu, N. Takahashi, S. Yoshizawa, and J. Nagumo, "Chaos and phase locking in normal squid axons," Phys. Lett. A **123**, 162–166 (1987).

[13] C. Morgan and A. Lazarow, "Immunoassay of insulin: two antibody system: plasma insulin levels of normal, subdiabetic and diabetic rats," Diabetes **12**, 115–126 (1963).

[14] O. K. Faber, C. Binder, J. Markussen, L. G. Heding, V. K. Naithani, H. Kuzuya, P. Blix, D. L. Horwitz, and A. H. Rubenstein, "Characterization of seven C-peptide antisera," Diabetes **27** (suppl. 1), 170–177 (1978).

[15] R. P. Eaton, R. C. Allen, D. S. Schade, K. M. Erickson, and J. Standefer, "Prehepatic insulin production in man: kinetic analysis using peripheral connecting peptide behavior," J. Clin. Endocrinol. Metab. **51**, 520–528 (1980).

[16] K. S. Polonsky, J. Licinio-Paixao, B. D. Given, W. Pugh, P. Rue, J. Galloway, and B. Frank, "Use of biosynthetic human C-peptide in the measurement of insulin secretion rates in normal volunteers and type I diabetic patients," J. Clin. Invest. **77**, 98–105 (1986).

[17] E. Van Cauter, F. Mestrez, J. Sturis, and K. S. Polonsky, "Estimation of insulin secretion rates from C-peptide levels: comparison of individual and standard kinetic parameters for C-peptide clearance," Diabetes **41**, 368–377 (1992).

[18] C. Kaas-Petersen, *PATH—User's Guide* (University of Leeds, Leeds, UK, 1987).

[19] E. Van Cauter, J. D. Blackman, D. Roland, J.-P. Spire, S. Refetoff, and K. S. Polonsky, "Modulation of glucose regulation and insulin secretion by circadian rhythmicity and sleep," J. Clin. Invest. **88**, 934–942 (1991).

[20] M. Byrne, J. Sturis, J. D. Blackman, K. S. Polonsky, and E. Van Cauter, "Decreased glucose tolerance during sleep may be partially mediated by GH, 74th Annual Meeting of the Endocrine Society, San Antonio, Texas, 1992, Abstract No. 40.

[21] N. M. O'Meara, J. Sturis, E. Van Cauter, and K. S. Polonsky, "Lack of control by glucose of ultradian insulin secretory oscillations in impaired glucose tolerance and in non-insulin-dependent diabetes mellitus," J. Clin. Invest. **92**, 262–271 (1993).

[22] C. Knudsen, J. Sturis, and J. S. Thomsen, "Generic bifurcation structures of Arnol'd tongues in forced oscillators," Phys. Rev. A **44**, 3503–3510 (1991).

[23] W. Vance and J. Ross, "A detailed study of a forced chemical oscillator: Arnol'd tongues and bifurcation sets," J. Chem. Phys. **91**, 7654–7670 (1989).

[24] M. A. Taylor and I. G. Kevrekidis, "Some common dynamic features of coupled reacting systems," Physica D **51**, 274–292 (1991).

[25] J. M. Gambaudo, "Perturbation of a Hopf bifurcation by an external time-periodic forcing," J. Differential Eqs. **57**, 172–199 (1985).

Discrete-time stimulation of the oscillatory and excitable forms of a FitzHugh–Nagumo model applied to the pulsatile release of luteinizing hormone releasing hormone

J. P. A. Foweraker, D. Brown, and R. W. Marrs
Department of Neurobiology, The Babraham Institute, Babraham Hall, Babraham,
Cambridge CB2 4AT, United Kingdom

(Received 11 May 1994; accepted for publication 7 December 1994)

A model for the pulsatile release of luteinizing hormone releasing hormone (LHRH) can be reduced to a FitzHugh–Nagumo model subject to regular and quasiregular (i.e., with slight random variation in the interstimulus interval), discrete-time stimulation. The relationship of output pulse frequency (OPF) to stimulus frequency is compared between the excitable and oscillatory forms of the model and discussed in the context of results from other pulse-driven model systems. Some examples of the changes in OPF caused by quasiregular and purely Poissonian stimuli are given for the excitable case. The unstimulated system frequently interacts with the stimulation in such a complex manner that the OPF bears little resemblance to the frequency of stimulation or of the unstimulated system. Furthermore, the inability of the oscillatory form of the model to allow complete suppression of output pulses for moderate stimulation frequencies suggests that the LHRH system can be more appropriately described by the excitable form of the model. © *1995 American Institute of Physics.*

I. INTRODUCTION

Luteinizing hormone (LH) secretion from the pituitary gland has the key function in all mammals of mediating neural control of ovulation. In intact animals a surge of LH is the main precursor of ovulation; at other times LH is released in intermittent small pulses, the frequency and amplitude of which are critical for follicular development. The pattern is partly determined by feedback from the ovary; in the ovariectomized (OVX) animal, ovarian feedback is abolished and LH is released in large amplitude pulses. This demonstrates that the intrinsic LH pulse generator is not dependent on feedback from the ovaries, although its action is modified by feedback. The amount and pattern of hypothalamic LH-releasing hormone (LHRH) release into the portal blood circulation in the brain, responsible in turn for LH release from the pituitary gland, is critically controlled by the activity of discrete populations of neurones within the hypothalamus.

It has been difficult to attribute a relative importance to the large number of neurotransmitters and neuromodulators which are involved in the regulation of LHRH neuronal activity. Nonetheless, it is generally acknowledged that the adrenergic neurotransmitters, adrenaline and noradrenaline, and the inhibitory amino acid, gamma-aminobutyric acid (GABA) are important physiological regulators of the pulsatile release of LHRH, and the model proposed by Brown *et al.*[1,2] includes components related to these. LHRH is released from LHRH cells in the hypothalamus [whose mean firing rate is represented by v in Eqs. (1) and (2)], and there is evidence that these cells have reciprocal connections with a population of GABA cells[3,4] (mean firing rate, w), which, possessing oestrogen receptors, mediate oestrogen feedback to the LHRH system in the intact animal. Adrenergic input is also critical to the functioning of this system, in that if this input is blocked, LHRH and LH pulses cease. Figure 1(a) (data from Terasawa *et al.*[5]) illustrates pulses of LHRH in the OVX monkey, and concomitant local concentrations of

norepinephrine (NE, an adrenergic input). Although the time resolution of the NE samples is rather poor because the measurements are near the limits of the assay sensitivity, the figure demonstrates that in general pulses of LHRH are preceded by NE pulses, although not all NE pulses result in LHRH pulses. Pulsatile adrenergic input is modeled as discrete increments in LHRH activity which vary randomly in magnitude and timing: instantaneous, positive perturbations of v, of size Δv which follow a lognormal distribution. They arrive at intervals Δt, which follow a negative exponential distribution with displaced origin, r, i.e., the intervals consist of a constant absolutely refractory period, r, followed by a variable period, which has a negative exponential distribution, mean τ, characteristic of a Poisson process. There is evidence of significant interactions between LHRH neurones,[6] modeled as a cubic polynomial in v in differential equation (1). Figure 1(b) (data from Robinson[7]) demonstrates, in microdialysis experiments in OVX ewes, that as LHRH is infused into the preoptic area of the hypothalamus, GABA concentrations rise, indicating that local rises in LHRH concentrations induce short term increases in GABA activity and release. This is represented in the model by GABA being subject to linear input from v, its activity declining exponentially in the absence of other influences. A slightly simplified version of the differential equation model of the continuous variables presented by Brown *et al.* is

$$\frac{dv}{dt} = s_0[-v(v-c)(v-1) - k_1 g + k_2 a], \tag{1}$$

$$\frac{dg}{dt} = b_0[k_3 a + k_4 v - k_5 g], \tag{2}$$

where $k_1 \ldots k_4$ are synaptic efficiencies, k_5 is the rate constant of the decay in GABA firing rate in the absence of stimulation, and s_0 and b_0 are rate-scaling constants. $k_1, k_4, k_5 \geq 0$, but k_2 and k_3 can take any sign. Both GABA and

(a)

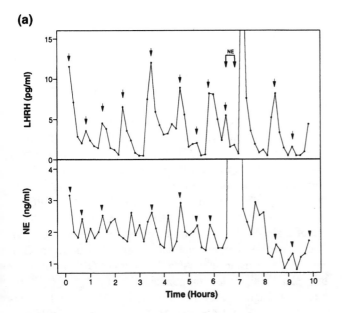

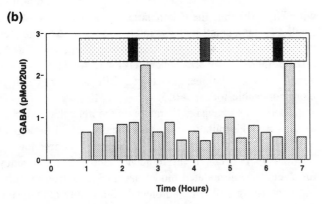

FIG. 1. (a) An example of the simultaneous measurement of *in vivo* release of LHRH and NE in a female rhesus monkey, data collected in 10 min fractions. NE release, like LHRH release was pulsatile. *Arrows* indicate LHRH pulses reported by PULSAR. *Arrowheads* indicate NE pulses that are synchronous with LHRH peaks, or precede LHRH peaks by 10 min. NE (10^{-6} M) infusion (*arrows joined by a bar*) for 20 min altered subsequent spontaneous NE release for approximately 2 h. Data from Terasawa *et al.*[5] (b) Experimental results showing that LHRH stimulates GABA release in the preoptic area (POA) in an individual ovariectomized ewe. The response of GABA (stippled bars) to infusion of 10^{-6} M LHRH into the POA via a microdialysis probe. LHRH was infused over a 20 min period on two occasions (black bars, top) with an intervening period of infusion of the LHRH molecule (amino acids 3–10; shaded bar, top). Between challenges, artificial cerebrospinal fluid was pumped round the probe (stippled bar). Samples were collected over 20 min periods and analyzed by high performance liquid chromatography with fluorescence detection. Data from Robinson.[7]

LHRH activity are subject to tonic influences of the adrenergic input, a, which can be excitatory or inhibitory. a is related to Δt and Δv by $a = qE[\Delta v/\Delta t]$, where q is a constant, and $E[\ ]$ denotes statistical expectation, or mean. There is a one-to-one relationship between pulses of LH and pulses of LHRH, and we restrict our attention to LHRH in the remainder of this paper.

Investigating this simplified form may reveal many of the original model's important attributes. Equations (1) and (2) can be simplified further by letting $w = g - k_3 a/k_5$, $I_{net} = a(k_2 - k_1 k_3/k_5)$ and rescaling:

$$\frac{dv}{dt} = \gamma[-v(v-\alpha)(v-1) - w + I_{net}], \qquad (3)$$

$$\frac{dw}{dt} = v - \beta w. \qquad (4)$$

This is a form of the Bonhoeffer–van der Pol (BVP) or FitzHugh–Nagumo model (FHN).[8,9] Here I_{net}, referred to as the *network current*, reflects the interpretation of the tonic adrenergic inputs by the LHRH/GABA network, and acts in the same way as an applied current in the BVP/FHN model. A substantial simplification in the work reported here is that the stimulus size Δv is taken to be a constant within any one model run; the effect of relaxing this restriction will be discussed elsewhere. The proportion of the mean interstimulus interval which is randomly varying throughout the simulation is $p_{stoch} = \tau/(r+\tau)$; the proportion constituting the constant refractory period therefore being $1 - p_{stoch} = r/(r+\tau)$. Much of the work in this paper deals with the case when the *time pattern* of the stimuli is *regular* ($p_{stoch} = 0$). The model with both Δt and Δv constant has the advantage that its qualitative behavior can be assessed using difference equation theory. Simulations with *quasiregular* (p_{stoch} small), or *Poissonian* ($p_{stoch} = 1$) stimulation patterns are included so that the effects of relaxing the constraint of a constant interstimulus interval slightly or totally can be assessed.

The motivation of the modeling exercise in this paper is as follows. Removal of the adrenergic input *in vivo* results in a loss of pulsatile secretion, but with time there is recovery of pulsatile output,[10,11] and, interestingly, cultured LHRH neurones *in vitro* can show quasipulsatile activity.[12] Thus there is biological data to suggest that the LHRH system *in vivo* may be an oscillatory system rather than an excitable system. To allow the system to oscillate in the absence of tonic adrenergic input we include an extra component in I_{net} so that $I_{net} = I_0 + a(k_2 - k_1 k_3/k_5)$, or, exhibiting the dependence on the mean frequency of stimulation, $E[1/\Delta t]$, $I_{net} = I_0 + dE[1/\Delta t]$, where $d [= (k_2 - k_1 k_3/k_5)q\Delta v]$ is a constant. Furthermore, in OVX rats, investigators have found that administration of either adrenergic receptor agonists or antagonists into the vicinity of the LHRH neurones results in a decrease to almost zero in LH pulse frequency.[13,14] Assuming that the antagonist reduces adrenergic input to near zero and that infusions of receptor agonists would greatly increase the frequency of receptor activation, this means that in our model system we require virtual abolition of LHRH pulses to result from both an increase and a decrease to zero in adrenergic input from some point over the range of possible adrenergic activity. The question then is: Could a stimulated oscillatory system model explain such experimental data as well as a stimulated excitable system model?

II. SIMULATION EXPERIMENTS

The parameters used were $\alpha = 0.2$, $\beta = 2.5$, $\gamma = 200$, and $d = 0$. The system is oscillatory for $0.0495 < I_{net} < 0.1745$ and so $I_{net} = 0.00$ (system excitable), $I_{net} = 0.05$ (system oscillating slowly), and $I_{net} = 0.10$ (system oscillating quickly) were chosen for the simulations in which Δt was constant, i.e., $p_{stoch} = 0$. Δv took values between 0.13 and 0.63 in steps of 0.02, and Δt between 0.01 and 0.99 in steps of 0.02. The effect of limited variability in the interstimulus interval, Δt, on the excitable system ($I_{net}=0.0$) was assessed by allowing p_{stoch} to take values 0.1 and 0.2, and for comparison a few simulations were carried out with $p_{stoch}=0.6$ and 1. The simulations were run, starting from (0,0), the stable equilibrium in the excitable case, for 10 time units (TU) before recordings were made. For the following 20 TU the number and times of the discrete stimuli, and any output pulses that occurred were recorded. For this purpose we arbitrarily define a pulse to occur when v becomes greater than 0.6, where there is no upwards crossing of this threshold in the previous 0.1 TU. The simulations were then carried out with a FORTRAN 77 program using NAG mark 15 numerical routines and running on a DECstation 5000 under ULTRIX. The differential equations were solved using Gear's method.

III. RESULTS

For $I_{net}=0.00$ [Figs. 2(a) and 3(a)] the system has an unforced OPF of 0 pulse/TU. For some physiologically plausible values of Δt the OPF=0, i.e., when $\Delta t>0.05$ and $\Delta v<0.25$, and when $\Delta t \in [0.065,0.09]$, $\forall \Delta v$. There is a nonmonotonic relationship between OPF and Δt, for constant $\Delta v>0.26$. As Δt increases, the OPF rises, then falls to zero, and then rises again. The main area of the graph where OPF>0 can be split into several zones—each delineated by a "cliff" running in an approximately negative exponential fashion of the form $\Delta v=0.25+c\,\exp(-k\Delta t)$. In each zone the OPF decreases in an approximately linear fashion with increasing Δt. There are complex transitional areas which exhibit cycles of very long period. Figure 3(a) is similar to Fig. 8 of Sato and Doi,[15] who worked with effectively the same excitable system except that their stimuli are not instantaneous, but occur over a brief time. In an earlier paper, Glass et al.[16] obtained a superficially similar return map to that of Sato and Doi using a one-dimensional difference equation derived from experimental data on cardiac impulses through the AV node. Glass et al. did not observe the chaotic behavior that Sato and Doi observed, although they only consider one stimulation rate. The results of Feingold et al.[17] are for negative stimuli applied to the control variable (our w) of a simpler excitable system model: the equivalent of the βw term in our Eq. (4) is absent. Their results are also phrased in terms of excited responses rather than output pulses. These differences of model and technique probably explain their substantially different results [cf. their Fig. 4 with our Fig. 3(a) and Sato and Doi's Fig. 8]. Simulations using our model and negative stimuli in w give approximately the same results as Feingold et al. with both $\beta=2.5$ and $\beta=0.0$. Takahashi et al.[18] obtained a similar diagram to Fig. 3(a) from experimental data.

The pulses for low values of Δt are "super-pulses" which are caused by the summation of the rapid stimuli. This phenomenon might not be seen physiologically, and would possibly be removed by changing the criteria for a pulse; alternatively it could be one stage in the LHRH surge generation. The area of OPF=0 for very low values of Δt, is due to super-threshold dynamic equilibria, or cross-threshold dynamic equilibria which do not satisfy the pulse criteria. Be-

cause their simulations cover a more restricted range of Δt, Sato and Doi did not observe these phenomena. The main area of OPF=0 is associated with the system settling into a subthreshold *dynamic equilibrium*[19]—so not allowing a pulse to be registered. Dynamic equilibria occur when there are no pulses, and the stimulated system is in a cycle of period 1. Sato and Doi also observed such regions of the $(\Delta v,\Delta t)$ plane in which there was no firing response to the stimuli.

When $I_{net}=0.05$ [Figs. 2(b) and 3(b)] the system has an unforced OPF of 1 pulse/TU and the OPF=0 only for very low values of Δt. Figure 2(b) is related to Fig. 2(a) in that it corresponds to a "filling in" of most areas where OPF=0 by the activity of the oscillator. Note that the area of OPF=0, for small Δt, has increased in size. The areas where OPF>2 are of a similar location and topology to those in Fig. 2(a). There remains a nonmonotonic relationship between OPF and Δt, for constant Δv. Also the range of OPF spanned by this relationship is less pronounced than for $I_{net}=0.00$, for a fixed Δv. Figures 2(c) and 3(c) ($I_{net}=0.10$) exhibit an unstimulated OPF of 1.4 pulse/TU. There are many similarities with Fig. 2(b), but there is a larger area with OPF=0 for small Δt, and a small increase in OPF for large Δt. The area where OPF>2 is similar to that in Fig. 2(b), and for $\Delta t>0.05$ there is no area where OPF<1. Again there is a nonmonotonic relationship between OPF and Δt which is more noticeable for $\Delta v>0.5$.

There is an extensive literature on theoretical approaches to, and model simulations of, periodically forced biological oscillators.[8,9,20–22] Perkel et al.[23] observed a nonmonotonic relationship between input frequency and firing frequency for a regularly stimulated model pacemaker neuron in *Aplysia*, contrasting with a monotonically increasing relationship for Poisson stimulation. Guevara et al.[24] assessed the effects of periodic pulse simulation of a BVP/FHN oscillator model in which they observed phase-locking and period-doubling bifurcations. Their unstimulated oscillator has three unstable equilibria, rather than one as here. Rajasekar and Lakshmanan[25,26] considered a similar system to ours but applied sinusoidal continuous time stimulation. Nomura et al.[27] applied inhibitory pulses of short duration to v in a model oscillator comparable to that in this paper, and observed phase-locked and nonlocked (quasiperiodic and chaotic) responses, and a nonmonotonic relation between output pulse and stimulus frequency. The phenomenon in which OPF=0 for very low Δt, high Δv is comparable to the rapid repetitive phase delay of Ypey et al.[28] and the 1:0 phase locking of Guevara and Glass[29] and Guevara et al.[30] Other studies using periodically forced Hodgkin–Huxley model oscillators include Guevara et al.,[24] Aihara et al.,[31] and Takabe et al.[32]

In order to clarify the results in Figs. 2 and 3 we examined the time series plots of v against t for three different values of I_{net} and for five different parameter combinations of Δv and Δt. The simulations were run for 2 TU to show the unstimulated behavior, and then for a further 8 TU stimulated. Six of these 15 time courses are depicted in Fig. 4. In Figs. 4(a), 4(c), and 4(e) the pulses are entrained by the stimuli, which does not happen in Figs. 4(b), 4(d), and 4(f). Figure 4(b) also shows a cycle of period 11, whilst Fig. 4(f) has a cycle of duration about 28 TU. In Figs. 4(c) and 4(e)

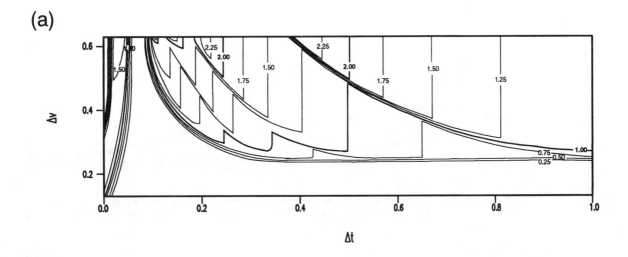

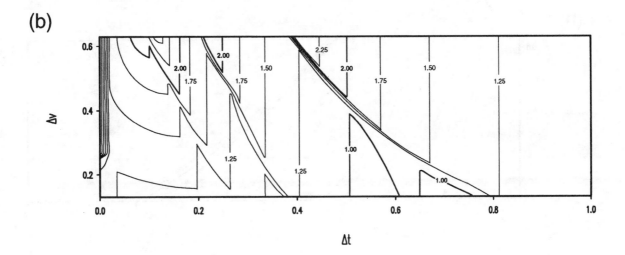

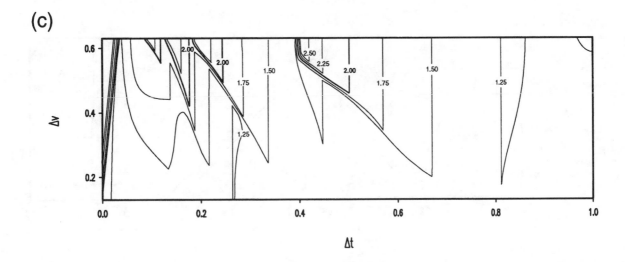

FIG. 2. Schematic contour diagram of output pulse frequency (OPF), the labels on the contours giving OPF in pulses per unit time, plotted against Δt and Δv. The parameter values used were $\alpha = 0.2$, $\beta = 2.5$, $\gamma = 200$ and (from top to bottom) (a) $I_{net} = 0.00$, (b) $I_{net} = 0.05$, and (c) $I_{net} = 0.10$. The figure is based on $\Delta t \in [0.01, 0.99]$ and $\Delta v \in [0.13, 0.63]$, both in steps of 0.02. Note the nonmonotonic relationship between OPF and Δt for constant Δv—including complete abolition of output pulses in (a) for $\Delta t \in [0.065, 0.09]$, $\forall \Delta v$.

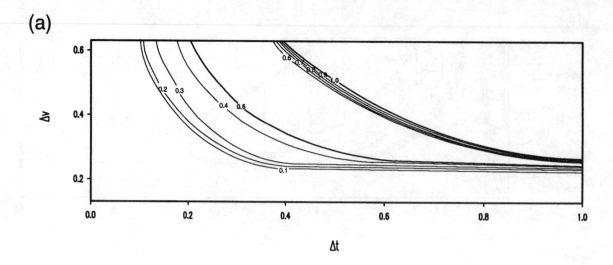

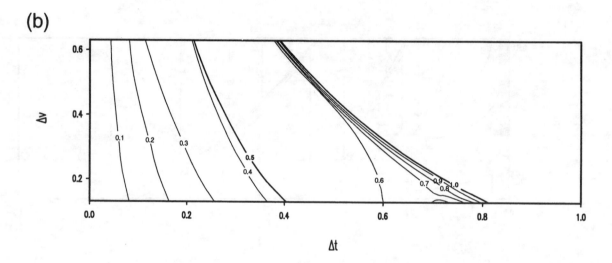

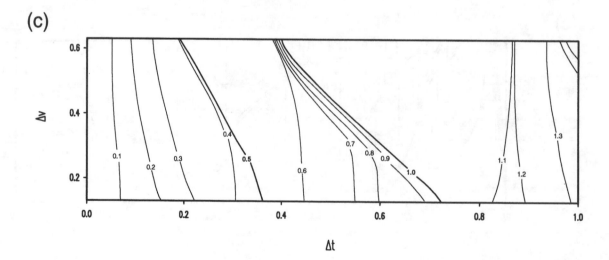

FIG. 3. Schematic contour diagram of ρ (contour labels=ρ=pulse frequency/stimulus frequency) plotted against Δt and Δv for (from top to bottom) (a) $I_{net}=0.00$, (b) $I_{net}=0.05$, and (c) $I_{net}=0.10$. Other parameters as in Fig. 1. There is a mostly monotonic relationship between ρ and Δt for constant Δv on all three graphs. $\rho>1$ only occurs then Δt is greater than the natural period of oscillation. In (a) there is no natural period, and so max(ρ)=1, $\forall \Delta t$, $\forall \Delta v$.

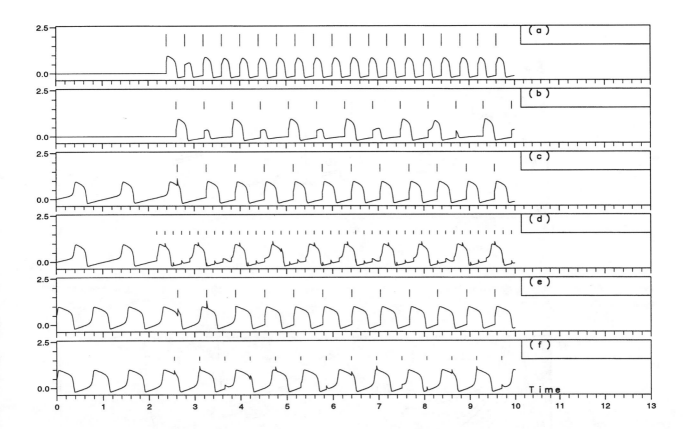

FIG. 4. Plot of the input stimuli (upper trace) and v (lower trace) against time for (a) $I_{net}=0.00$, $\Delta v=0.63$, and $\Delta t=0.40$; (b) $I_{net}=0.00$, $\Delta v=0.39$, and $\Delta t=0.61$; (c) $I_{net}=0.05$, $\Delta v=0.39$, and $\Delta t=0.63$; (d) $I_{net}=0.05$, $\Delta v=0.18$, and $\Delta t=0.18$; (e) $I_{net}=0.10$, $\Delta v=0.39$, and $\Delta t=0.63$; (f) $I_{net}=0.10$, $\Delta v=0.20$, and $\Delta t=0.55$. In (a), (c), and (e) there is pulse entrainment, but in (b), (d), and (f) there is not. (b) shows a cycle of period 11, and (f) has a cycle of duration about 28 TU.

the stimulation alters the OPF. Here the same values of Δv and Δt were used and the stimulated OPF is the same in both cases, although the natural OPF differs.

The adrenergic stimuli in the original model are quasi-regular. The effects on the model excitable system of increasing the random component in the interstimulus interval Δt are displayed in Fig. 5. For this degree of variability, the broad features remain the same as when $p_{stoch}=0$, but there are slight changes. The OPF$\neq$0 for all values of Δv, and $\Delta t \in [0.065,0.09]$; instead OPF=0 for $\Delta t \in [0.065,0.09]$ only for $\Delta v<0.35$, when $p_{stoch}=0.2$. The transitions between the different regions become more diffuse as p_{stoch} increases. The nonmonotonic relationship between OPF and Δt for constant Δv is less pronounced, eventually leading to the monotonic relationship observed by Brown et al.[2] (for $p_{stoch}=0$) in the excitable case. Perkel et al.[23] observed a similar phenomenon for an oscillator. Increasing the random component has reduced the maximum pulse frequency observed in our simulations from over 2.5 at $p_{stoch}=0$ to just over 2.0 at $p_{stoch}=0.2$. Figure 6 gives time courses for the parameter values in Figs. 4(a) and 4(b), but with $p_{stoch}=0.2$, 0.6, and 1.0. Comparison of Fig. 6 with Figs. 4(a) and 4(b) illustrates the transition from regular to quasiregular to Poissonian timing of stimuli. Figure 5 demonstrates that increasing randomness in the interstimulus interval reduces the OPF for many values of Δv and Δt. For the parameter values in

Figs. 6(a)–6(c), i.e., when $\Delta t=0.40$ and $\Delta v=0.63$, the reduction is much greater than in Figs. 6(d)–6(f). For values of $\Delta t \in [0.065,0.09]$ and higher values of Δv, on the other hand, increasing randomness increases OPF (Fig. 5).

IV. CONCLUSIONS

Previous studies[15,17,19,33] have shown that regularly stimulated excitable model systems, of various forms, frequently show a complex relationship between OPF and stimulus frequency. Many studies have shown that this is also the case for a model oscillatory system. The current simulations permit the comparison of excitable and oscillatory systems within the same model framework, and also introduce limited random variability in interstimulus timing.

One unexpected result of this comparison is that the excitable system can pulse more frequently than both oscillators, and the slow oscillator can pulse more frequently than the fast oscillator, when stimulated at the same rate and magnitude, for some parameter values. Also an increase in OPF as a result of stimulation occurs over a larger region of the $(\Delta t,\Delta v)$ plane for the slow oscillator. This is because the fast oscillator is in a refractory state for a greater proportion of each unstimulated cycle (about 50% compared to about 30% for the slow oscillator). The present results demonstrate

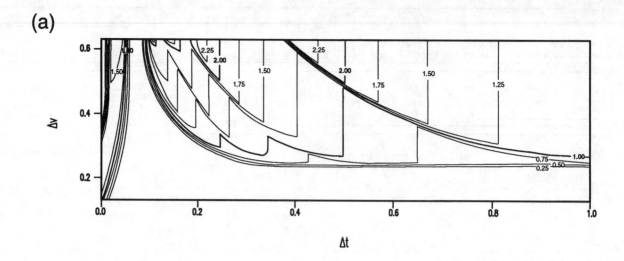

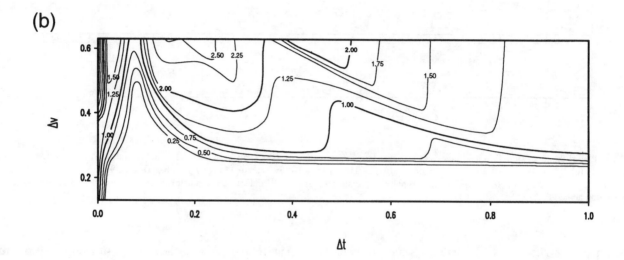

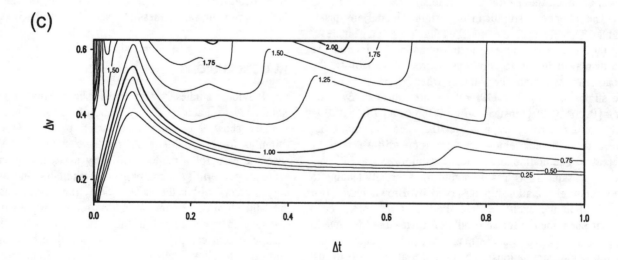

FIG. 5. Schematic contour diagram of output pulse frequency (OPF), contour labels giving OPF in pulses/unit time, plotted against Δt and Δv for (a) $p_{stoch}=0.0$, (b) $p_{stoch}=0.1$, and (c) $p_{stoch}=0.2$. The other parameter values, and the simulation grid are as in Fig. 1. Note the reduction in maximal OPF, the increasing diffuseness of the transitions from one zone of monotonicity to the other dnand the gradual removal of the zone of OPF=0 for $\Delta t \in [0.065, 0.09]$, $\forall \Delta v$.

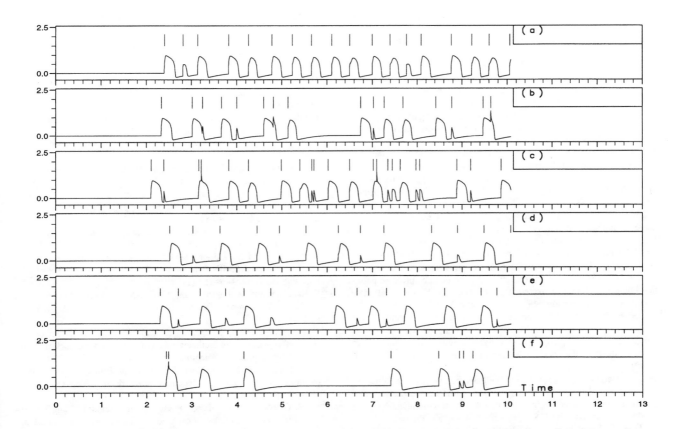

FIG. 6. Plot of the input stimuli (upper trace) and v (lower trace) against time for $I_{net}=0.00$, (a)–(c) $\Delta v=0.63$ and $\Delta t=0.40$, (d)–(f) $\Delta v=0.39$ and $\Delta t=0.61$, with (a) and (d) $p_{stoch}=0.2$, (b) and (e) $p_{stoch}=0.6$ and (c) and (f) $p_{stoch}=1.0$. Note that output pulse frequency (OPF) decreases with increasing p_{stoch}, and that in (a) and (d) [when compared with Figs. 4(a) and 4(b)] there is little change in either the OPF or the pulse waveform.

the relative importance of each of the stimulus parameters compared to I_{net} in determining the OPF, for some specific cases.

Some results are given for quasiregular stimulation patterns, demonstrating how the relationship between OPF and Δv and mean Δt changes as the degree of variability in the timing of the stimuli increases. Although exact regularity in output is lost by the introduction of any randomness in the stimulation pattern, some important features remain for low values of p_{stoch}, which are lost when $p_{stoch}=1$. The results are of general value to neurobiologists in showing that the output alone can sometimes give little information about the state of the system when not stimulated, or about the size and frequency of the neural stimuli.

Returning to the original application of this work, in female mammals, LHRH secretion is pulsatile throughout most of the reproductive cycle. This pulsatility is known to be dependent upon the adrenergic input in normal conditions, but the influence of this input appears paradoxical, in that increasing the input can either promote or suppress LHRH pulses depending upon the physiological condition. The non-monotonic change, and reduction to zero, of OPF with decreasing Δt (for a constant Δv), for an excitable system, appears to concur with experimental findings. The present results show that, as for an excitable system, a nonmonotonic relationship between stimuli and pulse output is possible when the system forms an oscillator—but that the reduction to zero frequency of output pulses that occurs in the excit-

able system does not occur in the oscillatory system, except at rates of stimulation which for the LHRH system are unrealistically high. The reduction to zero frequency also occurs with moderate sized stimuli when the stimuli applied to an excitable system are quasiregular, but not when they are completely random. Work is in progress on the effects of quasiregular stimulation on the oscillatory system. However, it seems unlikely that a slight degree of stochasticity in the stimuli will cause a substantial change in the stimulus–OPF relationship. One explanation that renders the above simulation results and the findings of Leonhardt et al.[11] compatible is that there is a degree of reorganization in the LHRH network when the cells are deprived of stimuli for a long time.

ACKNOWLEDGMENTS

The authors thank Gareth Leng and Allan Herbison for helpful discussion, and the referee for constructive comment and criticism. J.P.A.F. is supported by an MRC research studentship and by Jesus College, Cambridge.

[1] D. Brown, A. E. Herbison, G. Leng, and R. W. Marrs, "A mathematical model for the interaction between luteinizing hormone-releasing hormone (LHRH), GABA and noradrenaline cells in the rat," J. Phys. **446**, 67P (1992).
[2] D. Brown, A. E. Herbison, J. E. Robinson, R. W. Marrs, and G. Leng, "Modelling the LHRH pulse generator," J. Neurosci. **63**, 869–879 (1994).
[3] H. Jarry, H. A. Perschl, and W. Wuttke, "Further evidence that preoptic anterior hypothalamic GABAergic neurons are part of the GnRH pulse and surge generator," Acta Endocrinol **118**, 573–578 (1988).

[4] C. Leranth, N. J. MacLusky, H. Sakamoto, M. Shanbrough, and F. Naftolin, "Glutamic acid decarboxylase-containing axons synapse on LHRH neurons in the rat medial preoptic area," Neuroendocrinology **40**, 536–539 (1985).

[5] E. Teresawa, C. Krook, D. L. Hei, M. Gearing, N. J. Schultz, and G. A. Davis, "Norepinephrine is a possible neurotransmitter stimulating pulsatile release of luteinizing hormone releasing hormone in the rhesus monkey," Endocrinology **123**, 1808–1816 (1988).

[6] T. Funabashi, R. Hashimoto, and F. Kimura, "Luteinizing hormone releasing hormone released in the medial preoptic area controls its own secretion," Neuroendocrinology **52** (Suppl. 1), 167 (1990).

[7] J. E. Robinson, "The inhibitory amino-acid neurotransmitter gamma-aminobutyric acid and the control of luteinizing hormone-releasing hormone secretion in sheep," J. Reproduct. Fertility **49** (Suppl.), *Proceedings of the 4th International Symposium on Reproduction in Domestic Ruminants* (in press, 1995).

[8] R. FitzHugh, "Impulses and physiological states in theoretical models of nerve membranes," Biophys. J. **1**, 445–466 (1961).

[9] J. S. Nagumo, S. Arimoto, and S. Yoshizawa, "An active pulse transmission line simulating nerve axon," Proc. IRE **50**, 2061–2071 (1962).

[10] G. J. Kokoris, N. Y. Lam, M. Ferin, A. Silvermans, and M. J. Gibson, "Transplanted gonadotrophin-releasing hormone neurons promote pulsatile luteinizing hormone secretion in congenitally hypogonadal male mice," Neuroendocrinology **48**, 45–52 (1988).

[11] S. Leonhardt, H. Jarry, G. Falkstein, J. Palmer, and W. Wuttke, "LH release in ovariectomized rats is maintained without noradrenergic neurotransmission in the preoptic/anterior hypothalamic area: extreme functional plasticity of the GnRH pulse generator," Brain Res. **562**, 105–110 (1992).

[12] W. C. Wetsel, M. M. Valença, I. Merchenthaler, Z. Liposits, F. J. López, R. I. Weiner, P. L. Mellon, and A. Negro-Vilar, "Intrinsic pulsatile secretory activity of immortalized luteinizing hormone-releasing hormone-secreting neurons," Proc. Natl. Acad. Sci. USA **89**, 4149–4153 (1992).

[13] H. Jarry, S. Leonhardt, and W. Wuttke, "A norepinephrine-dependent mechanism in the preoptic-anterior hypothalamic area but not in the mediobasal hypothalamus is involved in the regulation of gonadotropin-releasing hormone pulse generator in ovariectomised rats," Neuroendocrinology **51**, 337–344 (1990).

[14] R. V. Gallo and R. E. Leipheimer, "Medial preoptic area involvement in norepinephrine-induced suppression of pulsatile luteinizing hormone release in ovariectomised rats," Neuroendocrinology **40**, 345–361 (1985).

[15] S. Sato and S. Doi, "Response characteristics of the BVP neuron model to periodic pulse inputs," Math. Biosci. **112**, 243–259 (1992).

[16] L. Glass, M. R. Guevara, and A. Shirer "Universal bifurcation and the classification of cardiac arrhythmias," Ann. NY Acad. Sci. **504**, 168–178 (1987).

[17] M. Feingold, D. L. Gonzalez, O. Piro, and H. Viturro, "Phase locking, period doubling, and chaotic phenomena in externally driven excitable systems," Phys. Rev. A **37**, 4060–4063 (1988).

[18] N. Takahashi, Y. Hanyu, T. Musha, R. Kubo, and G. Matsumoto, "Global bifurcation structure in periodically stimulated giant axons of squid," Physica D **43**, 318–334 (1990).

[19] D. Brown, J. P. A. Foweraker, and R. W. Marrs, "Dynamic equilibria and oscillations of a periodically forced excitable system," Chaos, Solitons Fractals (in press, 1995).

[20] L. Glass and M. C. Mackey, *From Clocks to Chaos: The Rhythms of Life* (Princeton University Press, Chichester, England, 1988).

[21] A. T. Winfree, *The Geometry of Biological Time* (Springer-Verlag, New York, 1980).

[22] F. C. Hoppensteadt, *An Introduction to the Mathematics of Neurons* (Cambridge University Press, Cambridge, 1986).

[23] D. H. Perkel, J. H. Schulman, T. H. Bullock, G. P. Moore, and J. P. Segundo, "Pacemaker neurons: Effects of regularly spaced synaptic input," Science **145**, 63–67 (1964).

[24] M. R. Guevara, L. Glass, M. C. Mackey, and A. Shrier, "Chaos in neurobiology," IEEE Trans. Syst. Man. Cyber. **SMC-13**, 790–798 (1983).

[25] S. Rajasekar and M. Lakshmanan, "Period-doubling bifurcation, chaos, phase-locking and devil's staircase in a Bonhoeffer–van der Pol oscillator," Physica D **32**, 146–152 (1988).

[26] S. Rajasekar and M. Lakshmanan, "Period-doubling route to chaos for a BVP oscillator with periodic external force," J. Theor. Biol. **133**, 473–477 (1988).

[27] T. Nomura, S. Sato, S. Doi, J. P. Segundo, and M. D. Stiber, "A Bonhoeffer–van der Pol oscillator model of locked and non-locked behaviours of living pacemaker neurons," Biol. Cybern. **69**, 429–437 (1993).

[28] D. L. Ypey, W. P. M. Van Meerwijk, and G. de Bruin, "Suppression of pacemaker activity by rapid repetitive phase delay," Biol. Cybern. **45**, 187–194 (1982).

[29] M. R. Guevara and L. Glass, "Phase-locking, period-doubling bifurcations and chaos in a mathematical model of a periodically driven oscillator: A theory for the entrainment of biological oscillators and the generation of cardiac dysrhythmias," J. Math. Biol. **14**, 1–23 (1982).

[30] M. R. Guevara, A. Shrier, and L. Glass, "Phase-locked rhythms in periodically stimulated heart cell aggregates," Am. J. Physiol. **254**, H1–H10 (1988).

[31] K. Aihara, G. Matsumoto, and Y. Ikegaya, "Periodic and non-periodic responses of periodically forced Hodgkin–Huxley oscillator," J. Theor. Biol. **109**, 249–269 (1984).

[32] T. Takabe, K. Aihara, and G. Matsumoto, "Response characteristics of the Hodgkin–Huxley equations to pulse-train stimulation," Trans. Inst. Elect. Inf. Commun. Eng. **J71-A**, 744–750 (1988).

[33] J. P. A. Foweraker, D. Brown, and R. W. Marrs, "Regular stimulation of a pulse generator," in *Proceedings of the V Rencontres de Blois–'Chaos and Complexity'*, edited by J. Trân Thanh Vân (Editions Frontières, in press).

Mechanisms of stochastic phase locking

André Longtin
Département de Physique, Université d'Ottawa, 150 Louis Pasteur, Ottawa, Ontario, K1N 6N5, Canada

(Received 3 June 1994; accepted for publication 21 September 1994)

Periodically driven nonlinear oscillators can exhibit a form of phase locking in which a well-defined feature of the motion occurs near a preferred phase of the stimulus, but a random number of stimulus cycles are skipped between its occurrences. This feature may be an action potential, or another crossing by a state variable of some specific value. This behavior can also occur when no apparent external periodic forcing is present. The phase preference is then measured with respect to a time scale internal to the system. Models of these behaviors are briefly reviewed, and new mechanisms are presented that involve the coupling of noise to the equations of motion. Our study investigates such stochastic phase locking near bifurcations commonly present in models of biological oscillators: (1) a supercritical and (2) a subcritical Hopf bifurcation, and, under autonomous conditions, near (3) a saddle-node bifurcation, and (4) chaotic behavior. Our results complement previous studies of aperiodic phase locking in which noise perturbs deterministic phase-locked motion. In our study however, we emphasize how noise can induce a stochastic phase-locked motion that does not have a similar deterministic counterpart. Although our study focuses on models of excitable and bursting neurons, our results are applicable to other oscillators, such as those discussed in the respiratory and cardiac literatures. © *1995 American Institute of Physics.*

I. INTRODUCTION

Biological oscillators exhibit a variety of dynamical behaviors that can be accessed experimentally through changes in the physicochemical parameters describing their internal and external environments. The oscillation may be endogeneous to the system, such as for a pacemaker cell. The system may be normally quiescent, but excitable: if sufficiently perturbed, it will become activated and then return to its resting state. The system may exhibit bursting, in which periods of activity, such as neural firing or the secretion of insulin from pancreatic beta cells, alternate with periods of quiescence. The same system may exhibit all these behaviors in different parameter ranges. Periodic forcing causes a competition between time scales of the system proper and that of the stimulation. Simple or complex phase-locked motion, or chaotic motion can then ensue. The mathematical models for these systems undergo bifurcations as parameters are varied, and one can associate these qualitative changes in motion with those observed experimentally. Further, in the context of dynamical diseases, bifurcations can correlate with the onset of pathology. The goal of these comparisons between data and models is to help build mathematical models with better predictive capabilities. This is possible because certain behaviors and bifurcations are characteristic signatures of certain kinds of nonlinearities.

Noise is traditionally seen as a nuisance that blurs or smears out known patterns of behavior. We like to think that, were the noise to disappear, the predictable pure pattern would be restored. While it is true that this can happen, it is also true that noise can move bifurcation points, or induce dynamical behaviors with no deterministic counterpart. These noise-induced transitions[1] are especially important near bifurcation points. Noise is often present in large amounts in physiological systems, but even in minute amounts it can significantly alter the observed behaviors (Sec. VI). It is useful then to view noise sources as important dynamical components that must be appropriately coupled to the other equations of motion. Further, the characteristics of noise such as probability density, intensity, and bandwidth must be viewed as parameters on equal footing with the deterministic parameters of the system.

The present study discusses mechanisms by which noise can produce stochastic phase locking in autonomous and periodically forced systems. This pattern is found in the vicinity of bifurcations where different dynamical behaviors coexist, as well as of bifurcations where they do not coexist. Bifurcation points and multistability are crucial concepts of dynamical diseases, thus the relevance of our study to this topic. Each mechanism studied here is found to have its own signature in the distribution of times between the events of interest. Other signatures, such as those associated with the return maps of interevent times, will be discussed elsewhere. We illustrate our findings on various neuron models in the vicinity of bifurcations commonly found in models of biological oscillators.

A. Stochastic phase locking or "skipping"

Many types of neurons exhibit stochastic phase locking or "skipping." Figure 1 is one possible simulation of the behavior of a skipping neuron using the Fitzhugh–Nagumo model (FHN) in the excitable regime (see Sec. III). The membrane voltage oscillates in response to a periodic current. Broadband noise is also driving this system. Near the peak of this noisy oscillation, action potentials or "spikes" are sometimes seen. The neuron may skip an integer number of cycles of the oscillation before spiking again. The multimodal histogram of interspike intervals (ISIH), seen in Fig. 1(B), is a characteristic signature of skipping. Because of the phase preference, the interspike intervals (ISIs) are grouped at integer multiples of the oscillation period T_0. The ISIH also contains information on the amplitude and frequency of

 1054-1500/95/5(1)/209/7/$6.00 © 1995 American Institute of Physics

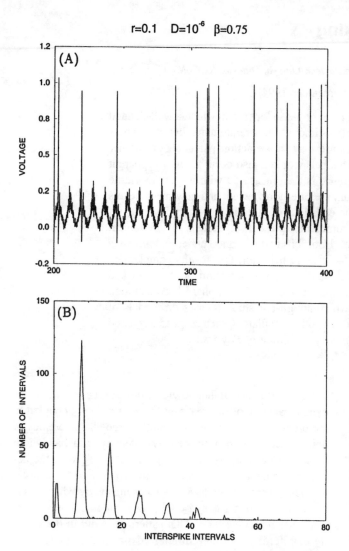

$r=0.1 \quad D=10^{-6} \quad \beta=0.75$

FIG. 1. Time series (upper panel) from low-frequency forcing of the Fitzhugh–Nagumo equation with periodic and stochastic forcing [Eqs. (1)–(3)]. The noiseless solution is a fixed point; an increase in b_0 brings on a limit cycle through a supercritical Hopf bifurcation. The ISIH peaks (lower panel) are at integer multiples of the driving period. Parameters are $a=0.5$, $b=0.12$, $d=1.0$, $r=0.1$, $\beta=0.75$, and $\epsilon=0.005$. Solutions for all the figures were obtained using a fixed step fourth-order Runge–Kutta method. The integration time step here is 0.005; 1000 steps were discarded as transients. A spike is counted when the positive going solution crosses the threshold value of 0.5. The ISIH was constructed from five realizations of 5×10^5 time steps.

the oscillation.[2] The peak widths are proportional to the noise intensity D. The rate of decay of the peak heights depends sensitively on D and the forcing amplitude. Also, when this amplitude increases, the ISIs get shorter, since the voltage spends more time near the spiking threshold during each stimulus cycle. The first peak in the ISIH is not always the highest, nor is it necessarily present, especially if the frequency is high (see Fig. 2). Spike generation is, in fact, determined by the amount and duration of the depolarization produced at the axon hillock.

Origins of skipping may be arbitrarily divided into two categories: autonomous and nonautonomous. The nonautonomous case applies when there is periodic forcing. This has been reported in a variety of systems, such as auditory

fibers,[3,4] mammalian mechanoreceptor afferents,[5] visual cortical neurons,[6] and crayfish mechanoreceptors.[7] When the driving frequency is not too high, the peaks of these ISIHs are "tunable," lining up at the integer multiples of the driving period. In the autonomous case, there is no obvious external periodic forcing, although firings may be synchronized to an internal (autonomous) oscillation of the membrane potential. Examples include shark multimodal sensory cells[8] and neurons in the cat lateral geniculate nucleus.[9] All these ISIHs are robust features of the neurons under nonpathological conditions.

Various forms of stochastic phase locking are also seen in the populations of cells involved in the generation of the cardiac and respiratory rhythms, especially in diseased states (see Refs. 11 and 12 for a review). In one example of mechanical ventilation, the number of phrenic bursts per ventilator cycle can alternate randomly between one and two. This would produce a histogram of intervals between phrenic bursts, with one peak at half the pump period and another at the pump period. The mechanisms studied in this paper may shed more light on such behaviors.

In our study, the stimulus and noise are modeled as currents that cause voltage fluctuations. Our results can be understood by knowing how the noiseless system bifurcates when a constant bias current increases. In the case of FHN (Sec. III), there is a supercritical Hopf bifurcation at a current value I_H, beyond which the neuron fires repetitively. If the total bias current is not constant, but rather fluctuates due to periodic and stochastic forcing then there exist time intervals during which the total bias exceeds I_H. Thus, depending on the activation rate constants and the distance between the voltage and the spiking threshold when $I>I_H$, the excitable s system can produce one or more spikes.

In Sec. II we review earlier modeling studies of skipping behavior. In Sec. III we study skipping in the FHN model near a supercritical Hopf bifurcation, and examine the tunability of the ISIH. In Sec. IV we look at skipping near the subcritical Hopf bifurcation in the Morris–Lecar equations. Skipping without periodic forcing is studied in the autonomous Hindmarsh–Rose model in Sec. V. Skipping in the vicinity of a period-doubling route to chaos is studied in the Plant model of slow-wave bursting in Sec. VI. In Sec. VII we briefly discuss the relevance of stochastic resonance (SR) when skipping is present. The paper concludes in Sec. VIII.

II. PREVIOUS MODELS OF SKIPPING

A simple model for skipping is simply the convolution of a Gaussian process, which accounts for the width of the peaks, and of a discrete Poisson process, which accounts for the skipping. To our knowledge, the earliest model of skipping is the integrate-and-fire (IF) model of Gerstein and Mandelbrot.[3] It accounted for the skipping response of primary auditory neurons to "clicks" of sound (short pulses of broadband noise). In this model, the periodic stimulus modulates the bias of the random walk of the voltage toward the threshold. Deletion models[10] have also been proposed for multimodal ISIHs such as those of Ref. 9. These models are based on the effect of individual synaptic events, and tend to produce multimodal ISIHs whose structure degrades with increasing ISI. Glass et al.[11] have reported that a simple IF oscillator with periodic input and noise can have patterns with irregular skipped beats. Descriptions of skipping based on stochastic point processes (in which there are no dynamical variables) can be found, in the context of auditory data, in Ref. 13. Dynamical modeling of skipping in auditory neurons has been done using stochastic Fitzhugh–Nagumo equations[14] and stochastic Hodgkin–Huxley-type equations.[15] Modeling of skipping in the context of bistability, excitability, and stochastic resonance (see Sec. VII) has been reported in Refs. 16–18, and 2.

Skipping can occur in completely deterministic models as well, when the dynamics are chaotic. This is the case for the forced Duffing equation.[16] The histogram of times between successive crossings from a given well to the other well in this double-well motion exhibits peaks near but not exactly at integer multiples of the driving period. The alignment with the multiples of T_0 gets better at larger ISIs. This is probably due to inertia and finite damping, since with infinite damping the peaks do line up.[2] While this example is not a good model for an excitable neuron, it indicates what to expect when a bistable neural system with higher-order dynamics is periodically forced.

III. THE FITZHUGH–NAGUMO EQUATIONS AND TUNABILITY

The skipping neuron can often be "tuned" to the external frequency.[4] This is illustrated in Fig. 1, which is a simulation of the stochastic Fitzhugh–Nagumo model[19] in the excitable regime:

$$\epsilon \frac{dv}{dt} = v(v-a)(1-v) - w + \eta(t),$$ (1)

$$\frac{dw}{dt} = v - dw - (b + r \sin \beta t),$$ (2)

$$\frac{d\eta}{dt} = -\lambda \eta + \lambda \xi(t),$$ (3)

where $\langle \xi(t) \rangle = 0$ and $\langle \xi(t)\xi(s) \rangle = 2D\,\delta(t-s)$. We chose the exponentially correlated Ornstein–Uhlenbeck process $\eta(t)$ for the noise throughout this paper, because its variance $D\lambda$ and correlation time $\tau_c = \lambda^{-1}$ can be controlled. The power spectrum of $\eta(t)$ is flat up to the cutoff frequency λ. The ISIHs are constructed from many different realizations of the stochastic process in Eqs. (1)–(3) (using a different seed for each realization). Equations (1)–(2) are taken from Ref. 19, in which the periodic forcing is on the slow variable. The ensuing behavior is qualitatively similar to that obtained by forcing the fast variable if the frequency is less than the relaxation rate of the fast variable ϵ.

The periodic forcing alone cannot produce spikes for the parameters in Fig. 1. If the bias b were increased, the model would bifurcate to a limit cycle of period 0.77 through a supercritical Hopf bifurcation. The effect of this limit cycle can already be seen with low-frequency forcing, as in Fig. 1(A), where two spikes ride one of the crests of the low-frequency modulation around the fixed point. Such multiple firings produce the peak at small ISIs. At higher forcing fre-

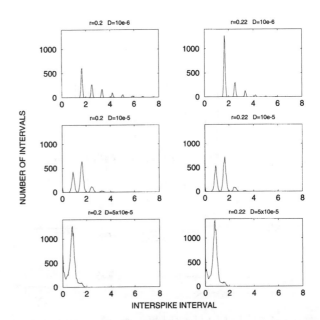

FIG. 2. Effect of phase locking on tunability: high-frequency forcing near a supercritical Hopf bifurcation. Multimodal ISIHs from the numerical integration of the FHN system with periodic and stochastic forcing [Eqs. (1)–(3)]. The simulation parameters are as in Fig. 1, except for r and β. The left panels, for a forcing amplitude $r=0.2$ characterize the noise-induced limit cycle. The right panels, for $r=0.22$, characterize the perturbed limit cycle, which has period 1.675 s when $D=0$. This is twice the forcing period of 0.837 s ($\beta=7.5$), i.e., the solution is a 2:1 phase locking. The model is also tunable, but the first peak is suppressed at low noise.

quencies, the time scale of the limit cycle and that of the forcing can compete, leading to phase-locked spiking solutions.[19,14,15] Note that phase-locked solutions can also arise even if the nonforced system is excitable.[20] Figure 2 shows two sets of ISIHs as the noise is increased. The frequency is ten times greater than in Fig. 1. The deterministic motion underlying the right panels is a 2:1 phase-locked solution (one spike for every two cycles of the stimulus), while that underlying the left panels is a fixed point modulated by the small periodic forcing (i.e., no spiking). With noise, there is not much difference between these sub- and superthreshold cases, except at zero noise, where the former gives an empty ISIH and the latter a sharp peak at the period 1.675 of the 2:1 phase-locked solution (not shown).

IV. MORRIS–LECAR EQUATIONS

The Morris–Lecar equations (see Ref. 21) are a hybrid of the Hodgkin–Huxley and FHN equations. We study the behavior, with stochastic and periodic forcing, of the fast voltage variable $v(t)$ in the vicinity of a subcritical Hopf bifurcation, where a fixed point and limit cycle (repetitive firing) coexist. Without noise $(D=0)$ and periodic forcing $(r=0)$, $v(t)$ goes to the fixed point or travels along the limit cycle, depending on the initial conditions. With $D>0$, the behaviors shown in Figs. 3(B)–3(D) do not depend on the initial conditions. Rather than choose a low frequency, for which the behavior is similar to that in Fig. 1, we focus on the vicinity of the phase-locked regime. For $r=0.015$ and $D=0$, the motion is phase locked with a very large period [Fig. 3(A)]. The presence of noise [Figs. 3(B)–3(C)] deletes

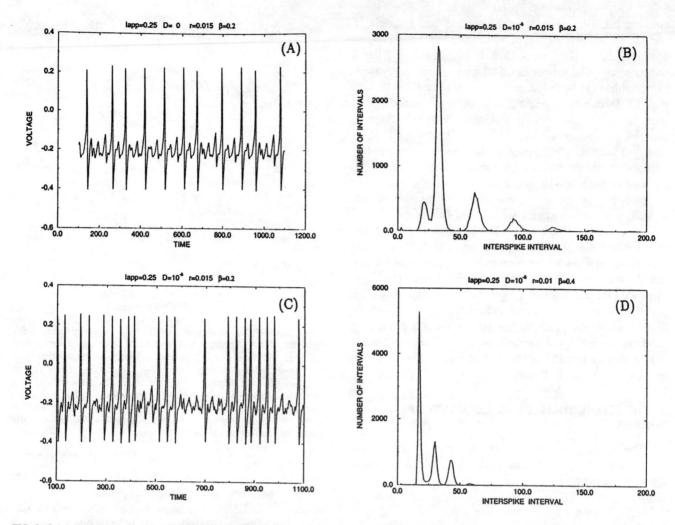

FIG. 3. Subthreshold forcing near a subcritical Hopf bifurcation: time series and ISIHs for the Morris–Lecar equations. The current $I=0.25$ is chosen, such that, in the absence of periodic and stochastic forcing, a limit cycle LC1 (repetitive firing) and a fixed point coexist. (A) A periodic phase-locked solution of high period (perhaps chaotic) when $D=0$ for forcing amplitude $r=0.015$ and angular frequency $\beta=0.2$ (period is 31.4). (B)–(C) ISIH and time series for the same parameters as in (A), but $D=10^{-5}$. The ISIH is multimodal, with peaks at integer multiples of 31.4. The small peak at 20.9 corresponds to the period of the limit cycle LC1. (D) Here $r=0.01$ and $\beta=0.4$ (forcing period 15.7). The underlying noiseless motion is a 5:3 solution of period 78.5. The peaks at 17.1, 30.15, 43.2, and 58.3 are near the multiples of 15.7, but appear perturbed by LC1. Parameters are as in Ref. 21: $v_1=-0.01$, $v_2=0.15$, $v_3=0$, $v_4=0.3$, $\bar{g}_{Ca}=1.1$, $\bar{g}_K=2.0$, $\bar{g}_L=0.5$, $v_K=-0.7$, $v_L=-0.5$, and $\phi=2$. Integration time step is 0.05, $\tau_c=0.01$, and the spiking threshold is 0.1. Integration involves 100 realizations of 220 000 time steps for $\beta=0.2$ and 50 realizations for $\beta=0.4$.

some spikes and induces others, the result being the familiar multimodal ISIH with peaks at multiples of the driving period T_0. There is also another peak in the flank of the T_0 peak, due to the presence of the limit cycle. In other words, sometimes the forcing brings this system into its limit cycle behavior, which may then impose its own time scale on the spiking. When $r=0.01$, the noiseless motion is a small modulation of the fixed point at the same frequency β; the ISIH with noise is like Fig. 3(B) but the limit cycle peak is more prominent and the perturbed phase-locked motion less prominent (not shown). If the frequency is then doubled [Fig. 3(D)], tunability is more degraded, presumably due to closeness of the limit cycle and forcing periods.

V. HINDMARSH–ROSE MODEL OF BURSTING

In this and the next section, we investigate how skipping can arise in the presence of noise, but without periodic stimulation. This possibility is examined in one of many models of bursting neurons: the Hindmarsh–Rose model:[22]

$$\frac{dx}{dt}=y-ax^3+bx^2+I-z+\eta(t), \qquad (4)$$

$$\frac{dy}{dt}=c-dx^2-y, \qquad (5)$$

$$\frac{dz}{dt}=r[s(x-x^*)-z]. \qquad (6)$$

This model is studied with stochastic forcing of the fast variable $x(t)$. A transition from one to three singular points occurs through a saddle-node bifurcation as I increases. At the same time, the system goes from fixed point to bursting to pacemaker activity. Bursting occurs for a given I because the adaptation current z causes a modulation of the nullclines, such that either one or three singular points coexist. The

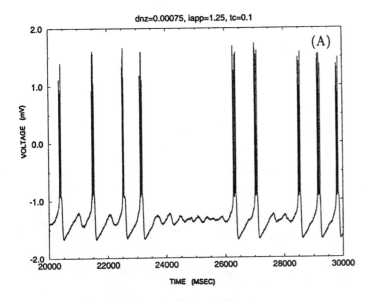

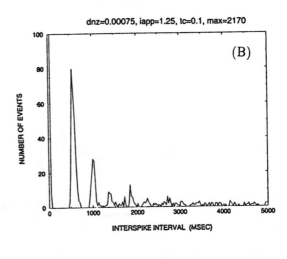

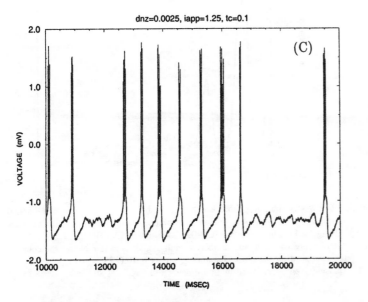

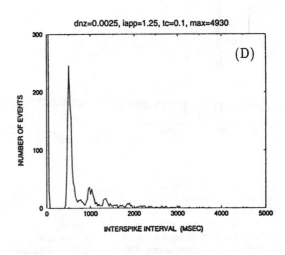

FIG. 4. Skipping near a saddle-node bifurcation in the Hindmarsh–Rose model Eqs. (4)–(6) of bursting behavior. Here there is only stochastic forcing. With $D=0$, the solution is a fixed point with complex eigenvalues having a negative real part. This explains the small oscillations seen (when $D>0$) between the larger waves. (A)–(B) Time series and corresponding ISIH for the noise level $D \equiv dnz = 7.5 \times 10^{-4}$. (C)–(D) The same as in (A)–(B), but $D = 2.5 \times 10^{-3}$. The peaks are at integer multiples of the period of the nearby deterministic bursting pattern. For large D, counts are concentrated in the first mode. The counts in the first bins are due to the short ISIs inside the bursts. The maximum of these bins is indicated above the panel. Parameters are $a=1.0$, $b=3$, $c=1$, $d=5$, $s=4$, $r=0.001$, $I=1.25$, and $x^*=-1.6$. The integration time step is 0.05, and the spike threshold is 1.0. Five realizations of 5.5×10^6 time steps were used to construct the ISIHs.

skipping patterns seen in Fig. 4 are possible when I is set at a value near but below that for the onset of bursting. The noise induces skipping between active and quiescent phases of the bursting pattern. Since the induced behavior is bursting, multiple spikes appear on top of each wave that has reached the threshold. The small oscillations seen between the bursts are a consequence of the complex eigenvalues with negative real part characterizing the behavior around the fixed point near -1.4. An increase in noise concentrates the probability into the first bins. This autonomous system thus behaves in many ways like the periodically driven systems above.

VI. PLANT'S "SLOW-WAVE BURSTER" MODEL

Chaos can appear in models for bursting cells. In the chaotic regime, the ISIs are distributed continuously rather than discretely. A bit of noise can smooth out the ISIH structure into a multimodal ISIH. This is illustrated here in Plant's model[23] for slow-wave bursting, originally proposed to explain the firing behavior of the R-15 pacemaker neuron of Aplysia. Its autonomous five-dimensional dynamics are significantly more complicated than the other models studied up to now in this paper. The equations and parameters used can be found in Ref. 23. Again, the fast variable is forced by a

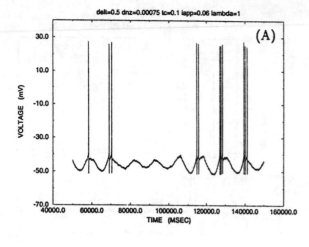

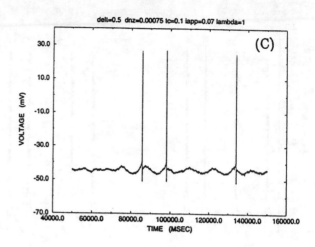

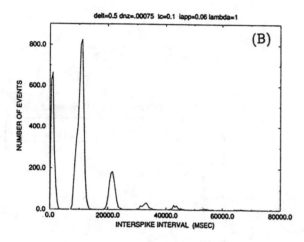

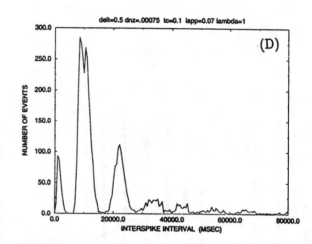

FIG. 5. Stochastic forcing near a chaotic regime: skipping in the Plant model of slow-wave bursting. Stochastic forcing with $D=7.5\times10^{-4}$ is present. (A)–(B) Time series and ISIH for the applied current $I_{app}=0.06$. When $D=0$, the solution is a period-doubled version of a solution having only one spike per burst. When $D>0$, the ISIH peaks are at integer multiples of the slow-wave underlying the bursting behavior. (C)–(D) The same as (A)–(B), but $I_{app}=0.07$. The noiseless solution here appears chaotic to the accuracy of our simulation (in double precision). Again the ISIH is multimodal, as in (B). Notice the counts in the first bins, corresponding as in Fig. 4 to the ISIs in the brief active phases induced by the noise. Parameters are as in Ref. 23; $\tau_c=0.1$, and the spike threshold is 10. Ten realizations of 4×10^6 integration steps (minus 5×10^4 transient steps) were used, with a time step of 0.5.

bias current and noise. The bursting mechanism here is different from that of the Hindmarsh–Rose model. But these systems are similar in that they can exhibit simple limit cycle motion, the time scale of which governs the skipping. Skipping can arise when the parameters are chosen such that the motion belongs to a period-doubling route to chaos. For $I_{app}=0.06$ and $D=0$, the ISIH has two close sharp peaks characteristic of the first period-doubled solution. As D increases (not shown), the peaks broaden, then merge; then peaks at integer multiples of this peak appear, and the number of short ISIs increases. At higher values of D, the probability bunches up into the first peak (which is also wider). This beavhior is similar to that of the noisy FHN system with low-frequency forcing, when the underlying deterministic behavior is a limit cycle (i.e., as in Fig. 1, but with a larger value of b). We find also that if I_{app} changes to 0.07, skipping

is again seen, but the peaks are wider. Abrupt transitions to other ISIHs can be seen as I_{app} increases beyond 0.07.

VII. STOCHASTIC RESONANCE

All the systems studied above may, due to their stochastic switching properties, exhibit stochastic resonance (SR). This is an nonlinear effect in which the presence of a deterministic oscillation in the state variable is enhanced by noise. This presence can be measured, e.g., by the power spectrum of $V(t)$, from which a signal-to-noise ratio (SNR) can be extracted. As D increases from zero, the SNR goes through a maximum (at the "resonance"), leading to the paradoxical notion that an increase in noise can increase the SNR. This is possible if the deterministic forcing cannot by itself induce the neuron to fire (i.e., it is subthreshold). Hence, without noise, no firings occur. As D increases, more firings occur, and they are more correlated with the small driving signal over a certain range of D. If the noise becomes too strong, this correlation decreases. Skipping is not SR, nor is it a sufficient condition for SR. SR has been suggested to occur in real neurons in Ref. 24; it was studied in the context of excitable models in Refs. 17 and 18, and was shown to occur experimentally in Ref. 7.

VIII. CONCLUSION

Skipping can occur with or without external periodic forcing, depending on the regimes of neural activity that can be "accessed" through noise (fixed point, excitable, pacemaker, and bursting). It is somewhat striking that it appears in the vicinity of so many noisy bifurcations; this may underlie its ubiquity in neurobiology. The best way to uncover its mechanism in an experimental setting is probably to vary system parameters (as is the case to demonstrate chaos in any system). The different ISIHs thus obtained are characteristic of the underlying dynamics. For example, as the applied current is changed in Plant's model, the ISIH structure can change drastically. This is not the case for the FHN model near a Hopf bifurcation.

Our study of skipping was not intended to be comprehensive. It is, first of all, limited to situations where the noise and deterministic oscillation bring the soma voltage closer to the spiking threshold. Spikes can also arise out of postinhibitory rebound, and skipping may occur when rebound events are deleted from a periodic pattern of such events. And pacemaker activity at a noisy inhibitory synapse[25] can produce skipping. The insights our study offers into skipping will potentially be useful for the interpretation of this and other physiological data. For example, in the cardiac arrhythmia known as concealed bigeminy,[12] there is a putative 2:1 entrainment between the sinus and ectopic rhythms. Fluctuations in refractory time are thought to cause skipping in the ectopic rhythm. The results of Secs. III–IV indicate that this could also occur if the origin of the 2:1 entrainment were noise induced rather than deterministic. The study of stochastic phase locking has[11] and will continue to benefit from the powerful concepts found in the theory of circle maps. Moreover, we suspect there exists a deeper connection between resonances in circle maps and stochastic resonance, as both involve the interaction of specific time scales.

ACKNOWLEDGMENTS

The author thanks Leon Glass for pointing out the possible relevance of this study to certain cardiac arrhythmias.

The author gratefully acknowledges support by NSERC (Canada), and by NIMH (USA) through Grant No. 1-R01-MH47184-01.

[1] W. Horsthemke and R. Lefever, *Noise-Induced Transitions. Theory and Applications in Physics, Chemistry, and Biology*, Springer Series in Synergetics (Springer-Verlag, Berlin, 1984), Vol. 15.

[2] A. Longtin, A. Bulsara, D. Pierson, and F. Moss, "Bistability and the dynamics of periodically forced sensory neurons," Biol. Cybern. **70**, 569 (1994).

[3] G. L. Gerstein and B. Mandelbrot, "Random walk models for the spike activity of a single neuron," Biophys. J. **4**, 41 (1964).

[4] J. Rose, J. Brugge, D. Anderson, and J. Hind, "Phase-locked response to low frequency tones in single auditory nerve fibers of the squirrel monkey," J. Neurophysiol. **30**, 769 (1967).

[5] W. Talbot, I. Darian-Smith, H. Kornhuber, and V. Mountcastle, "The sense of flutter-vibration: Comparison of the human capacity with response patterns of mechanoreceptive afferents for the monkey hand," J. Neurophysiol. **31**, 301 (1968).

[6] R. M. Siegel, "Non-linear dynamical system theory and primary visual cortical processing," Physica D **42**, 385 (1990).

[7] J. K. Douglass, L. Wilkens, E. Pantazelou, and F. Moss, "Noise enhancement of information transfer in crayfish mechanoreceptors by stochastic resonance," Nature **365**, 337 (1993).

[8] H. A. Braun, H. Wissing, K. Schäfer, and M. C. Hirsch, "Oscillation and noise determine signal transduction in shark multimodal sensory cells," Nature **367**, 270 (1994).

[9] T. Ogawa, P. O. Bishop, and W. R. Levick, "Temporal characteristics of responses to photic stimulation by single ganglion cells in the unopened eye of the cat," J. Neurophysiol. **6**, 2 (1966).

[10] G. Sampath and S. K. Srinivasan, *Stochastic Models for Spike Trains of Single Neurons*, Lecture Notes in Biomathematics (Springer-Verlag, Berlin, 1977), Vol. 16.

[11] L. Glass, C. Graves, G. A. Petrillo, and M. C. Mackey, "Unstable dynamics of a periodically driven oscillator in the presence of noise," J. Theor. Biol. **86**, 455 (1980).

[12] L. Glass, A. L. Goldberger, M. Courtemanche, and A. Shrier, "Nonlinear dynamics, chaos and complex cardiac arrhythmias," Proc. R. Soc. London Ser. A **413**, 9 (1987).

[13] D. H. Johnson, "The response of single auditory-nerve fibers in the cat to single tones: Synchrony and average discharge rate." Ph.D. thesis, Massachusetts Institute of Technology, Cambridge, MA, 1974.

[14] I. J. Hochmair-Desoyer, E. S. Hochmair, H. Motz, and F. Rattay, "A model for the electrostimulation of the nervus acusticus," Neuroscience **13**, 553 (1984).

[15] H. Motz and F. Rattay, "A study of the application of the Hodgkin–Huxley and the Frankenhaeuser–Huxley model for electrostimulation of the acoustic nerve," Neuroscience **18**, 699 (1986).

[16] A. Longtin, "Deterministic and stochastic dynamics of periodically forced neurons," *Center for Nonlinear Studies Newsletter*, Los Alamos National Laboratory preprint LA-UR-92-163, Jan. 1992, Vol. 74, pp. 1–19.

[17] A. Longtin, "Stochastic resonance in neuron models," J. Stat. Phys. **70**, 309 (1993).

[18] D. R. Chialvo and V. Apkarian, "Modulated noisy biological dynamics: Three examples," J. Stat. Phys. **70**, 375 (1993).

[19] J. C. Alexander, E. J. Doedel, and H. G. Othmer, "On the resonance structure in a forced excitable system," SIAM J. Appl. Math. **50**, 1373 (1990).

[20] M. Feingold, D. L. Gonzalez, O. Piro, and H. Viturro, "Phase locking, period doubling, and chaotic phenomena in externally driven excitable systems," Phys. Rev. A **37**, 4060 (1988).

[21] J. Rinzel and G. B. Ermentrout, "Analysis of neural excitability and oscillations," in *Methods in Neuronal Modeling*, edited by C. Koch and I. Segev (MIT Press, Cambridge, MA, 1989).

[22] J. L. Hindmarsh and R. M. Rose, "A model of neuronal bursting using three coupled first order differential equations," Proc. R. Soc. London Ser. B **221**, 87 (1984).

[23] R. E. Plant, "Bifurcation and resonance in a model for bursting nerve cells," J. Math. Biol. **11**, 15 (1981).

[24] A. Longtin, A. Bulsara, and F. Moss, "Time-interval sequences in bistable systems and the noise-induced transmission of information by sensory neurons," Phys. Rev. Lett. **67**, 656 (1991).

[25] A. F. Kohn, A. Freitas da Rocha, and J. P. Segundo, "Presynaptic irregularity and pacemaker inhibition," Biol. Cybern. **41**, 5 (1981).

AUTHOR INDEX

SUBJECT INDEX